# Walkable Neighborhoods

# Walkable Neighborhoods

## The Link between Public Health, Urban Design, and Transportation

Special Issue Editors

**Koichiro Oka**
**Mohammad Javad Koohsari**

MDPI • Basel • Beijing • Wuhan • Barcelona • Belgrade

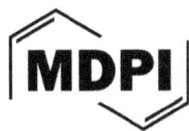

*Special Issue Editors*
Koichiro Oka
Waseda University
Japan

Mohammad Javad Koohsari
Waseda University
Japan

*Editorial Office*
MDPI
St. Alban-Anlage 66
4052 Basel, Switzerland

This is a reprint of articles from the Special Issue published online in the open access journal *International Journal of Environmental Research and Public Health* (ISSN 1660-4601) from 2018 to 2019 (available at: https://www.mdpi.com/journal/ijerph/special_issues/walkable_neighborhoods).

For citation purposes, cite each article independently as indicated on the article page online and as indicated below:

LastName, A.A.; LastName, B.B.; LastName, C.C. Article Title. *Journal Name* **Year**, *Article Number, Page Range.*

**ISBN 978-3-03921-930-8 (Pbk)**
**ISBN 978-3-03921-931-5 (PDF)**

Cover image courtesy of Koichiro Oka and Mohammad Javad Koohsari.

# Contents

# About the Special Issue Editors

**Koichiro Oka** is a faculty member at the Faculty of Sport Sciences at Waseda University, Japan. His research focuses on health impacts and determinants of physical activity and sedentary behaviour as well as interventions to promote active behaviours. He is the vice-president of the Japanese Association of Exercise Epidemiology, and on the editorial boards of the Japanese Journal of Behavioral Medicine, and the Japanese Journal of Health Education and Promotion.

**Mohammad Javad Koohsari** is an Assistant Professor of Urban Design and Health at the Faculty of Sport Sciences, Waseda University, Japan. As an urban designer, his research focuses on how built environment attributes can contribute to population health, especially in the context of super-aged societies. He is currently on the editorial boards of the Annals of Behavioral Medicine and Journal of Architectural & Planning Research.

## Preface to "Walkable Neighborhoods"

It is now widely recognized that individual-based motivational interventions alone are not sufficient to address the global pandemic of physical inactivity (lack of exercise and too much sitting time). There has been a growing interest in the effect the physically built environment can have on people's active behaviors. The fundamental assumption is that surrounding physical environments can support active behaviors among a large number of people with long-term effects. This topic has received much attention over the last decade, mainly in the three fields of urban design, public health, and transportation. This Special Issue aims to provide multidisciplinary and evidence-based state-of-the-art research on how the locations where people live impact their active behaviors and health outcomes.

**Koichiro Oka and Mohammad Javad Koohsari**
*Guest Editors*

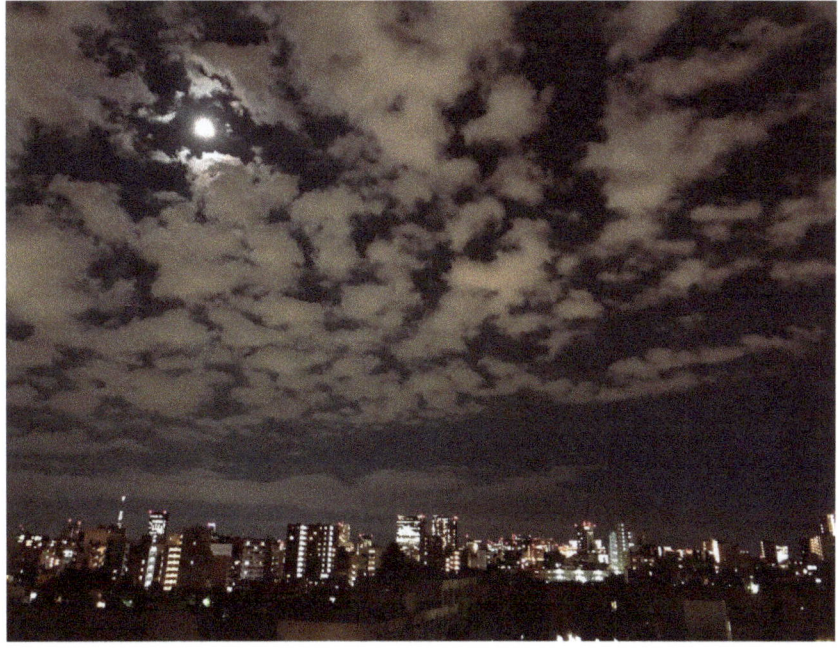

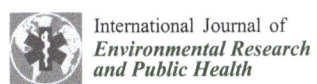

International Journal of
*Environmental Research
and Public Health*

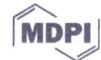

*Commentary*

# Activity-Friendly Built Environments in a Super-Aged Society, Japan: Current Challenges and toward a Research Agenda

**Mohammad Javad Koohsari [1,2,3,*], Tomoki Nakaya [4] and Koichiro Oka [1]**

[1]  Faculty of Sport Sciences, Waseda University, Saitama 359-1192, Japan; koka@waseda.jp
[2]  Behavioural Epidemiology Laboratory, Baker Heart and Diabetes Institute, Melbourne 3004, Australia
[3]  Mary MacKillop Institute for Health Research, Australian Catholic University, Melbourne 3000, Australia
[4]  Graduate School of Environmental Studies, Tohoku University, Sendai City 980-0845, Japan;
     tomoki.nakaya.c8@tohoku.ac.jp
*  Correspondence: Javad.Koohsari@baker.edu.au; Tel.: +81-4-2947-7189

Received: 1 September 2018; Accepted: 18 September 2018; Published: 19 September 2018

**Abstract:** There is a growing recognition of the role of built environment attributes, such as streets, shops, greenways, parks, and public transportation stations, in supporting people's active behaviors. In particular, surrounding built environments may have an important role in supporting healthy active aging. Nevertheless, little is known about how built environments may influence active lifestyles in "super-aged societies". More robust evidence-based research is needed to identify how *where* people live influences their active behaviors, and how to build beneficial space in the context of super-aged societies. This evidence will also be informative for the broader international context, where having an aging society will be the inevitable future. This commentary sought to move this research agenda forward by identifying key research issues and challenges in examining the role of built environment attributes on active behaviors in Japan, which is experiencing the longest healthy life expectancy, but rapid "super-aging", with the highest proportion of old adults among its population in the world.

**Keywords:** urban design; active living; aging; physical activity; sedentary behavior; age-friendly environments

---

## 1. Built Environments, Physical Inactivity, and Aging

Physical inactivity (defined as lack of exercise and prolonged sitting time) is one of the leading risk factors for most chronic diseases [1,2]. For example, a systematic review using meta-analysis found an inverse relationship between physical activity and type 2 diabetes [3]. Another recent meta-analysis review of 47 studies demonstrated the association between too much sitting time with chronic disease risk, regardless of time spent in physical activity [4]. Nevertheless, the rate of physical inactivity has been constantly increasing across the world over the last decades [5]. For instance, a study using pooled data from 76 countries found one in five adults in the world is physically inactive [6].

Motivating individuals to make lifestyle changes is important in promoting physical activity and reducing sedentary behavior [7]. However, since people's daily active behaviors are highly habitual (not involving conscious decisions), such interventions targeting individual motivation may not be totally effective [8]. There is a growing recognition of the role of built environment attributes, such as streets, shops, workplaces, greenways, parks, and public transportation stations, in supporting people's active behaviors [9,10]. For instance, an international study using data from 14 cities worldwide found built environment attributes, including higher residential density, well-connected street network, availability of public transport, and higher number of parks, to be positively associated with adults' physical activity [11]. The fundamental assumption is that even if the effects of built environment interventions on each person's behavior is small, the overall population effect can be large, and these effects may be sustained over a relatively long-term period [12].

The world population is aging, with the number of persons aged 60 or over expected to be more than double by 2050, compared to 2017, and the number of super-aged societies has been continually increasing [13]. According to the United Nations, a super-aged society refers to a society where more than 20% of their total population is aged 65 years and older. People's ability to be active and their mobility gradually declines as they age; because of their declining physical function [14]. Older adults may be interested in doing physical activity, but their physical function may substantially limit their mobility. Therefore, their surrounding immediate environment may play an important role in supporting healthy active aging [15,16]. While few studies exist in other regions [17,18], there are many studies examining associations of environmental attributes with active behaviors conducted in developed societies in New Worlds, such as the United States, Canada, and Australia (which are characterized by a Western colonization history, high car dependency, and large proportions of relatively young immigrants). In particular, little is known about how such attributes may influence active lifestyle in super-aged, non-anglosphere societies, such as Japan and Germany [15,19]. For example, in a recent systematic review of built environment attributes related to older adults' active travel, only one study (out of 42) was conducted in Japan (and no studies were from Germany) [19]. More robust evidence-based research is needed to identify how *where* people live influences their active behaviors, and how to build beneficial space in the context of super-aged societies. This evidence will also be informative for the broader international context, where having an aging society will be the inevitable future.

This commentary sought to move this research agenda forward by identifying key research issues and challenges in examining the role of built environment attributes on active behaviors in Japan, which is experiencing the longest healthy life expectancy, but rapid "super-aging", with the highest proportion of old adults among its population in the world.

## 2. Key Issues in Activity-Friendly Built Environment Research in Japan

Although the Japanese are the healthiest population in the world, the rate of physical inactivity is increasing in Japan, following the global trend. For instance, according to a study using a nationally representative sample of Japanese adults, the number of adults' daily walking steps has gradually decreased since approximately 1998–2000 [20]. Japanese adults also reported the highest amount of sitting time per day among 20 countries [21]. In addition, Japan is already a super-aged society with 26.6% of its total population aged 65 years and over in 2015 [22]. Therefore, promoting physical activity has become one of the major public health targets in Japan. "Health Japan 21"—the national plan for health promotion—emphasizes the importance of environments for supporting an active and healthy lifestyle [23].

Several studies conducted in Asian countries examined how environmental attributes can influence active behaviors [24–26]. Similarly, the associations between built environment attributes and active behaviors have been investigated in several previous studies in Japan [27–34]. For instance, several perceived environmental measures, including residential density, access to shops, sidewalk availability, and availability of bike lanes, were found to be positively associated with adults' physical activity in two areas in Japan [28]. Another study found objective measures of population density and the presence of parks to be positively associated with Japanese older adults' leisure physical activity [33]. And, a recent Japanese study found that residents who lived in areas with well-connected streets were likely to report more walking and less driving, compared with those who lived in less-connected areas [31]. These studies shed light on better understanding the environmental correlates of active behaviors in Japan. They especially provide preliminary evidence about the importance of perceived neighborhood attributes in supporting an active lifestyle. The identified set of influential environmental attributes are somewhat like those reported in the United States, Canada, and Australia. Nevertheless, there are several issues about activity-friendly built environments in Japan—as a super-aged society—which need to be investigated.

## 2.1. Shrinking Cities: An Active Living Opportunity or a Threat?

The Shrinking Cities International Research Network [35] defined a shrinking city as "a densely populated urban area with a minimum population of 10,000 residents that has faced population losses in large parts for more than two years and is undergoing economic transformations with some symptoms of a structural crisis" [36]. Japan's population has been continually declining since 2005. Except for a few metropolitan areas (such as Tokyo, Osaka, and Nagoya), many other parts of Japan, especially small towns and rural areas, are experiencing severe shrinking. As an emerging research agenda in urban design and planning, shrinking cities may produce many new challenges [37,38]. In relation to activity-friendly neighborhoods, urban shrinking means that Japanese cities and towns can become far less dense and eventually unable to sustain enough facilities to support daily lives, such as retail stores and public transportation, in the near future. Higher residential density has been consistently found to be associated with people's active behaviors [11,39]. For example, a Japanese study found the average physical activity levels in Japanese cities to be positively correlated with their urban population density [40]. Therefore, managing urban shrinking can potentially be a future issue for walkability in Japan.

At the same time, urban shrinking may create a new opportunity to reshape built environments as more walkable, since newly available vacant houses and spaces will emerge over the entire city region [41]. A key issue in using these newly available spaces in cities will be "land use mix", referring to having a variety of destinations such as homes, shops, parks, schools, offices, and train stations within a given area. Previous studies have identified land use mix as one of the main neighborhood walkability features [42,43]. The underlying assumption is that those people who live in an area with a high level of land use mix may have better opportunities to be active within their area. This indicates that encouraging land use mix in neighborhood (re)development plans can be key for supporting an active lifestyle. In the context of the United States, the unwalkable residential suburbs, which are occupied by only single-family houses, emerged through the Euclidian zoning system, which allows exclusively single land use for designated zones. Due to the lack of a rigid regulation scheme, Japanese suburbs have occasionally developed unintended mixed land use of various residential zones with commercial, industrial, and agricultural zones in relatively small areas in the age of urban sprawl. However, uncontrolled mixed land use development is not necessarily beneficial for health. For instance, it may increase noise and crime risks, and the emerged landscape is likely to be chaotic and aesthetically less attractive. How to control suburbanization and how to manage the use of newly available (but sporadically) emerging new spaces in existing built-up areas for creating opportunities that support an active lifestyle is vital for the future of shrinking cities.

In response to urban shrinking, Japanese local and national governments are now encouraging compact city policies. The policy may keep enough population density in residential areas to sustain urban facilities, which are an important element of walkability. It may also reduce car dependency of residents by sustaining public transportation service. Compact city may be a response to urban shrinking in cities where already experiencing shrinking; and it may not be a solution to avoid urban shrinking in other areas. In addition, while compact city policies have been widely advocated across the world, their health effects have not been fully examined [44]. Future research is needed to identify challenges and opportunities raised by urban shrinking in super-aged societies in relation to activity-friendly neighborhoods.

## 2.2. Extreme Levels of Environmental Attributes

Apart from land use mix, several differences exist in built environment attributes influencing active life between Japan and Western societies. For example, slope is an environmental attribute that Japanese cities have in extreme levels compared to the United States., Canadian, and Australian cities.

About three-quarters of the national land of Japan is mountains, and the residential areas are limited to only four percent of the national land [45]. Slope is one of the typical features of Japanese cities and suburbs. It is not uncommon to see steep slopes (greater than 25 percent), even in central parts of Japanese cities (Figure 1). Some previous studies have shown the positive effects of slope on type 2 diabetes, assumingly through vigorous physical activity [46,47]. However, slope (and subsequently stairs) has been identified as one of the barriers for the elderly to be physically active within their neighborhoods [48–50]. Most previous studies examining accessibility measures of built environments, such as access to shops, train stations, and parks, in relation with active behaviors, did not take into account the slope factor [50]. Another extreme level of environmental attribute in Japanese cities is residential density. For instance, the city of Nagoya in Japan has a population density of 7080 persons per square kilometer [51], whereas the population density of Melbourne (the most dense capital city in Australia) is only 450 people per square kilometer [52].

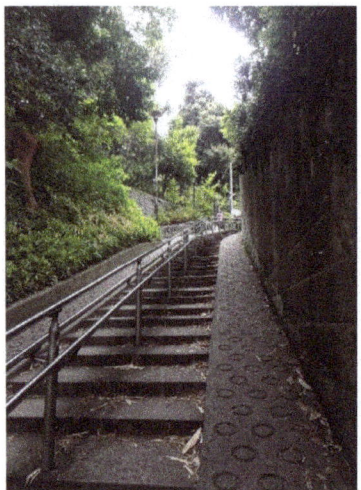 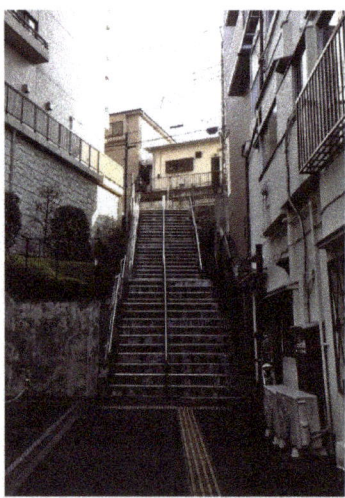

**Figure 1.** Steep slopes in the central parts of Tokyo, Japan (source: authors).

The relationship between environment and active behavior may not be always linear: there may be specific levels (thresholds) over which the effects of a built environment attribute on a behavior may change, especially among the elderly [53,54]. For example, there may be specific amounts of slope or residential density beneficial for elderly active behaviors and health. Nevertheless, most evidence on the importance of built environments on active behaviors comes from Western countries with relatively less extreme levels of environmental attributes [17,18]. This suggests that it is not clear how extreme levels of these environmental attributes may shape elderly's active behaviors. Investigating the effects of built environments on active behaviors in Japan can provide the international field with an opportunity to identify the optimal values of these environmental attributes for supporting an active aging life.

*2.3. Exposures to Environments: Time/Place in Active Behaviors*

Not only levels but also the way people are exposed to environments or use surrounding environmental opportunities can be distinctively different between societies. In particular, temporality is an important issue in investigating the relationships between environmental attributes and active behavior [55,56]. People are exposed to different types of environments in daily life depending on their mobility status. Consequently, their active behaviors are influenced not only by their immediate residential environment, but also by a broader environmental context. There are several reasons why the temporality in the relationships between environment and behavior may be more important in the context of Japan compared with other regions. First, safety from crime is relatively higher in Japan than other industrialized societies [57]. Since there is a low crime rate even at night-time, time restrictions for walking outside are minimal in Japan. Second, since most convenience stores in Japan are open 24 h a day and 7 days a week, there are still people walking to their local convenience stores even at midnight. Finally, Japan benefits from an efficient public transportation system that includes trains and buses, especially within urban areas. This efficient public transport system enhances the elderly's mobility and enables them to travel far from their homes (and be exposed to a wide range of environments) in their daily life. Therefore, future studies in Japan need to include time-specific measures of environment and active behaviors.

*2.4. Health Disparities, Environmental Equity, and Activity-Friendly Urban Design*

Reducing health disparities is now a major goal of public health across the world [58]. Health disparities across regions are increasing in Japan. A recent study published in *Lancet* has shown widening life expectancies and clear variations of disease burden across the Japanese prefectures [59]. Larger health disparities may also exist at a smaller areal level in Japan [60]. Several previous studies showed an association between physical activity levels and socioeconomic status (SES): more disadvantaged people are likely to be less physically active [61,62]. For example, a systematic review found people with high SES were more active than those with low SES during leisure time [61]. Mitigating the physical activity gap between low and high SES areas can be an important step in reducing the health disparity, especially among elderly [63]. Inequitable distribution of environmental attributes supporting physical activity (e.g., commercial destinations, parks, and well-connected streets) across low and high SES areas may be one of the reasons for this gap. Several previous studies showed those who lived in more deprived areas have less walkable built environment attributes [64,65]. For instance, a national study conducted in Germany found a significant positive association between income level and the amount of urban green space [65]. However, some studies found either no SES disparities or clear patterns in access to walkable neighborhood attributes [66,67]. For example, a recent national study conducted in the United States found a complex relationship between SES and walkable neighborhood attributes: those who lived in more disadvantaged areas, or in areas with more educated people, had better environmental attributes conducive to walking [66].

Nevertheless, there are few studies yet to investigate whether disadvantaged people have poorer walkable neighborhood attributes in Japan. For example, access to parks was found to be poorer for disadvantaged areas in Yokohama City, Japan, compared with affluent areas [68]. Another recent Japanese study found deprived neighborhoods to be less walkable in terms of population density, street density, and access to commercial concentrations [69]. However, little is known if changes in such environmental attributes could alter the health disparity. Considering the life course epidemiological approach, past environmental disparities may contribute to health disparity in later life [70]. Identifying both historical and geographical patterns between differing SES areas with walkable neighborhood attributes will guide urban design interventions to reduce the physical activity gap between these areas, and ultimately reduce the health disparities across regions.

## 3. Conclusions: Toward a Research Agenda

There has been a growing body of research examining how built environment attributes can influence active behaviors. We have identified key issues and challenges providing robust evidence-based research on the role of the surrounding physical environment on people's active life in the context of a super-aged society. To summarize, the following issues need to be investigated in future studies:

- explore challenges and opportunities that shrinking cities will have on active behaviors;
- identify optimal levels of environmental attributes, such as residential density and slope, needed to support healthy active aging;

- understand time/place in the elderly's active behaviors (the way elderly are exposed to environments or use surrounding environmental opportunities); and
- examine disparities in the distribution of activity-friendly environmental attributes.

In this commentary, our focus was only on walking, as the most common type of physical activity, especially among older adults. There are other types of physical activities, such as exercise, which may be of interest for elderly. Understanding how built environments may influence exercise among elderly requires further research. Cross-disciplinary research, between urban design/planning, sport sciences, public health, transport, geography, and gerontology, is needed to build evidence on how to build, retrofit, and sustain activity-friendly built environments in the context of a super-aged society.

**Author Contributions:** M.J.K., K.O. and T.N. conceived the idea and drafted the paper. All authors contributed to the writing and assisted with the interpretation. All authors have read and approved the final manuscript.

**Funding:** M.J.K. was supported by a JSPS Postdoctoral Fellowship for Research in Japan (#17716) from the Japan Society for the Promotion of Science. T.N. was supported by Japan Society for the Promotion of Science KAKENHI Grant Number JP15H02964 for this research. K.O. was supported by the MEXT-Supported Program for the Strategic Research Foundation at Private Universities, 2015–2019 the Japan Ministry of Education, Culture, Sports, Science and Technology (S1511017).

**Conflicts of Interest:** The authors declare no conflict of interest.

## References

1. Booth, F.W.; Roberts, C.K.; Laye, M.J. Lack of exercise is a major cause of chronic diseases. *Compr. Physiol.* **2012**, *2*, 1143–1211. [PubMed]
2. Owen, N.; Healy, G.N.; Matthews, C.E.; Dunstan, D.W. Too much sitting: The population-health science of sedentary behavior. *Exerc. Sport Sci. Rev.* **2010**, *38*, 105–113. [CrossRef] [PubMed]
3. Aune, D.; Norat, T.; Leitzmann, M.; Tonstad, S.; Vatten, L.J. *Physical Activity and the Risk of Type 2 Diabetes: A Systematic Review and Dose–Response Meta-Analysis*; Springer: New York, NY, USA, 2015.
4. Biswas, A.; Oh, P.I.; Faulkner, G.E.; Bajaj, R.R.; Silver, M.A.; Mitchell, M.S.; Alter, D.A. Sedentary time and its association with risk for disease incidence, mortality, and hospitalization in adults: A systematic review and meta-analysis. *Ann. Intern. Med.* **2015**, *162*, 123–132. [CrossRef] [PubMed]
5. Ng, S.W.; Popkin, B.M. Time use and physical activity: A shift away from movement across the globe. *Obes. Rev.* **2012**, *13*, 659–680. [CrossRef] [PubMed]
6. Dumith, S.C.; Hallal, P.C.; Reis, R.S.; Kohl, H.W. Worldwide prevalence of physical inactivity and its association with human development index in 76 countries. *Prev. Med.* **2011**, *53*, 24–28. [CrossRef] [PubMed]
7. Doyle, Y.; Furey, A.; Flowers, J. Sick individuals and sick populations: 20 years later. *J. Epidemiol. Community Health* **2006**, *60*, 396–398. [CrossRef] [PubMed]
8. Marteau, T.M.; Hollands, G.J.; Fletcher, P.C. Changing human behavior to prevent disease: The importance of targeting automatic processes. *Science* **2012**, *337*, 1492–1495. [CrossRef] [PubMed]
9. Sallis, J.F.; Floyd, M.F.; Rodríguez, D.A.; Saelens, B.E. Role of built environments in physical activity, obesity, and cardiovascular disease. *Circulation* **2012**, *125*, 729–737. [CrossRef] [PubMed]
10. Sallis, J.F.; Owen, N. Ecological models of health behavior. In *Health Behavior Theory*; Glanz, K., Rimer, B.K., Viswanath, K., Eds.; Jossey-Bass: San Francisco, CA, USA, 2015; pp. 43–64.
11. Sallis, J.F.; Cerin, E.; Conway, T.L.; Adams, M.A.; Frank, L.D.; Pratt, M.; Salvo, D.; Schipperijn, J.; Smith, G.; Cain, K.L. Physical activity in relation to urban environments in 14 cities worldwide: A cross-sectional study. *Lancet* **2016**, *387*, 2207–2217. [CrossRef]
12. Chokshi, D.A.; Farley, T.A. Changing behaviors to prevent noncommunicable diseases. *Science* **2014**, *345*, 1243–1244. [CrossRef] [PubMed]
13. United Nations Population Division. *World Population Prospects: The 2017 Revision—Key Findings and Advance Tables*; Working Paper No. ESA/P/WP/248; United Nations Population Division: New York, NY, USA, 2017.
14. Milanović, Z.; Pantelić, S.; Trajković, N.; Sporiš, G.; Kostić, R.; James, N. Age-related decrease in physical activity and functional fitness among elderly men and women. *Clin. Interv. Aging* **2013**, *8*, 549–556. [CrossRef] [PubMed]

15. Kerr, J.; Rosenberg, D.; Frank, L. The role of the built environment in healthy aging: Community design, physical activity, and health among older adults. *J. Plan. Lit.* **2012**, *27*, 43–60. [CrossRef]
16. Rosso, A.L.; Auchincloss, A.H.; Michael, Y.L. The urban built environment and mobility in older adults: A comprehensive review. *J. Aging Res.* **2011**, *2011*, 816106. [CrossRef] [PubMed]
17. Koohsari, M.J.; Sugiyama, T.; Sahlqvist, S.; Mavoa, S.; Hadgraft, N.; Owen, N. Neighborhood environmental attributes and adults' sedentary behaviors: Review and research agenda. *Prev. Med.* **2015**, *77*, 141–149. [CrossRef] [PubMed]
18. Sugiyama, T.; Neuhaus, M.; Cole, R.; Giles-Corti, B.; Owen, N. Destination and route attributes associated with adults' walking: A review. *Med. Sci. Sports Exerc.* **2012**, *44*, 1275–1286. [CrossRef] [PubMed]
19. Cerin, E.; Nathan, A.; Van Cauwenberg, J.; Barnett, D.W.; Barnett, A. The neighbourhood physical environment and active travel in older adults: A systematic review and meta-analysis. *Int. J. Behav. Nutr. Phys. Act.* **2017**, *14*, 15. [CrossRef] [PubMed]
20. Inoue, S.; Ohya, Y.; Tudor-Locke, C.; Tanaka, S.; Yoshiike, N.; Shimomitsu, T. Time trends for step-determined physical activity among Japanese adults. *Med. Sci. Sports Exerc.* **2011**, *43*, 1913–1919. [CrossRef] [PubMed]
21. Bauman, A.; Ainsworth, B.E.; Sallis, J.F.; Hagströmer, M.; Craig, C.L.; Bull, F.C.; Pratt, M.; Venugopal, K.; Chau, J.; Sjöström, M. The descriptive epidemiology of sitting: A 20-country comparison using the International Physical Activity Questionnaire (IPAQ). *Am. J. Prev. Med.* **2011**, *41*, 228–235. [CrossRef] [PubMed]
22. Ministry of Internal Affairs and Communication. *Statistical Handbook of Japan 2015*; Statistics Bureau, Ministry of Internal Affairs and Communication: Tokyo, Japan, 2015.
23. Ministry of Health Labor and Welfare. *Health Japan 21 (The Second Term)*; Ministry of Health Labor and Welfare: Tokyo, Japan, 2012.
24. Cerin, E.; Lee, K.-Y.; Barnett, A.; Sit, C.H.P.; Cheung, M.-C.; Chan, W.-M. Objectively-measured neighborhood environments and leisure-time physical activity in Chinese urban elders. *Prev. Med.* **2013**, *56*, 86–89. [CrossRef] [PubMed]
25. Ying, Z.; Ning, L.D.; Xin, L. Relationship between built environment, physical activity, adiposity, and health in adults aged 46–80 in Shanghai, China. *J. Phys. Act. Health* **2015**, *12*, 569–578. [CrossRef] [PubMed]
26. Feng, J. The influence of built environment on travel behavior of the elderly in urban China. *Transp. Res. Part D Trans. Environ.* **2017**, *52*, 619–633. [CrossRef]
27. Liao, Y.; Sugiyama, T.; Shibata, A.; Ishii, K.; Inoue, S.; Koohsari, M.J.; Owen, N.; Oka, K. Associations of perceived and objectively measured neighborhood environmental attributes with leisure-time sitting for transport. *J. Phys. Act. Health* **2016**, *13*, 1372–1377. [CrossRef] [PubMed]
28. Inoue, S.; Murase, N.; Shimomitsu, T.; Ohya, Y.; Odagiri, Y.; Takamiya, T.; Ishii, K.; Katsumura, T.; Sallis, J.F. Association of physical activity and neighborhood environment among Japanese adults. *Prev. Med.* **2009**, *48*, 321–325. [CrossRef] [PubMed]
29. Ishii, K.; Shibata, A.; Oka, K. Environmental, psychological, and social influences on physical activity among Japanese adults: Structural equation modeling analysis. *Int. J. Behav. Nutr. Phys. Act.* **2010**, *7*, 61. [CrossRef] [PubMed]
30. Inoue, S.; Ohya, Y.; Odagiri, Y.; Takamiya, T.; Ishii, K.; Kitabayashi, M.; Suijo, K.; Sallis, J.F.; Shimomitsu, T. Association between perceived neighborhood environment and walking among adults in 4 cities in Japan. *J. Epidemiol.* **2010**, *20*, 277–286. [CrossRef] [PubMed]
31. Koohsari, M.J.; Sugiyama, T.; Shibata, A.; Ishii, K.; Liao, Y.; Hanibuchi, T.; Owen, N.; Oka, K. Associations of street layout with walking and sedentary behaviors in an urban and a rural area of Japan. *Health Place* **2017**, *45*, 64–69. [CrossRef] [PubMed]
32. Koohsari, M.J.; Sugiyama, T.; Shibata, A.; Ishii, K.; Hanibuchi, T.; Liao, Y.; Owen, N.; Oka, K. Walk Score® and Japanese adults' physically-active and sedentary behaviors. *Cities* **2018**, *74*, 151–155. [CrossRef]
33. Hanibuchi, T.; Kawachi, I.; Nakaya, T.; Hirai, H.; Kondo, K. Neighborhood built environment and physical activity of Japanese older adults: Results from the Aichi Gerontological Evaluation Study (AGES). *BMC Public Health* **2011**, *11*, 657. [CrossRef] [PubMed]
34. Inoue, S.; Ohya, Y.; Odagiri, Y.; Takamiya, T.; Kamada, M.; Okada, S.; Oka, K.; Kitabatake, Y.; Nakaya, T.; Sallis, J.F. Perceived neighborhood environment and walking for specific purposes among elderly Japanese. *J. Epidemiol.* **2011**, *21*, 481–490. [CrossRef] [PubMed]

35. Wiechmann, T. What are the problems of shrinking cities? lessons learned from an international comparison. In *The Future of Shrinking Cities-Problems, Patterns and Strategies of Urban Transformation in a Global Context*; University of California, Berkeley: Berkeley, CA, USA, 2007; pp. 5–16.

36. Hollander, J.B.; Pallagst, K.; Schwarz, T.; Popper, F.J. Planning shrinking cities. *Prog. Plan.* **2009**, *72*, 223–232.

37. Martinez-Fernandez, C.; Audirac, I.; Fol, S.; Cunningham-Sabot, E. Shrinking cities: Urban challenges of globalization. *Int. J. Urban Reg. Res.* **2012**, *36*, 213–225. [CrossRef] [PubMed]

38. Pallagst, K. The planning research agenda: Shrinking cities—A challenge for planning cultures. *Town Plan. Rev.* **2010**, *81*, i–vi. [CrossRef]

39. Christiansen, L.B.; Cerin, E.; Badland, H.; Kerr, J.; Davey, R.; Troelsen, J.; van Dyck, D.; Mitáš, J.; Schofield, G.; Sugiyama, T.; et al. International comparisons of the associations between objective measures of the built environment and transport-related walking and cycling: IPEN adult study. *J. Transp. Health* **2016**, *3*, 467–478. [CrossRef] [PubMed]

40. Oba, T.; Matsunaka, R.; Nakagawa, D.; Inoue, K. Analysis of the Relationship between Urban Characters and Physical Activity Levels Based on the Travel Behavior Data. *J. City Plan. Inst. Jpn.* **2013**, *48*, 73–81. (In Japanese)

41. Aiba, S. *Folding a City: Urban Planning to Design Population Declining Age (Toshi wo Tatamu: Jinko Gensyo Jidaiwo Dezainsuru Toshikeikaku)*; Kaden-sha: Tokyo, Japan, 2015. (In Japanese)

42. Frank, L.D.; Sallis, J.F.; Saelens, B.E.; Leary, L.; Cain, K.; Conway, T.L.; Hess, P.M. The development of a walkability index: Application to the Neighborhood Quality of Life Study. *Br. J. Sports Med.* **2010**, *44*, 924–933. [CrossRef] [PubMed]

43. Owen, N.; Cerin, E.; Leslie, E.; Coffee, N.; Frank, L.D.; Bauman, A.E.; Hugo, G.; Saelens, B.E.; Sallis, J.F. Neighborhood walkability and the walking behavior of Australian adults. *Am. J. Prev. Med.* **2007**, *33*, 387–395. [CrossRef] [PubMed]

44. Krupp, J.; Acharya, K. *Up or out?: Examining the Trade-offs of Urban Form*; The New Zealand Initiative: Wellington, New Zealand, 2014.

45. Ministry of Land Infrastructure Transport and Tourism. Land and Climate of Japan. Available online: http://www.mlit.go.jp/river/basic_info/english/land.html (accessed on 29 August 2018).

46. Villanueva, K.; Knuiman, M.; Koohsari, M.J.; Hickey, S.; Foster, S.; Badland, H.; Nathan, A.; Bull, F.; Giles-Corti, B. People living in hilly residential areas in metropolitan Perth have less diabetes: Spurious association or important environmental determinant? *Int. J. Health Geogr.* **2013**, *12*, 59. [CrossRef] [PubMed]

47. Fujiwara, T.; Takamoto, I.; Amemiya, A.; Hanazato, M.; Suzuki, N.; Nagamine, Y.; Sasaki, Y.; Tani, Y.; Yazawa, A.; Inoue, Y.; et al. Is a hilly neighborhood environment associated with diabetes mellitus among older people? Results from the JAGES 2010 study. *Soc. Sci. Med.* **2017**, *182*, 45–51. [CrossRef] [PubMed]

48. Rantakokko, M.; Wilkie, R. The role of environmental factors for the onset of restricted mobility outside the home among older adults with osteoarthritis: A prospective cohort study. *BMJ Open* **2017**, *7*. [CrossRef] [PubMed]

49. Rantakokko, M.; Mänty, M.; Iwarsson, S.; Törmäkangas, T.; Leinonen, R.; Heikkinen, E.; Rantanen, T. Fear of moving outdoors and development of outdoor walking difficulty in older people. *J. Am. Geriatr. Soc.* **2009**, *57*, 634–640. [CrossRef] [PubMed]

50. Edwards, N.; Dulai, J. Examining the relationships between walkability and physical activity among older persons: What about stairs? *BMC Public Health* **2018**, *18*, 1025. [CrossRef] [PubMed]

51. Nagoya City. Statistical Sketch of Nagoya. Available online: http://www.city.nagoya.jp/en/page/0000014120.html (accessed on 28 August 2018).

52. Australia Bureau of Statistics. *Regional Population Growth, Australia, 2014–2015*; Catalogue No. 3218.0; Australia Bureau of Statistics: Canberra, Australia, 2016.

53. Koohsari, M.J.; Badland, H.; Giles-Corti, B. (Re)Designing the built environment to support physical activity: Bringing public health back into urban design and planning. *Cities* **2013**, *35*, 294–298. [CrossRef]

54. Kaczynski, A.T.; Potwarka, L.R.; Smale, B.J.; Havitz, M.E. Association of parkland proximity with neighborhood and park-based physical activity: Variations by gender and age. *Leis. Sci.* **2009**, *31*, 174–191. [CrossRef]

55. Kwan, M.-P. The limits of the neighborhood effect: Contextual uncertainties in geographic, environmental health, and social science research. *Ann. Am. Assoc. Geogr.* **2018**, 1–9. [CrossRef]

56. Kwan, M.-P. The uncertain geographic context problem. *Ann. Am. Assoc. Geogr.* **2012**, *102*, 958–968. [CrossRef]

57. Dijk, J.V.; Kesteren, J.V.; Smit, P. *Criminal Victimisation in International Perspective*; Boom Juridische Uitgevers: Den Haag, The Netherlands, 2007.

58. World Health Organization. *10 Facts on Health Inequities and Their Causes*; World Health Organization: Geneva, Switzerland, 2017.

59. Nomura, S.; Sakamoto, H.; Glenn, S.; Tsugawa, Y.; Abe, S.K.; Rahman, M.M.; Brown, J.C.; Ezoe, S.; Fitzmaurice, C.; Inokuchi, T. Population health and regional variations of disease burden in Japan, 1990–2015: A systematic subnational analysis for the Global Burden of Disease Study 2015. *Lancet* **2017**, *390*, 1521–1538. [CrossRef]

60. Nakaya, T. 'Geomorphology' of Population Health in Japan: Looking through the Cartogram Lens. *Environ. Plan. A* **2010**, *42*, 2807–2808. [CrossRef]

61. Beenackers, M.A.; Kamphuis, C.B.; Giskes, K.; Brug, J.; Kunst, A.E.; Burdorf, A.; van Lenthe, F.J. Socioeconomic inequalities in occupational, leisure-time, and transport related physical activity among European adults: A systematic review. *Int. J. Behav. Nutr. Phys. Act.* **2012**, *9*, 116. [CrossRef] [PubMed]

62. Farrell, L.; Hollingsworth, B.; Propper, C.; Shields, M.A. The socioeconomic gradient in physical inactivity: Evidence from one million adults in England. *Soc. Sci. Med.* **2014**, *123*, 55–63. [CrossRef] [PubMed]

63. Frieden, T. *Strategies for Reducing Health Disparities—Selected CDC-Sponsored Interventions, United States, 2014*; Foreword; MMWR Supplements; U.S. Department of Health and Human Services: Atlanta, GA, USA, 2014; Volume 63, p. 1.

64. Riggs, W. Inclusively walkable: Exploring the equity of walkable housing in the San Francisco Bay Area. *Local Environ.* **2016**, *21*, 527–554. [CrossRef]

65. Wüstemann, H.; Kalisch, D.; Kolbe, J. Access to urban green space and environmental inequalities in Germany. *Landsc. Urban Plan.* **2017**, *164*, 124–131. [CrossRef]

66. King, K.E.; Clarke, P.J. A disadvantaged advantage in walkability: Findings from socioeconomic and geographical analysis of national built environment data in the United States. *Am. J. Epidemiol.* **2014**, *181*, 17–25. [CrossRef] [PubMed]

67. Gullón, P.; Bilal, U.; Cebrecos, A.; Badland, H.M.; Galán, I.; Franco, M. Intersection of neighborhood dynamics and socioeconomic status in small-area walkability: The Heart Healthy Hoods project. *Int. J. Health Geogr.* **2017**, *16*, 21. [CrossRef] [PubMed]

68. Yasumoto, S.; Jones, A.; Shimizu, C. Longitudinal trends in equity of park accessibility in Yokohama, Japan: An investigation into the role of causal mechanisms. *Environ. Plan. A* **2014**, *46*, 682–699. [CrossRef]

69. Koohsari, M.J.; Hanibuchi, T.; Nakaya, T.; Shibata, A.; Ishii, K.; Liao, Y.; Oka, K.; Sugiyama, T. Associations of neighborhood environmental attributes with walking in Japan: Moderating effects of area-level socioeconomic status. *J. Urban Health* **2017**, *94*, 847–854. [CrossRef] [PubMed]

70. Pearce, J.; Shortt, N.; Rind, E.; Mitchell, R. Life course, green space and health: Incorporating place into life course epidemiology. *Int. J. Environ. Res. Public Health* **2016**, *13*, 331. [CrossRef] [PubMed]

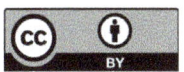

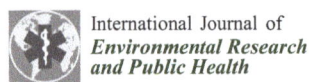

International Journal of
*Environmental Research
and Public Health*

*Commentary*

# A Case Study of a Natural Experiment Bridging the 'Research into Policy' and 'Evidence-Based Policy' Gap for Active-Living Science

**Paula Hooper [1,*], Sarah Foster [2] and Billie Giles-Corti [2]**

[1]  Australian Urban Design Research Centre, School of Design, The University of Western Australia, Perth 6009, Australia
[2]  Centre for Urban Research, RMIT University, Melbourne 3000, Australia
*   Correspondence: paula.hooper@uwa.edu.au

Received: 10 May 2019; Accepted: 6 July 2019; Published: 10 July 2019

**Abstract:** The translation of research into tangible health benefits via changes to urban planning policy and practice is a key intended outcome of academic active-living research endeavours. Conversely, policy-makers and planners identify the need for policy-specific evidence to ensure policy decisions and practices are informed and validated by rigorously established evidence. In practice, however, these two aspirations rarely meet and a research-translation gap remains. The RESIDE project is a unique longitudinal natural experiment designed to evaluate the health impacts of the 'Liveable Neighbourhoods' planning policy, which was introduced by the Western Australian Government to create more walkable suburbs. This commentary provides an overview and discussion of the policy-specific study methodologies undertaken to quantitatively assess the implementation of the policy and assess its active living and health impacts. It outlines the key research-translation successes and impact of the findings on the Liveable Neighbourhoods policy and discusses lessons learnt from the RESIDE project to inform future natural experiments of policy evaluation.

**Keywords:** natural experiment; built environment; urban design; policy evaluation; active living; liveability; Australia

---

## 1. Introduction

Government policy and planning initiatives determine the way cities, towns and neighbourhoods are developed and configured. They also play a vital role in creating and shaping the environments that support or undermine residents' health [1] and their ability to be safely and conveniently physically active [2,3]. Creating healthy, active communities is recognized as a global priority from both environmental sustainability and health perspectives [2,4]. However, achieving this laudable goal is not without challenges. It requires the involvement (and commitment) of multiple sectors beyond health, including urban planning and design, property development, construction, and finance, each with competing priorities and pressures.

Over the last 15 years, a comprehensive body of research has documented the impact of the design of the built environment on residents' active-living behaviours [5–8]. The translation of active-living research into tangible health benefits via changes to urban planning policy and practice is a key intended outcome of these academic endeavours [9]. At the same time, enlightened policy-makers and planners regularly affirm the need for "evidence-based policy and practice" to ensure their policy decisions and practices are informed and validated by rigorously established evidence. In practice, these two aspirations are rarely met and a research-translation gap remains between the ambitions of public health and urban planning on the one hand and the on-ground delivery of healthy, active communities on the other. With an increasing awareness and acceptance of the need for health-enhancing planning interventions, it is essential to understand why this research-translation gap remains. One explanation relates to the type of health-related evidence that is needed by planners and (planning) policy-makers in order for it to be utilized and applied [6]. This raises the question, is all evidence equal? Allender and colleagues [10] have argued that 'evidence-based' public health recommendations to planners and policy-makers are usually made without any obvious links to existing policies or legislation. Moreover, public health evidence rarely (if ever) provides quantifiable, evidence-based information about the potential health impacts of urban planning policies and decisions [10,11]. This has led to calls for public health research to be better aligned with current and future policy environments [6,12], and for science to more effectively guide city planning policy and practice [13]. However, if science is to inform policy, it must match the policies that it aims to influence [13]. Studies that develop policy surveillance measures and investigate and evaluate planning policy processes and implementation are well placed to bridge the translation gap [13,14]. Such research can provide a better, more nuanced understanding of how policies are implemented, how much of the policy has been delivered (i.e., the 'dose' of the policy intervention) and allow more accurate quantification of its impacts on active-living behaviours [14]. In particular, case studies and evaluations of urban planning policies, undertaken in partnership with planning professionals, are needed to identify the policies (or parts thereof) that produce desirable health-related outcomes [13–15].

To date, the public health evidence has mainly been cross-sectional in nature and the field has largely focused on the need for longitudinal natural experiment studies to evaluate policy implementation and as a way of understanding the impact of population-level policies on health outcomes [16]. A growing number of case studies and research papers now exist which compare new areas developed under different design principles or alternate planning movements or theories such as New Urbanism or Smart Growth and compare the health outcomes of residents [17–19]. These studies have typically measured and characterized the built environment with regards to how it relates to New Urbanist principles or planning policies [19,20]. However, to our knowledge, no studies have explicitly assessed or quantified the implementation of specific planning policies or design codes and empirically evaluated their impact on health-promoting behaviours and positive wellbeing outcomes. This is despite calls for studies of this type [6].

In addition to prospective study designs, greater emphasis is needed to identify which aspects of the policy produce desirable health-related outcomes [6,10,13–15,21]. This requires additional emphasis on process evaluation. Policy evaluation enables detailed assessment and quantification of which components of a policy were implemented as intended (in order to assess the 'dose' of the policy implementation), which components of the policy are the most influential active living ingredients, and which have no observable impacts. Without process evaluation, it is impossible to know whether positive effects (e.g., desirable active living or health behaviours) are the result of the policy intervention itself, and it is also impossible to establish whether a lack of observed outcomes is due to policy failure or inadequate policy implementation [22].

Few public health studies have measured policy implementation using policy-specific measures monitored over time, and assessed their impact on health-supportive behaviours [21]. Planning academics have also lamented the dearth of studies that quantitatively assess the implementation of policy to determine to what degree urban development policies and guidelines have been implemented as intended, how this relates to the intended planning goals, and to assess the on-ground outcomes [23,24]. Indeed, much of the literature about the implementation of planning theory concentrates on examining planning documents, processes, or decisions [18], not what is actually implemented in reality in communities and neighbourhoods.

State and local governments in jurisdictions around the world, including North America and Australia, are seeking to implement urban planning policies designed to shift growth away from low density, automobile-oriented development [6]. While evidence from across the globe in different settings is an important input which informs local decision-making, policy-makers often prioritize local evidence that directly relates to the planning and policy context [9]. Different jurisdictions in different contexts implement different policies and, as a result, produce different outcomes [25]. Hence, creating context-specific, local, policy-relevant evidence on the implementation of local policies is both important and timely.

## 2. RESIDE—A Natural Experiment of a New Urban Planning Policy

In 1998, when the State Government introduced the Liveable Neighbourhoods Community Design Guidelines policy (LN), a unique opportunity arose to collaborate with policy-makers and practitioners to evaluate the health impacts of an urban policy reform in situ through a longitudinal natural experiment study design. [26]. Liveable Neighbuorhoods was a response to conventional planning policies and practices implemented through the 1970s and the 1990s that had facilitated suburban sprawl and motor vehicle dependency across Perth, the capital city of Western Australia. The LN policy embraced emerging New Urbanism planning concepts [27] that provided an alternative approach to suburban neighbourhood design. LN has promoted a structure of walkable neighbourhoods where community facilities and services are (ideally) accessed by walking, cycling, and public transport through an efficient, interconnected movement network.

In 2003, with the support of key local policy-makers and advocates, the RESIDential Environments project (RESIDE) began with the aim of assessing the impact of LN on the desired policy outcomes including walking, cycling and public transport use, sense of community, safety from crime, and mental health.

All "liveable" and "conventional" developments that were under construction across the Perth metropolitan region with land sold for housing during the RESIDE recruitment period (in 2003) were included in the study. The Western Australian Department of Planning, Lands and Heritage (formerly the Department of Planning) categorized new development applications it received as either 'liveable' (i.e., aspiring to meet many of the LN requirements), 'hybrid' (i.e., meeting some but not all of the LN requirements), or 'conventional' (approved under the old policy). A total of 74 new developments (19 LN, 11 hybrid, and 44 conventional) [28] were selected for inclusion in the longitudinal study based on their stage of development, size, and location (e.g., distance to the ocean). The majority were being constructed on greenfield sites (i.e., previously unused or undeveloped land areas that had been rezoned, typically from urban deferred or rural to urban land uses and projects). Others were being constructed in brownfield areas (existing urban zones being redeveloped, sometimes following rezoning from industrial or other non-residential use).

The Water Corporation was approached to assist with the study. They invited all households that purchased house and land packages in the 74 developments ($n = 10,193$) to participate in the study [28]. To be eligible, customers had to be $\geq 18$ years of age; proficient in English; building a home in the selected development and planning to move into that home by December 2005; and they had to indicate that they were willing to complete three surveys and wear a pedometer for one week on three separate occasions over a five-year period. Only one eligible person was selected at random from each household [28]. The University of Western Australia's Human Research Ethics Committee provided ethics approval (#RA/4/1/479). Participants completed a postal survey on four occasions: Time 1 (T1), at baseline in 2003–2005 during construction of their new home and before relocation ($n = 1813$; 33.4% response rate); Time 2 (T2) in 2004–2006, approximately one year after relocation to their new home ($n = 1465$); Time 3 (T3) in 2006–2008, approximately three years after relocating ($n = 1229$); and Time 4 (T4) in 2011–2012, about six to nine years after relocating ($n = 565$) [29].

The mean age of the study population at baseline ($n = 1813$) was 40 years. Sixty percent were female, 82% were married or living with a partner, and 49% had children living at home. Just under one quarter of the sample (23%) had a bachelor's degree or higher, 43% had professional or managerial-administrator occupations, and 25% lived in households that earned AUD$90,000 or more per year. A large proportion of participants (43%) worked 39–59 hours per week and almost all (98%) had access to a motor vehicle [28,29].

This commentary provides a case study overview and discussion of the key lessons from the RESIDE project. It focuses on the policy-specific methodology and analyses that ensured RESIDE findings resonated with the local planning industry, and our research-translation efforts and their subsequent impacts on the LN policy. In discussing RESIDE we will also reflect on the three domains of evidence-based policy identified by Brownson and colleagues [15] and five key strategies identified as being essential to close the active-living research-translation gap [9]. The alignment between these domains and translation strategies is outlined in Table 1.

**Table 1.** Criteria for assessing the policy-relevant research-translation efforts of the RESIDE project.

| Three Domains of Evidence-Based Policy [15] | Strategies for Closing the Active-Living Research-Translation Gap [9] |
|---|---|
| ▪ Process—to understand approaches to enhance the likelihood of policy adoption. | ▪ Understand the 'policy world' we want to change.<br>▪ Establish links and research agendas jointly with policy-makers and practitioners.<br>▪ Apply policy-relevant study designs (e.g., quantifying policy implementation) that evaluate policy reform. |
| ▪ Content—to identify specific policy elements that are likely to be effective. | ▪ Identify reasons for implementation (or non-implementation). |
| ▪ Outcomes—to document the potential impact of policy. | ▪ Quantifying policy impacts on health.<br>▪ Highlight specific policy implications. |

## 3. Understanding the 'Policy World' for Liveable Neighbourhoods

In earlier work [9], we highlighted the critical need for active-living researchers to understand the 'policy world' in which decisions are made, and which active-living researchers are trying to influence. Similarly, Gagnon and Bellefleur [30] argue that public health researchers need to be familiar with the science of public policy-making in order "to better understand potential intervention contexts". Research-translation opportunities, therefore, need to be understood in the context of politics and public policymaking processes. Policy frameworks developed in the public policy and political science fields are used in a range of disciplines to analyze agenda-setting and policy-making. The Multiple Streams Framework originally developed by Kingdon [31] is an agenda-setting theory focused on how major policy change comes about. It posits that three elements contribute to policy change: a problem stream consisting of the issues that policy-makers and citizens want addressed; a politics stream comprising the factors that affect policy-makers' willingness to make a decision, including pressure group campaigns and political ideology; and a policy stream made up of ideas for feasible policy solutions [31]. According to this theory, policy change is possible when these streams align at critical moments in time, opening a 'window of opportunity' with the help of one or more policy entrepreneurs (individuals or organizations) who act as power brokers and manipulators of preferences.

The introduction of the LN policy was the result of a 'window of opportunity' where, in accordance with Kingdon's three streams theory of policy development, there was convergence between the problem, policy, and politics [31]. First, the problem of unsustainable suburban development and sprawl (the problem stream) was recognized and perceived as an issue of pressing importance for the future sustainability of Perth by policy-and decision-makers. Second, a proposal for an alternative policy solution promoting more sustainable design principles to those currently in operation was introduced via the global advocacy efforts of the Congress of New Urbanism (the policy stream). Finally, there was a supportive political climate and a willingness to trial a new approach (the politics stream) from the State Government, the Western Australian Planning Commission and the Department of Planning, plus growing awareness for the need of a different planning approach among the more enlightened property developers, through the advocacy and educational efforts of Council of New Urbanism [27]. The convergence of the three streams opened a policy window [31], allowing the trial of a new policy—the Liveable Neighbourhoods design guide.

The first edition of the new LN policy instrument was introduced in 1998 as a trial voluntary design code to be implemented by developers. The policy underwent extensive public and industry consultation before being adopted for full implementation in 2002 (as Edition 2) by the Western Australian Planning Commission as its preferred policy for assessing and approving all new greenfield and infill development applications in Western Australia.

In 2013, a decade after the RESIDE team first surveyed its cohort of participants and 15 years after the introduction of the LN policy, a comprehensive review of the LN policy was announced by the West Australian Department of Planning. This presented the opening of the policy window for the results from RESIDE to inform and influence the LN policy.

## 4. Establish Links and Joint Research Agendas with Policymakers and Practitioners

A partnership with the Department of Planning was formed in the planning stages of RESIDE, which was instrumental in galvanizing the Department's support for the project. Departmental officials were involved in selecting the developments for inclusion in the study, and later, a multi-sector advisory board was established to oversee and advise on the direction of RESIDE as it progressed. Throughout the study, Department of Planning staff received regular project updates. As a result, they were privy to results prior to publication and were able to provide feedback to the RESIDE study team. This process helped researchers to articulate the planning and policy implications of their research, and embed these in the 'so what' messaging and communication of the findings. Further, key supporters of the project from the Department provided opportunities for RESIDE researchers to present updates and findings to Department staff. This was essential in generating ongoing exposure and keeping the project on the Department's agenda.

Whilst the LN was highly regarded internationally as an effective local interpretation of New Urbanism, and despite the (then) Minister for Planning stating, in his foreword of the 2000 (second) edition of the guidelines, that *"the ability to measure their on-ground performance will further refine the policy"* [26], by 2003 there had been no formal evaluation of the policy. Therefore, in addition to assessing the health and wellbeing outcomes of the LN policy, a key interest of the policy partners within the Department was the assessment of which aspects of the policy were (or were not) being implemented and were (or were not) most effective. Upon the commencement of the review of the LN policy in 2013, and as a consequence of the ongoing collaboration and communication with the Department of Planning, there was, therefore, considerable interest in identifying which, if any, of the multitude of design features addressed in the policy were the 'key performance indicators or "non-negotiable" requirements for enhancing health'.

## 5. Quantify Policy Implementation and Delivery

In order to accurately assess the impacts of the LN policy on the health behaviours of residents and evaluate whether the policy was achieving its intended outcomes, it was essential to determine the degree to which the on-ground implementation had occurred (i.e., the 'dose' of the policy intervention that had been delivered). Hence, a novel aspect of the RESIDE project was the inclusion of a process evaluation to measure and quantify the levels of on-ground delivery of the policy in a subset of 36 of the 74 housing developments. The 19 LN developments were matched with 17 of the 44 conventionally designed developments by their stage of development (i.e., the proportion of the gross development area that had been constructed), size, and location (i.e., distance from the ocean). The varied sizes provided an opportunity to investigate how the LN policy was being applied at different scales of development and at which scale (or scales) the policy produced the greatest impacts.

Although RESIDE was a longitudinal study, the process evaluation of the policy implementation was cross-sectional in design. The majority of the housing developments selected for inclusion in the RESIDE project were being built on greenfield sites (i.e., previously undeveloped land). Because of the lack of any existing infrastructure on these sites and the timelines required for the construction of the developments from scratch, the timing of the process evaluation was chosen to coincide with the third time point of RESIDE data collection—i.e., five to six years post the commencement of the RESIDE study and approval of the housing developments. This allowed for the greatest amount of construction to have occurred within the study housing developments.

The process evaluation was designed to understand how much of the policy and what specific design requirements were (or were not) being adopted and implemented, and whether any dissappointing observed health and wellbeing outcomes were due to shortcomings of the policy principles, or failure to implement the policy [32,33]. The process evaluation used spatial measures tailored to quantify the urban design features required by the policy [32]. A total of 43 requirements were measured across four policy elements:

(1) Community design *n* = 13: These requirements determined the provision, location, and configuration of neighbourhood centres to create a hub of diverse destinations that attract people to a variety of activities. Objective measures of design features included land-use mix, number of destinations, design and configuration of activity centres, and presence of schools;

(2) Movement network *n* = 15: These requirements aimed to produce a highly interconnected street system aimed at reducing travel distances to local centres, schools, public transport links and other destinations, and adequate infrastructure for pedestrians and cyclists. Objective measures of design features included street connectivity, cul-de-sac lengths and block sizes, footpath networks and public transport;

(3) Lot layout *n* = 7: These requirements focused on higher residential densities to create more compact urban development and encourage the provision of a mixture of residential lot sizes to facilitate housing variety, choice and affordability, and to cater for increasingly diverse household types. Objective measures of design features included residential density, average area, and mix of residential lot sizes;

(4) Public parkland *n* = 8: These requirements aimed for a minimum contribution of 10% of the gross subdivisible land area to be provided as public parkland (Western Australian Planning Commission 2000) and specify different park types based on size and catchment areas to provide for a range of uses and activities. Objective measures of design features included the number and area of public parkland, distance to parks, and the assets and amenities within the parkland.

Policy compliance was defined as the degree to which the LN standards or requirements were reflected in the 'on-ground' construction of the developments. A simple scoring system was developed to quantify the extent to which the 43 measurable requirements had been implemented as intended by the LN [32]. The level of compliance for each element (defined as the degree to which the developments met the LN standards within that element) and overall LN compliance was calculated as the percentage of the maximum policy implementation score attainable.

The findings revealed that none of the developments had implemented the full suite of requirements as intended by the policy [32] and indeed, across all new developments, overall the LN policy was only half implemented, with overall compliance averaging just 46% (range: 30–60%) across the 36 developments [32]. Percentage compliance scores for each of the four elements were also well below full implementation: community design 27% (0–67%); movement network 48% (37–59%); lot layout 52% (19–88%); and public parkland 48% (30–60%) [32].

Figure 1 identifies the policy targets for seven design requirements from the LN policy that were found to be supportive of health behaviours [32–36]. It also plots the measured levels of on-ground compliance in each of the 36 RESIDE housing developments that were included in the process evaluation [32]. The results were presented in this way to the Department of Planning to clearly represent the levels of implementation being achieved versus the policy target and aspiration, and how this differed between design requirements.

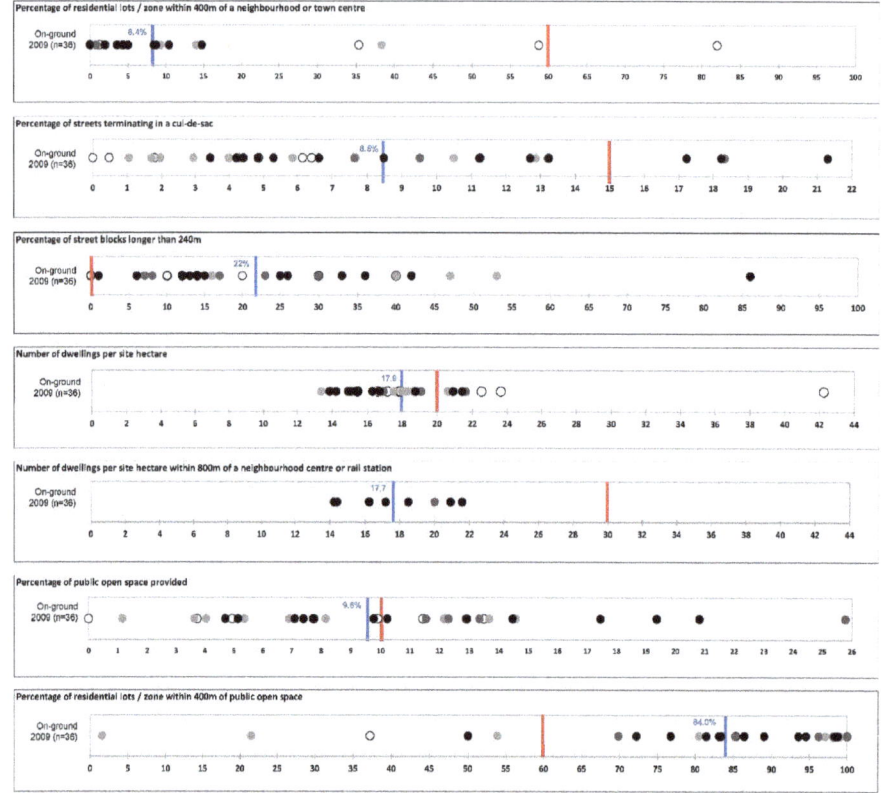

**Figure 1.** Compliance scores on selected design requirements measured in 36 housing developments on-the-ground in 2009 and approved development applications in 2015. Top = on-ground 2009 (*n* = 36): ○ Small subdivision ≤60 hectare (*n* = 8); ◉ Large subdivision >60 hectares ≤100 hectares (*n* = 10); ● Structure plan >100 hectares ≤300 hectares (*n* = 5); ● Regional master plan >300 hectares (*n* = 13); Indicates the Liveable Neighbourhoods policy target for the respective design feature; | Indicates the average level of compliance across the 36 housing developments.

## 6. Quantify Policy Impacts on Health-Related Outcomes

Despite incomplete implementation of the policy, analyses were also undertaken to determine if greater on-ground implementation of the policy was associated with positive health and wellbeing outcomes. The results revealed a strong dose–response relationship between policy compliance and four health-related outcomes, suggesting that new communities built in accordance with the LN policy principles and design features have the potential to promote the health and wellbeing of residents by creating neighbourhoods that encourage transport and recreational walking and have a stronger sense of community where residents feel safer [32,34–36]. For every 10% increase in levels of overall policy compliance, the odds of RESIDE participants walking for transport in the neighbourhood increased by 53% [32]; the odds of having a higher sense of community increased by 21% [35]; low psychological distress (i.e., better mental health) increased by 14% [35]; and the odds of being a victim of crime decreased by 40% [34]. Furthermore, a series of analyses unpacked the policy further to identify which of the specific design requirements from each of the policy elements were most strongly associated with walking [36], sense of community, mental health [35] and reports of safety or being a victim of crime [34]. Additional analyses also investigated which of the specific design features from the four policy elements showed the strongest associations with these four outcomes [32,34–36]. Other RESIDE analyses have also shown the design of the neighbourhoods to be positively associated with public transport use [37] and cycling [38].

## 7. Understand the Barriers and Facilitators to Policy Implementation

The results of the process evaluation revealed incomplete levels of implementation and compliance with the LN policy in that the totality of on-ground built form outcomes intended by the LN was at the time, not evident. This raised questions as to why incomplete implementation had occurred. Because the planning principles underpinning the LN differed from the conventional planning policies and development and engineering practices of the time, problems were experienced when implementing the LN.

Working with the project advisory board and key personnel from the Department of Planning, considerable efforts were made to identify and understand the barriers or factors that limited or acted as obstacles to the implementation of the LN. This was also an essential step in helping to determine whether principle or practice gaps were affecting its success. Conversely, it also helped to identify the factors or approaches that enhanced the likelihood of policy adoption and implementation.

For example, the construction of housing developments is generally sequenced, and the order in which land and infrastructure are developed appears to be dictated by several factors, including a balance between marketing or sales purposes and economic considerations. Developers appear to regard public open space as an important aesthetic feature that is instrumental to land sales and as such is typically installed early [39,40]. In contrast, community infrastructure such as neighbourhood centers, health services, schools, and public transport are often delayed until there is a sufficient critical mass of residents to warrant these services being provided [29,41,42]. The longitudinal component of the study allowed these changes in the new developments to be identified, tracked, and explained over time.

The LN policy document is also complex. It contained 128 different requirements and significant amounts of duplication within and across the four elements, which proved to be daunting and difficult for developers to understand and apply [43].

Furthermore, development proposals submitted for assessment and approval under the LN policy required additional compulsory information compared with the conventional policies. This was a significant disincentive for developers and resulted in their reluctance to submit proposals using the new LN policy, which also created difficulties for officials assessing and approving the applications [43].

Many of the LN design requirements directly contradicted existing conventional policies and engineering standards. Whilst LN was meant to prevail in instances of conflict, the voluntary nature of the guide meant it had no legal standing or precedence over the existing Local Government Authority planning schemes. It was, therefore, vulnerable to negotiation and to the compromising of LN standards. As a result, many of the LN features approved for development may not have been implemented on the ground. The inconsistencies between the state-sanctioned LN and LGA planning schemes were identified as a major barrier to developers adopting and implementing the LN policy (UDIA 2005; Jones 2010; STAC 2012).

Finally, given the time taken to construct the new developments, the six years between the commencement of the RESIDE project (in 2003) to the time of evaluation (in 2009) was a relatively short time period. This is likely to have contributed to many of the developments being incomplete at the time of evaluation. This was an important consideration not to be overlooked when designing future natural experiment studies of policy implementation.

The findings indicated that the policy was worthy of wider dissemination, but a greater emphasis on policy implementation was needed. The identified policy implementation gap highlighted the importance of process evaluation and the need for longitudinal study design. It also highlighted the value of undertaking research in partnership with policy-makers within local contexts [9–11].

## 8. Highlight Specific Policy Implications

When undertaking case studies or natural experiment evaluations of planning policies and practices in partnership with policy-makers and practitioners, outputs that are directly relevant to the policy and its implementation are needed to help partners gauge the health impact of their current policies and practices. When presenting updates and results to our industry advisory board, we were consistently challenged to reflect on the findings and identify the policy significance in terms of being able to communicate 'what bit of what policy would we change and what should it be changed to?'

RESIDE's process evaluation study provided policy-specific empirical evidence that showed that when implemented as intended, the LN policy could positively impact a range of health and wellbeing outcomes and produce outcomes that were aligned with the policy's overall objectives. Through the quantification of policy implementation with tailored spatial measures and the longitudinal tracking of the built environments over time, the RESIDE process evaluation project highlighted important gaps in the implementation of LN design features. Without this knowledge, it was impossible to judge whether the observed associations with health outcomes (or lack of) were due to the ineffectiveness of the policy principles or a failure to implement the policy on the ground.

This data resonated with the Department of Planning, which was keenly interested in the policy-specific measures of implementation as they both illustrated and confirmed how well the policy was being implemented and the potential promise of the policy principles. For the first time, the process evaluation armed the Department of Planning with the objective evidence they needed to assist in reviewing a planning policy and its processes. Importantly, it enabled them to gauge current levels of LN implementation and identify what aspects of the policy were (or were not) being delivered on the ground.

In direct response to their interests and jointly established research questions, we were able to identify the specific design requirements shown to be important for health and wellbeing outcomes, derived from analyses examining individual policy requirements [32–36]. The empirically based submissions were also important in terms of preventing policy regression (i.e., health-promoting requirements were not removed from the policy). Specifically, policy advocates needed a highly regarded, policy specific, and well-understood evidence-base to help preserve the design requirements that had been shown to consistently and positively influence health-enabling or health-promoting behaviours. This was an important outcome of the RESIDE project and a direct result of the policy-specific nature of the measurement and analyses undertaken.

## 9. Undertaking Policy-Relevant Research and Natural Experiments—Lessons Learned

The long-term partnership between researchers and policy-makers from the Department of Planning was paramount to the success of the RESIDE research-translation. Throughout the study, Department of Planning staff received regular project updates, ensuring they were privy to results prior to publication, and provided feedback to the RESIDE study team. This process helped researchers to understand and articulate the planning and policy implications of their research and embed these in the 'so what' messaging and communication of the research findings.

Another crucial success factor was understanding the planning and development processes. Concerted efforts were made to work with our industry partners to understand the development and construction processes of the local planning system. Indeed, the relevance of research findings and their applicability to a local context have been identified as important enablers of research uptake among policy-makers (Oliver et al. 2014). The guidance provided by the partners was essential in helping the research team to understand (1) the different stages of the 'policy pipeline'—that is, the different stages of approval a development application goes through; (2) the relevant authorities responsible for the approval of a development application at each of stage of the process (i.e., local government versus state government); and (3) which specific design requirements were assessed and approved at each stage of the process and at different scales of development (e.g., regional masterplan, structure plan, or subdivision). This knowledge was essential in alerting the researchers to the challenges that practitioners face throughout the development application process, whilst simultaneously helping and enabling the research team to credibly frame, contextualise, and communicate the policy-relevance of the findings when presenting to the policy-makers and planning practitioners. Further, it was apparent that different aspects of policy compliance were the responsibility of different authorities, and it was important to understand this to tailor targeted messages to specific groups. Other lessons learned were an understanding of the complexity of the process of developing policy and delivering outcomes on the ground in communities, and a recognition of the number of actors involved in the policy pipeline. With our industry partners, we attempted to conceptualize this process in what we've termed 'the leaky pipe' of the policy pipeline process (see Figure 2).

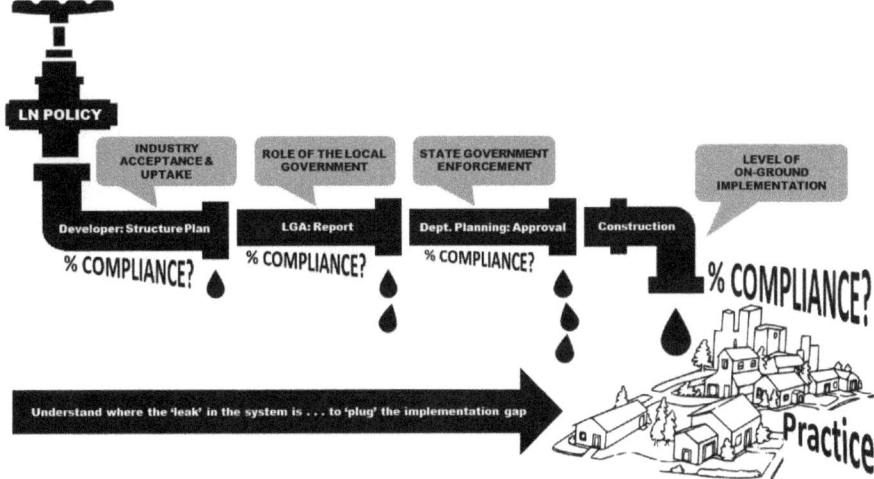

**Figure 2.** The 'leaky pipe' of the policy pipeline process for the Liveable Neighbourhoods Community Design policy in Perth, Western Australia.

The concept of the 'leaky pipe' in policy evaluation studies is important, because if policies are to be fully implemented and studies are to be established to identify where leakages occur between a policy and its on-the-ground delivery, it is essential that researchers understand what agencies or authorities are responsible for the approval and enforcement of different design features within the policy. Moreover, understanding the policy pipeline could help with the translation of active-living and public health research findings by going beyond simply identifying that a policy was not working to identifying where in the policy implementation pipeline leakages were occurring. This would enable specificity in the messaging by highlighting the aspects of the policy that are important for positive health impacts. Moreover, if different organizations are responsible for different design features, it may be necessary to communicate and target research findings to the specific authorities and agencies responsible for these design requirements at different stages of the approvals process.

In an ideal world, there should be an increase in policy compliance at each stage of the policy pipeline, as the different authorities uphold and enforce the intent (and implementation) of the policy. But at each stage, there is also the potential for 'leakage' (e.g., failure to implement parts of the policy). Hence, research is needed to understand and identify how much and what specific features of the policy are being approved and enforced at each stage of the process, to enable any leakages to be 'plugged' or resolved to ensure full policy implementation. Moreover, if the custodians of the policy (in our case, the Department of Planning) wish to close the gap between policy and implementation, they need to exercise greater oversight of development applications as they move through each stage of the pipeline process and identify and stem any leakages.

Our process evaluation provided a benchmark of the on-ground delivery of the LN policy for the Department of Planning; however, they have since embarked on an ongoing (in-house) monitoring program to track LN policy uptake. In partnership with department planners, we identified the design requirements from the LN policy that had been shown (from RESIDE) to be important for the health and wellbeing outcomes that they were directly responsible for enforcing. These were adopted by the Department of Planning in 2016 as 'performance indicators' to provide a framework for the assessment of future development applications against the LN policy. This consistent capture of policy-specific data by the Department was also the basis for an ongoing monitoring and evaluation framework for the LN policy, and a cross-check of how well (and how much of) the policy was being adopted and enforced at the last point in the pipeline before construction.

A final lesson learned from RESIDE was the need to benchmark and quantify the levels of compliance against the policy aspirations and targets at different stages of the policy pipeline. This is important to explain findings related to the intended policy outcomes versus those actually being realized. It would also assist in translating research findings, ensuring that different authorities are appropriately targeted to assist in avoiding leakages between policy and delivery on the ground. Future process evaluations of policy implementation could seek to quantify the levels of compliance with the policy at the different stages of the policy pipeline with the aim of identifying where leaks in the system are occurring and to gain an understanding of the barriers to, or facilitators of, compliance and implementation.

## 10. Conclusions

This paper demonstrated how policy-relevant research and natural experiments can be undertaken and disseminated to policy-makers to positively impact policy. The longitudinal natural experiment approach adopted by RESIDE allowed time for sufficient development to unfold. This, coupled with a process evaluation to quantify the dose of the LN policy being evaluated, helped to bridge the gap between active-living research and its application for evidence-based (or informed) planning policy. Evidence-informed planning and better monitoring of urban policy implementation [32] can help assess progress towards maintaining and strengthening the health and liveability of cities. The development and regular measurement of spatial indicators to benchmark and monitor the implementation of policies designed to create healthy, liveable communities is essential to ensure the policies aimed at creating these environments are fulfilled.

**Author Contributions:** P.H. conceived, conceptualized, and led the development and writing of the paper with input and assistance from S.F. and B.G.-C. P.H. led the methodology and analyses reported in the paper under the supervision of B.G.-C. P.H. prepared the original draft of the manuscript with substantial subsequent input and editing from S.F. and B.G.-C. All authors have approved the final manuscript. The RESIDE project was conceptualized, led and overseen by B.G.-C., who was responsible for all project funding acquisition as listed below.

**Funding:** All funding bodies are gratefully acknowledged. RESIDE was funded by grants from the Western Australian Health Promotion Foundation (Healthway) (#11828) and the Australian Research Council (ARC) (#LP0455453) and supported by an Australian National Health and Medical Research Council (NHMRC) Capacity Building Grant (#458688). The first author was supported by a Healthway Research Fellowship (#32992) and an NHMRC CRE in Healthy Liveable Communities (#1061404); SF is supported by an ARC Discovery Early Career Researcher Award (DE160100140); BGC is supported by an NHMRC Senior Principal Research Fellow Award (#1107672).

**Acknowledgments:** The following GIS team (Kimberley Van Niel, Nick Middleton, Sharyn Hickey, Bridget Beasley, and Bryan Boruff) are gratefully acknowledged for their assistance and advice in the development of the GIS measures in this study. Spatial data were based on information provided by, and with the permission of, the Western Australian Land Information Authority and the Department of Planning. Destination data were purchased from the Sensis (Yellow Pages). Hayley Christian, Jacinta Francis, Claire Lauritsen, and Roseanne Barnes coordinated RESIDE survey data collections.

**Conflicts of Interest:** The authors declare no conflict of interest.

# References

1. Chandrabose, M.; Rachele, J.N.; Gunn, L.; Kavanagh, A.; Owen, N.; Turrell, G.; Giles-Corti, B.; Sugiyama, T. Built environment and cardio-metabolic health: Systematic review and meta-analysis of longitudinal studies. *Obes. Rev.* **2019**, *20*, 41–54. [CrossRef] [PubMed]
2. Giles-Corti, B.; Vernez-Moudon, A.; Reis, R.; Turrell, G.; Dannenberg, A.L.; Badland, H.; Foster, S.; Lowe, M.; Sallis, J.F.; Stevenson, M.; et al. City planning and population health: A global challenge. *Lancet* **2016**, *388*, 2912–2924. [CrossRef]
3. Stevenson, M.; Thompson, J.; de Sá, T.H.; Ewing, R.; Mohan, D.; McClure, R.; Roberts, I.; Tiwari, G.; Giles-Corti, B.; Sun, X.; et al. Land use, transport, and population health: Estimating the health benefits of compact cities. *Lancet* **2016**, *388*, 2925–2935. [CrossRef]
4. United Nations. Sustainable development goals. In *Goal 11: Make Cities Inclusive, Safe, Resilient and Sustainable*; UN: New York, NY, USA, 2016.
5. Ding, D.; Gebel, K. Built environment, physical activity, and obesity: What have we learned from reviewing the literature? *Health Place* **2012**, *18*, 100–105. [CrossRef] [PubMed]
6. Durand, C.P.; Andalib, M.; Dunton, G.F.; Wolch, J.; Pentz, M.A. A systematic review of built environment factors related to physical activity and obesity risk: Implications for smart growth urban planning. *Obes. Rev.* **2011**, *12*, e173–e182. [CrossRef] [PubMed]
7. Mayne, S.L.; Auchincloss, A.H.; Michael, Y.L. Impact of policy and built environment changes on obesity-related outcomes: A systematic review of naturally occurring experiments. *Obes. Rev.* **2015**, *16*, 362–375. [CrossRef] [PubMed]
8. Smith, M.; Hosking, J.; Woodward, A.; Witten, K.; MacMillan, A.; Field, A.; Baas, P.; Mackie, H. Systematic literature review of built environment effects on physical activity and active transport—An update and new findings on health equity. *Int. J. Behav. Nutr. Phys. Act.* **2017**, *14*, 158. [CrossRef] [PubMed]
9. Giles-Corti, B.; Sallis, J.F.; Sugiyama, T.; Frank, L.D.; Lowe, M.; Owen, N. Translating active living research into policy and practice: One important pathway to chronic disease prevention. *J. Public Health Policy* **2015**, *36*, 231–243. [CrossRef] [PubMed]
10. Allender, S.; Cavill, N.; Parker, M.; Foster, C. 'Tell us something we don't already know or do!' The response of planning and transport professionals to public health guidance on the built environment and physical activity. *J. Public Health Policy* **2009**, *30*, 102–116. [CrossRef]
11. Oliver, K.; Innvar, S.; Lorenc, T.; Woodman, J.; Thomas, J. A systematic review of barriers to and facilitators of the use of evidence by policymakers. *BMC Health Serv. Res.* **2014**, *14*, 2. [CrossRef]
12. Orton, L.; Lloyd-Williams, F.; Taylor-Robinson, D.; O'Flaherty, M.; Capewell, S. The use of research evidence in public health decision making processes: Systematic review. *PLoS ONE* **2011**, *6*, e21704. [CrossRef] [PubMed]
13. Sallis, J.F.; Bull, F.; Burdett, R.; Frank, L.D.; Griffiths, P.; Giles-Corti, B.; Stevenson, M. Use of science to guide city planning policy and practice: How to achieve healthy and sustainable future cities. *Lancet* **2016**, *388*, 2936–2947. [CrossRef]
14. Sallis, J.; Story, M.; Lou, D. Study Designs and Analytic Strategies for Environmental and Policy Research on Obesity, Physical Activity and Diet. *Am. J. Prev. Med.* **2009**, *36*, S72–S77. [CrossRef] [PubMed]
15. Brownson, R.C.; Jones, E. Bridging the gap: Translating research into policy and practice. *Prev. Med.* **2009**, *49*, 313–315. [CrossRef] [PubMed]
16. Craig, P.; Cooper, C.; Gunnell, D.; Haw, S.; Lawson, K.; Macintyre, S.; Ogilvie, D.; Petticrew, M.; Reeves, B.; Sutton, M.; et al. Using natural experiments to evaluate population health interventions: New Medical Research Council guidance. *J. Epidemiol. Community Health* **2012**, *66*, 1182–1186. [CrossRef] [PubMed]
17. Gordon, D.L.A.; Tamminga, K. Large-scale Traditional Neighbourhood Development and Pre-emptive Ecosystem Planning: The Markham Experience, 1989–2001. *J. Urban Des.* **2002**, *7*, 321–340. [CrossRef]
18. Grant, J. Theory and Practice in Planning the Suburbs: Challenges to Implementing New Urbanism, Smart Growth, and Sustainability Principles. *Plan. Theory Pract.* **2009**, *10*, 11–33. [CrossRef]
19. Trudeau, D. A typology of New Urbanism neighborhoods. *J. Urban. Int. Res. Placemaking Urban Sustain.* **2013**, *6*, 113–138. [CrossRef]
20. Sohmer, R.R.; Lang, R.E. From seaside to Southside: New urbanism's quest to save the inner city. *Hous. Policy Debate* **2000**, *11*, 751–760. [CrossRef]

21. Sallis, J.; Bauman, A.; Pratt, M. Environmental and Policy Interventions to Promote Physical Activity. *Am. J. Prev. Med.* **1998**, *15*, 379–397. [CrossRef]

22. Dehar, M.; Casswell, S.; Duignan, P. Formative and Process evaluation of health promotion and disease prevention programs. *Eval. Rev.* **1993**, *17*, 204–220. [CrossRef]

23. Brody, S.D.; Carrasco, V.; Highfield, W.E. Measuring the Adoption of Local Sprawl: Reduction Planning Policies in Florida. *J. Plan. Educ. Res.* **2006**, *25*, 294–310. [CrossRef]

24. Talen, E. Do Plans Get Implemented? A Review of Evaluation in Planning. *J. Plan. Lit.* **1996**, *10*, 248–259. [CrossRef]

25. Arundel, J.; Lowe, M.; Hooper, P.; Roberts, R.; Rozek, J.; Higgs, C.; Giles-Corti, B. *Creating Liveable Cities in Australia*; Centre for Urban Research; RMIT University: Melbourne, Australia, 2017.

26. Western Australian Planning Commission. *Liveable Neighbourhoods: A Western Australian Government Sustainable Cities Initiative*, 2nd ed.; Western Australian Planning Commission: Perth, Australia, 2000.

27. CNU. Congress for the New Urbanism. 1997. Available online: http://www.cnu.org/ (accessed on 1 May 2019).

28. Giles-Corti, B.; Knuiman, M.; Timperio, A.; Van Niel, K.; Pikora, T.J.; Bull, F.C.; Shilton, T.; Bulsara, M. Evaluation of the implementation of a state government community design policy aimed at increasing local walking: Design issues and baseline results from RESIDE, Perth Western Australia. *Prev. Med.* **2008**, *46*, 46–54. [CrossRef] [PubMed]

29. Knuiman, M.W.; Christian, H.E.; Divitini, M.L.; Foster, S.A.; Bull, F.C.; Badland, H.M.; Giles-Corti, B. A Longitudinal Analysis of the Influence of the Neighborhood Built Environment on Walking for Transportation: The RESIDE Study. *Am. J. Epidemiol.* **2014**, *180*, 453–461. [CrossRef]

30. Gagnon, F.; Bellefleur, O. Influencing public policies: Two (very good) reasons to look toward scientific knowledge in public policy. *Can. J. Public Health* **2014**, *106* (Suppl. 1), eS9–eS11.

31. Kingdon, J. *Agendas, Alternatives, and Public Policies*, 2nd ed.; Pearson: New York, NY, USA, 2003.

32. Hooper, P.; Giles-Corti, B.; Knuiman, M. Evaluating the implementation and active living impacts of a state government planning policy designed to create walkable neighborhoods in Perth, Western Australia. *Am. J. Health Promot.* **2014**, *28* (Suppl. 3), S5–S18. [CrossRef]

33. Hooper, P.; Knuiman, M.; Bull, F.; Jones, E.; Giles-Corti, B. Are we developing walkable suburbs through urban planning policy? Identifying the mix of design requirements to optimise walking outcomes from the 'Liveable Neighbourhoods' planning policy in Perth, Western Australia. *Int. J. Behav. Nutr. Phys. Act.* **2015**, *12*, 63. [CrossRef]

34. Foster, S.; Hooper, P.; Knuiman, M.; Bull, F.; Giles-Corti, B. Are liveable neighbourhoods safer neighbourhoods? Testing the rhetoric on new urbanism and safety from crime in Perth, Western Australia. *Soc. Sci. Med.* **2015**, *164*, 150–157. [CrossRef]

35. Hooper, P.; Foster, S.; Knuiman, M.; Giles-Corti, B. Testing the Impact of a Planning Policy Based on New Urbanist Planning Principles on Residents' Sense of Community and Mental Health in Perth, Western Australia. *Environ. Behav.* **2018**. [CrossRef]

36. Hooper, P.; Foster, S.; Knuiman, M.; Giles-Corti, B. The building blocks of a 'Liveable Neighbourhood': Identifying the key performance indicators for walking of an operational planning policy in Perth, Western Australia. *Health Place* **2015**, *36*, 173–183. [CrossRef] [PubMed]

37. Badland, H.; Hickey, S.; Bull, F.; Giles-Corti, B. Public transport access and availability in the RESIDE study: Is it taking us where we want to go? *J. Transp. Health* **2014**, *1*, 45–49. [CrossRef]

38. Beenackers, M.A.; Foster, S.; Kamphuis, C.B.; Titze, S.; Divitini, M.; Knuiman, M.; van Lenthe, F.J.; Giles-Corti, B. Taking Up Cycling After Residential Relocation: Built Environment Factors. *Am. J. Prev. Med.* **2012**, *42*, 610–615. [CrossRef]

39. Grose, M. Changing relationships in public open space and private open space in suburbs in south-western Australia. *Land. Urban Plan.* **2009**, *92*, 53–63. [CrossRef]

40. Grose, M. Practice wisdom from planners, developers, environmentalists, and other players finding the 'true debates' in suburban development in south-western Australia. *Aust. Plan.* **2010**, *47*, 26–36. [CrossRef]

41. Christian, H.; Knuiman, M.; Divitini, M.; Foster, S.; Hooper, P.; Boruff, B.; Bull, F.; Giles-Corti, B. A Longitudinal Analysis of the Influence of the Neighborhood Environment on Recreational Walking within the Neighborhood: Results from RESIDE. *Environ. Health Perspect.* **2017**, *125*, 077009. [CrossRef]

42. Giles-Corti, B.; Bull, F.; Knuiman, M.; McCormack, G.; Van Niel, K.; Timperio, A.; Christian, H.; Foster, S.; Divitini, M.; Middleton, N.; et al. The influence of urban design on neighbourhood walking following residential relocation: Longitudinal results from the RESIDE study. *Soc. Sci. Med.* **2013**, *77*, 20–30. [CrossRef]
43. Curtis, C.; Punter, J. Design-Led Sustainable Development: The Liveable Neighbourhoods Experiment in Perth, Western Australia. *Town Plan. Rev.* **2004**, *75*, 31–65. [CrossRef]

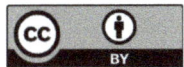

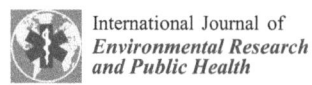

International Journal of
*Environmental Research
and Public Health*

*Article*

# Older Adults Using *Our Voice* Citizen Science to Create Change in Their Neighborhood Environment

Anthony G. Tuckett [1,2,*], Abbey Freeman [2], Sharon Hetherington [3], Paul A. Gardiner [4], Abby C. King [5] and On behalf of Burnie Brae Citizen Scientists [2,†]

[1]  Director, Postgraduate Coursework Programs (Nursing, Midwifery), The University of Queensland, St Lucia, QLD 4072, Australia
[2]  School of Nursing, Midwifery and Social Work, The University of Queensland, St Lucia, QLD 4072, Australia; a.freeman@uq.net.au
[3]  Healthy Connections Exercise Clinic, Burnie Brae Ltd., Chermside, QLD 4032, Australia; Hetherington.s@burniebrae.org.au
[4]  Centre for Health Services Research, Faculty of Medicine, The University of Queensland, St Lucia, QLD 4102, Australia; p.gardiner@uq.edu.au
[5]  Department of Health Research and Policy and Medicine, Stanford Prevention, Research Center, Stanford University School of Medicine, Palo Alto, CA 94305, USA; king@stanford.edu
\*  Corresponding: a.tuckett@uq.edu.au
†  On behalf of Burnie Brae Citizen Scientists, Burnie Brae Ltd., Chermside, QLD 4032, Australia; helleenpurdy@gmail.com

Received: 29 September 2018; Accepted: 26 November 2018; Published: 28 November 2018

**Abstract:** Physical activity, primarily comprised of walking in older adults, confers benefits for psychological health and mental well-being, functional status outcomes and social outcomes. In many communities, however, access to physical activity opportunities are limited, especially for older adults. This exploratory study engaged a small sample ($N = 8$) of adults aged 65 or older as citizen scientists to assess and then work to improve their communities. Using a uniquely designed mobile application (the Stanford Healthy Neighborhood Discovery Tool), participants recorded a total of 83 geocoded photos and audio narratives of physical environment features that served to help or hinder physical activity in and around their community center. In a facilitated process the citizen scientists then discussed, coded and synthesized their data. The citizen scientists then leveraged their findings to advocate with local decision-makers for specific community improvements to promote physical activity. These changes focused on: parks/playgrounds, footpaths, and traffic related safety/parking. Project results suggest that the *Our Voice* approach can be an effective strategy for the global goals of advancing rights and increasing self-determination among older adults.

**Keywords:** older adult; physical activity; social connectedness; physical environment; citizen science; Discovery Tool

---

## 1. Introduction

### 1.1. Population Ageing

In 2030 there will be 1 billion older adults globally (12% of the total population) [1]. Across the planet, the number of older adults is growing faster than the number of people in any other age group [2]. We can expect a 150% expansion of the population aged 65 and over in the next 35 years [1]. Worldwide the population 80 and over is projected to more than triple between 2015 and 2050 from 126.5 million to 446.6 million [1]. The WHO notes that reducing severe disability from disease and health conditions within this age cohort is one key to constraining health and social costs [3]. It is recommended that we need specifically targeted policies to address the needs of older adults to include housing, employment, health care, social protection and other forms of intergenerational support [2].

*1.2. Physical Activity*

For nearly all older adults, declining muscle mass, muscle strength and physical performance and increasing time spent sedentary are common pathways to disease, disability, falls risk, dependency and morbidity [4–7]. Consequent to this are the attendant care needs, community care costs and rising residential aged care uptake.

The evidence of the benefits of physical activity for the prevention and management of chronic conditions for older adults is well documented [6,8,9]. Pertinent to this study is the evidence that physical activity, primarily comprised of walking in older adults, confers benefits for psychological health and mental well-being (e.g., anxiety, depression, life satisfaction), functional status outcomes (e.g., sarcopenia, physical and cognitive function), and social outcomes (e.g., community involvement and social networks) [1,5,10,11]. Local environments can in turn affect physical activity levels. In addition to the effects of social aspects of the environment on physical activity, an extensive amount of evidence underscores the importance of physical environment features (e.g., intersection crossings, footpaths) on physical activity levels in different age groups.

*1.3. Social Connectedness*

Enhancing social participation is a central component of the WHO's response to concerns about population ageing [12]. In its many forms social connectedness (social networks, social integration, social embeddedness, human companionship) is vital for active ageing [13]. Social ties help humans build resilience in the face of various hardships and help to extend our lives. They can matter even more as we age when ill health increases, which can diminish opportunities for social engagement [14]. Those who have larger networks tend to have better health especially when the interaction with network members is frequent [15]. Generally speaking, adults who are more socially connected are healthier and live longer than their isolated peers; there is also a direct relationship between poor mental health and risk of dying which can be influenced by low quantity and quality of social relationships [16]. Social ties influence health behaviors and physical health [16].

Social connectedness and engagement can be affected by the surrounding physical environment in which older adults live. For example, proximity to parks and community centers can influence the amount of social engagement as well as physical activity that older adults obtain on a regular basis. Local community senior centers and volunteer organizations can play an important role in facilitating engagement with social activities. Social groups occurring in neighborhoods or at nearby community venues are typically 'cheap to run' (they do not require a trained other to manage them) and because of their contribution to better bio-psychological health and health behaviors across time, their capacity to build social connectedness can contribute to lower healthcare costs and greater quality of life [11,16].

*1.4. Physical Environment*

The associations between neighborhoods and health have been reported to be the strongest among adults around retirement age [17]. Furthermore, the positive impacts of walking on older adults' strength and flexibility supports the value of walking in warding off disability and extending older adults' capacity for independence and aging in place [18]. Planners and civil engineers are therefore groups that can contribute to ' … developing new and redeveloping existing communities to address the health, safety and mobility of older adults' [18] (p. 43). This latter sentiment is supported elsewhere: 'policy makers should consider how to provide both psychosocial and physical environment resources to support seniors' physical activity' [19] (p. 73). Hence, urban planners have been increasingly encouraged to incorporate into their designs walkable neighborhoods which by definition are characterized by mixed land use, interconnecting streets, convenient transit locations and compact communities [20]. What is currently less clear are the types of neighborhood features that would be particularly helpful for promoting regular walking among older adults across the continuum of mobility as people age. A valid and reliable approach for older adults to inform urban planners and policy-makers about older adults' needs related to their physical environment is through citizen science.

## 1.5. Citizen Science "by the People"

The *Our Voice* Citizen Science model is a community-based empowerment approach in which citizen scientists are trained and supported to become agents of change in their own communities [21]. In the "Discover" phase of this approach, citizen scientists use a simple mobile application called the Stanford Healthy Neighbourhood Discovery Tool (DT), to document local environmental features through geo-coded photographs, audio narratives, and walking routes. The DT is user-friendly across all levels of education and technology literacy, and has been operated successfully by persons ages 10 to 92. In the facilitated "Discuss" phase, citizen scientists review and analyze their own data in order to collectively identify and prioritize challenges. The group then moves into the "Activate" phase, brainstorming potential solutions and working with local community partners to develop and advocate for realistic, low-cost changes to local structures, policies and practices (see Figure 1). This process gives participants a "voice"—a means of telling their stories, building consensus, and motivating action. *Our Voice* blends the active participant engagement and ownership inherent in community-based participatory research with the standardized participant-based data collection methods that are a hallmark of citizen science. This approach allows citizen scientists to merge individual storytelling to represent collective experiences and advocate for changes that will impact both individuals and their communities.

Research has demonstrated that this approach works. Having older adults evaluate their neighborhoods and then meet with local and public sector decision makers for the purpose of bringing improvements to these neighborhoods is a viable approach [22]. Citizen science empowers older adults to participate more actively in local management decisions [23] and policy-making [23]. Accordingly, 'engaging older adult community residents in advocacy has the potential to achieve better local policy outcomes, improve [ ... ] physical activity environments, and provide direct benefit to the residents' physical health and well-being' [24]. As Miller [25] suggests, community development works best when social change is initiated from bottom-up support and actions. The approach lends itself to improved knowledge transfer impacting policy and action [26,27]. Specific to research with older adults as citizen scientists, Buman and his colleagues concluded that community-focused values and interests bought by the older adults themselves guarantees that policy decisions reflect the older adults' priorities and beliefs [24]. The purpose of this study was to apply the *Our Voice* citizen science model with older adults affiliated with the Burnie Brae community center, engaging and empowering those participants to document their lived experiences and drive positive changes in their local environment.

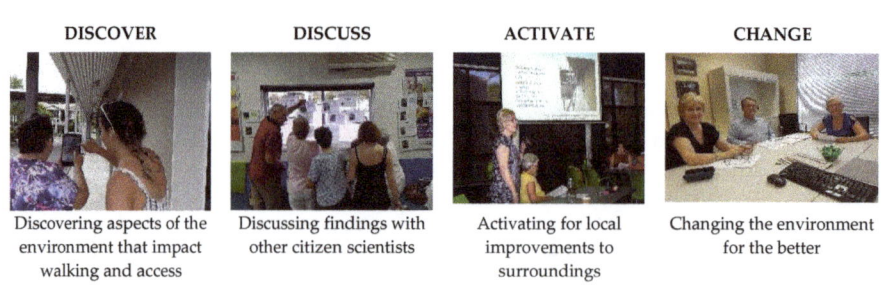

| DISCOVER | DISCUSS | ACTIVATE | CHANGE |
|---|---|---|---|
| Discovering aspects of the environment that impact walking and access | Discussing findings with other citizen scientists | Activating for local improvements to surroundings | Changing the environment for the better |

**Figure 1.** Our Voice Citizen Scientist framework (King et al., 2016) [21]. © Stanford University. All rights reserved.

Research questions

1.  What are the features that help or hinder access to a seniors' center?
2.  What are the features of the physical environment surrounding a seniors' center that help or hinder physical activity (walking)?
3.  In what ways can older adults acting as citizen scientists bring about changes to their local environment?

## 2. Methods

This study applied the *Our Voice* citizen science framework (Figure 1) [27]. *Our Voice* is a community partnership process aimed at better understanding community members' lived experiences—supporting outreach and action as a direct consequence of a collaborative research project [28].

Burnie Brae (the Chermside and District Senior Citizens Centre Incorporated, Queensland, Australia) is a large not-for-profit and charitable organization established in Brisbane (Australia) in 1984. It is Queensland's largest over 50's community center. Burnie Brae operates across four locations on the north side of Brisbane (Australia) and offers a wide range of activities to its membership base of more than 6000 (average age 69 years). The Burnie Brae Centre is adjacent to Burnie Brae Parklands—an area of approximately 3.91 hectares (0.0391 km$^2$). Based on an ongoing academic partnership, the Centre Executive invited the research to be undertaken.

Data were collected from January to March 2018. All citizen scientists gave their informed consent for inclusion before they participated in the study. The study was conducted in accordance with the Declaration of Helsinki, and the protocol was approved by the University of Queensland Human Research Ethic Committee (Approval number #2017000913) as well as approval through the Burnie Brae Research Administration Group (September 2017).

### 2.1. Participants and Recruitment

#### 2.1.1. Citizen Scientists

To be eligible to participate in this study, citizen scientists had to be members of the Burnie Brae, aged 65 years or older, English speaking, actively engaged in a range of social activities (e.g., volunteer gardening, attended the gymnasium and/or participating in organized social outings) and able to walk unaided (i.e., independent of walking aids of any kind). Participants were recruited from December 2017–January 2018 via posters displayed at Burnie Brae with further person-to-person invitations through the Burnie Brae subsidiary Healthy Connections Exercise Clinic. People registered their interest and attended a 60-min group face-to-face information session. At this information session they were given a detailed verbal explanation of the study (using a Power Point presentation) that included a YouTube © video (www.youtube.com/watch?v=sYcYXh51Bl0), safety instructions and instructions not to photograph persons' faces/identifiable features. Attendees were assessed for eligibility based on the inclusion/exclusion criteria with all found eligible. Citizen scientists were also provided a hard copy project information sheet and provided written informed consent and they also signed a photography release form.

#### 2.1.2. Researchers (Partner Facilitators)

Eight citizen scientists partnered with members of the research team and a research assistant in the implementation and emerging design of this research. All but one of the citizen scientists was female, and all were independently mobile and 65 years or over. Researchers AT and PG are active members of the Stanford University Citizen Science Global Research Network (CSGRN see: http://med.stanford.edu/ourvoice.html), AF is a senior undergraduate dual-degree nursing/midwifery scholar who undertook a short summer research internship and SH is a Burnie Brae researcher and Accredited Exercise Physiologist (AEP).

### 2.1.3. Enabling Actors (Decision Makers)

Burnie Brae Executives and the Member for Northgate-Brisbane City Council, were the purposefully targeted decision-makers. For Burnie Brae this included the Chief Executive Officer (CEO), the Chairman of the Board (COB) and the Operating Manager (OM). Municipal Councillor AA is the elected representative for the Brisbane City Council and has local jurisdiction over a Council Parks Team, the Transport Planning and Strategy Branch, and the Field Services Team responsible for repair and improvements to surrounding parklands, footpaths and roadways in the immediate neighborhood. The CEO, COB and OM were invited by AT to hear the findings and the CEO later also met with AT and the citizen science advocates (HP, NK) to reach an agreement on actions. Councillor AA was invited through the Chairman of the Board to attend a further hearing of findings and proposed solutions in the company of the citizen scientist pair (DW, CL) and Chairman of the Board and co-researchers AT and PG.

### 2.1.4. Discovery: Data Collection by Citizen Scientists

To discover aspects of the local neighborhood environment, the citizen scientists walked around the Burnie Brae center and the adjacent park. During these walks, the citizen scientists used the Stanford Healthy Neighborhood Discovery Tool (Version 1.9.6) (Stanford University, Palo Alto, CA, USA) application on a Nexus tablet. The Stanford Healthy Neighborhood Discovery Tool (DT) is a non-medical mobile application created by Stanford University. It is licensed for use by contributing research projects at outside institutions for the purpose of data collection only. The DT is designed for single use by community members to gather environmental photos (explicitly not to include identifiable persons), audio narratives, and GPS-tracked walking routes. Users also answer a brief 8-question survey that captures basic non-identifiable demographic information and assesses perceptions of the neighborhood environment [29]. This app is designed to record physical environment (neighborhood features) and building access points that citizen scientists perceived impacted walking or accessing their center [29]. Citizen scientists individually designated a feature as helpful or a hindrance on the DT app. by clicking on a green smiley face or red angry face after reviewing each image. Citizen scientists were accompanied by a trained member of the research team who provided verbal instructions on how to use the app. The accompanying trained member of the research team did not influence the data recorded but served as a silent observer to ensure the safety of the participant [30] and, where required, to provide technical support [31]. The neighborhood walk canvassed the outside building facilities and amenities, parking areas and surrounding Burnie Brae Park (http://www.brisparks.com.au/qld/chermside/burnie-brae-park). Four participants undertook the discovery phase of the study immediately following the information session, with the remaining four participants completing the walk within 3 days (*N* = 3) and 15 days (*N* = 1) of the information session, respectively (see Figure 1).

### Data Storage and Security

Data are uploaded to a password protected Discovery Tool Data Repository (DTDR) and stored on a secure server at the Stanford University School of Medicine. All data uploaded to the password-protected data repository are backed up with remote data storage servers. The servers are maintained by Stanford IT managers. Access to these data are managed by a Protocol Director. The data are kept securely within the Stanford University system for up to 30 years. Anonymous data are collected with the DT. No personal health information is recorded or stored. Data uploaded to the DTDR are not linked to individual participants. Any identifiable photos are immediately blurred or removed from the server. The audio narratives recorded on the DT are the only potentially-identifiable data that is stored in the DTDR. Project data collected using the DT and stored in the DTDR may be shared via a password-protected website only with those collaborators who have signed the DT License

Agreement and submitted and complied with an approved study protocol; and human subjects/ethics standards from their home institution.

## 2.2. Data Preparation by Research Team Members

All attendant geocoded narratives were transcribed and photographs downloaded and printed in high resolution color. These were then placed in named plastic sleeves corresponding to the citizen scientists (A–H). The day after the final walk (late January 2018) two members of the research team (AT, AF) met to prepare the data for the first community meeting where the data were discussed (see Figure 1). The research team relied on the initial 19 content elements derived from a previous developed coding schema [29,30]. It was deemed necessary to replace some code element terminology (for culturally specific reasons); to merge some code elements (to be specific to the neighborhood walk for this precinct) and remove some altogether (where no data were obviously forthcoming) (see Table 1).

**Table 1.** The coded elements used here to derive the three issues prioritized by the citizen scientists during the Discuss session, January 2018.

| Code Element [29,30] (N = 19) | Code Element (N = 10) |
| --- | --- |
| Parks/playgrounds | Parks/playgrounds |
| Traffic<br>Traffic related safety<br>Parking | Traffic related safety/Parking |
| Sidewalks | Footpaths |
| Mobility/Access issues | Mobility/Access issues |
| Amenities/destinations | Amenities/destinations |
| Crosswalks | Zebra crossing |
| Other | Other |
| Street features | Street features |
| Aesthetics | Pretty surroundings |
| Trash | Rubbish/litter/filth |
| Private residences | |
| Crime/security | |
| Graffiti | |
| Other people | |
| Footbridge | |
| Vacant lots | |
| Dogs | |

## 2.3. Discuss: Data Analysis by Citizen Scientists

After completion of the last walk and data preparation, the discuss phase was enacted and citizen scientists gathered to code their own data (see Figure 1). Co-researcher AT reiterated and further explained the process and facilitated the citizen scientist group.

Code element headings based on the validated coding schema comprising our revised 10 elements [29,30] were affixed to the walls of the meeting place. The citizen scientists assigned their photographs, paired with transcribed audio narratives, on the wall under the appropriate heading. In addition, the citizen scientists allocated positive data on one side of each element space and negative data on the other. The benefit of this was that it created an immediate visual impression of what the most frequently noted content element and hindrances were. Once each citizen scientist had completed their data assignment, the group walked around to each of the 10 content elements for the purpose of reaching consensus. The data from one citizen scientist, who was unable to attend this session, were not analyzed.

At this point the group nominated two citizen scientist advocates to be the group's representatives to take the findings and their solutions to the activate session (see Figure 1). One of the citizen science advocates (HP) led the discussion to prioritize three hindrances to walking and/or center access that they wanted addressed. Determinations by the citizen scientists of the most important barriers in their physical environment that hinder physical activity were facilitated by them tallying the negative data assignment (see Table 2). Finally, a collective brainstorming of solutions took place. Priorities and solutions were written on a whiteboard and recorded photographically and by the researcher taking notes of the session.

**Table 2.** The barriers and facilitators coded by citizen scientists at the Discuss session, ranked by total frequency, that hinder or help physical activity (walking) and access, January 2018.

| Coded Elements | Total | | Hinder | | Help | | Neutral | |
|---|---|---|---|---|---|---|---|---|
| | N | % | N | % | N | % | N | % |
| Parks/playgrounds | 24 | 33 | 9 | 13 | 14 | 19 | 1 | 1 |
| Footpaths | 12 | 17 | 6 | 8 | 5 | 7 | 1 | 1 |
| Pretty surroundings | 11 | 15 | 0 | 0 | 11 | 15 | 0 | 0 |
| Traffic related safety/Parking | 8 | 11 | 7 | 10 | 1 | 1 | 0 | 0 |
| Mobility/Access issues | 8 | 11 | 4 | 6 | 4 | 6 | 0 | 0 |
| Other | 5 | 7 | 1 | 1 | 3 | 4 | 1 | 1 |
| Amenities/destinations | 3 | 4 | 3 | 4 | 0 | 0 | 0 | 0 |
| Zebra crossings | 1 | 1 | 1 | 1 | 0 | 0 | 0 | 0 |
| Street features | 0 | 0 | 0 | 0 | 0 | 0 | 0 | 0 |
| Rubbish/litter/filth | 0 | 0 | 0 | 0 | 0 | 0 | 0 | 0 |

*2.4. Activate: Voicing the(ir) Needs and Prioritising Solutions by Citizen Scientists*

Two activate sessions were driven by the citizen scientists-activate session one was a public presentation open to the center membership and the eight citizen scientist co-researchers (see Figure 1); activate session two was a 'closed' citizen science presentation to the municipal council member. Activate session one took place in the first week of February and activate session two took place in third week of March, 2018.

At activate session one, the nominated citizen science advocates delivered a 55-minute, Power-Point presentation followed by a question and answer session. This session focused on the group's needs (N = 7), and their proposed solutions to improve the features of the physical environment surrounding their center to encourage physical activity (walking). The audience comprised the enabling actors, five citizen scientists and three members of the research team, and the research assistant. The citizen science advocates had input into the design of the Power-Point presentation; were provided a presentation script (based on the co-designed Power-Point presentation) in the days before the session and arrived on the day one hour before the session to practice their oral presentation and Power-Point skills with AF and AT. A week following this activate session one, the CEO of Burnie Brae met again with the two citizen science advocates and co-researcher AT to further discuss and commit to changing the physical environment features that needed improvement and over which the CEO had jurisdiction.

At activate session two, the nominated citizen science advocates were unavailable to attend due to prior commitments. Instead, citizen scientists DW and CL advocated for the group. With the change to the citizen scientists acting as the groups' advocates, the Power- Point presentation and question and answer session was co-delivered with AT. Present at this session were the municipal council member AA, Burnie Brae Chairman of the Board and co-researcher PG. The focus of the session was also the physical environment features that needed improvement and over which the Councillor had jurisdiction and thus responsibility through the municipal council. It was here that the Councillor committed to making the citizen scientists' proposed changes.

## 2.5. Change: Citizen Scientists Making a Real Difference

At the time of writing, the planning continues for the work related to Burnie Brae Centre access and the commitments to physical environment features that needed improvement, and over which Burnie Brae's CEO has jurisdiction. Councillor AA, as the elected representative for the Brisbane City Council, has instructed his Council Parks Team, the Transport Planning and Strategy Branch, and the Field Services Team responsible for repair and improvements to surrounding parklands, footpaths and roadways to commence work. Footpath repairs and have started. Line marking road works are completed. A derived outcome from this project has been the approval for the construction of a new toilet block and additional exercise equipment in the Park.

## 3. Results: Citizen Scientist Participation and Data Collected

Eight citizen scientists participated in this study. Most were women (87.5%, 7/8), and all were able to walk independently. All were 65 years or over. 87.5% (7/8) rated the app 'extremely useful' with the one other rating the app. 'somewhat useful'. All but one of the citizen scientists was contacted both by telephone and attended the information session. Seven attended the discuss session with five attending activate session 1 and two activate session 2 (see Figure 1).

The citizen scientists took a total of 83 photographs and recorded 83 audio commentaries of the photographs (9–11 photos/commentaries per citizen scientist) on an average walk duration of 18 min. Table 2 shows the number of images by coded elements from the discuss session. The three issues prioritized by the citizen scientists to advocate for were parks/playgrounds, footpaths, and traffic related safety/parking.

The following represents examples of the citizen scientists' findings and solutions under the three priority issues (features of the physical environment surrounding a senior's centre that hinder physical activity). Further audio-narratives that support these hindrances are provided in Table 3.

**Table 3.** Examples of audio narratives (hindrance) to physical activity (walking) and access made by citizen scientists using the Discovery Tool during the Discover sessions, January 2018.

| Coded Element | Quotations about Hindrances to Physical Activity (Walking) and Access (−, Negative) |
|---|---|
| Parks/playgrounds | "A tap or drinking bubbler would be nice in the park because if you do have children or people here for a small picnic there is no way of getting hold of water" "Been walking for a little while and noticed there are no seats in the park this far I can see" "This gravel path through the park where there is a little arbour and shrubs, it's great but there is some trimming that needs to be done so folks don't get caught up with it" |
| Footpaths | "Raised paving in the footpath (is) a trip hazard" "Seems to be a loose gravel path (and) can't quite see where it's heading; but maybe it wouldn't be a good (path) for people with walkers" "This pathway is too narrow for more than one person, but it may be difficult to widen it" |
| Traffic related safety/Parking | "I think the sign is misleading and (I am) not sure which side people would be designated to walk. An actual sign on the pathway would be beneficial" "Car park is always full; difficult for some people to be able to park in the car park" "This is the entrance from X street to the car park and the pedestrian entrance to the gymnasium (as well) everyone who goes (to the gym) has to walk up and down the hill; a zebra crossing down the hill would be useful; also traffic flow in-and-out is confusing for everyone" |

### 3.1. Parks/Playgrounds

Citizen scientist F and H recorded this environmental feature (Figure 2). Citizen scientist F narrated:

*"I'm finding when you get to the end of the gravel path, there is a sleeper (a heavy timber beam, especially one that is laid horizontally on the ground), I'm not too sure if it's supposed to be on a slope but one part is sticking out quite a bit that would cause some problem to people with walkers"*

The feature was evaluated as a safety risk. During the discuss phase (see Figure 1) the citizen scientist group proposed that the nominated citizen scientist advocates investigate the purpose of this feature with Council, with a view to having it removed. When the advocate pair presented their finding at the community meeting and met with the Burnie Brae Chief Executive Officer, the issue was dealt with by Centre Grounds and Maintenance to make the hazard more visible as it could not be removed.

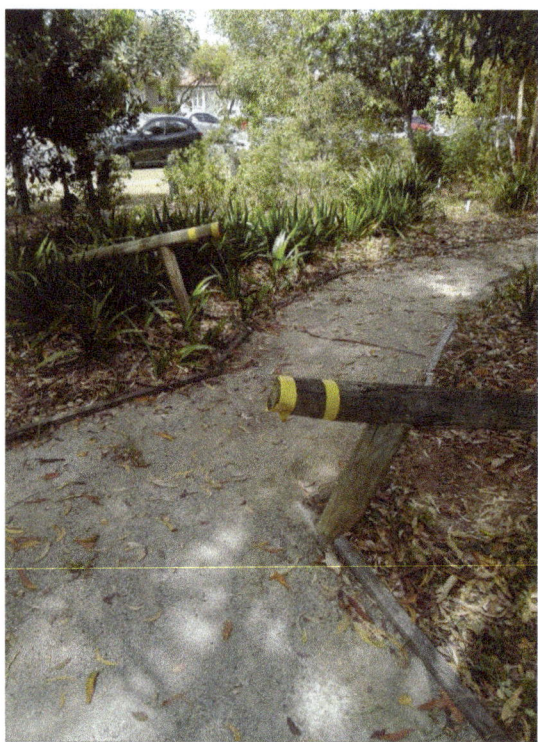

**Figure 2.** The sleeper.

Citizen scientist C recorded this feature (Figure 3) and citizen scientist F cautioned where these facilities do exist 'you just have to be a little bit careful walking onto the cement slab':

*"More covered shade over the tables, there is three other tables, which would make it more convenient for a picnic and make it more pleasant"*

Whilst other citizen scientists recorded favorably the shaded areas that do exist, the group felt that there remains a need to build more shaded shelter. This was a priority taken to the municipal Councillor.

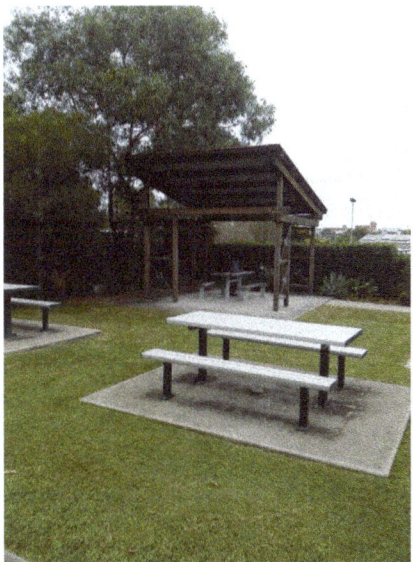

**Figure 3.** Shade.

Citizen scientist H noted the outside shade areas for a different reason (Figure 4), concerned about the impact on walking around Burnie Brae Park:

*"This is a photo of urine stench, don't know how it gets there or how to keep it away but it is very unpleasant"*

It was recommended to the Burnie Brae Executive by the citizen scientist advocates that the group's solution was to demand the municipal council to spray and clean the area regularly. However, the Executive group acknowledged the problem as a Centre issue and directed Grounds & Maintenance to clean and disinfect the area.

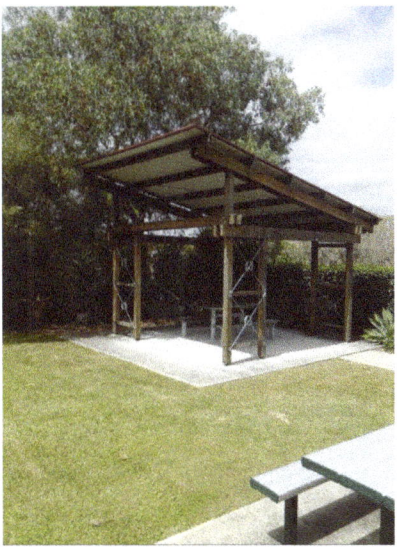

**Figure 4.** Urine stench.

### 3.2. Footpaths

Citizen scientist B recorded Figure 5. In contrast, it was the case that citizen scientists A and H agreed that the shared pathway (bike/pedestrian) in the park was a facilitator for their walking; and citizen scientist C recorded an impression of 'safe pathways'. However, for citizen scientist B:

*"Seems to be a loose gravel path, can't quite see where it's heading, but maybe it wouldn't be a good idea for people with walkers"*

The group supported this as an issue and proposed that signage be placed to alert persons that the path was a loose surface. At activate session one (1) the Executive group explained that the nature of the surface meant it was prone to scuffing. However, the CEO agreed that signage could be posted to alert persons that the path surface was loose (see Figure 1).

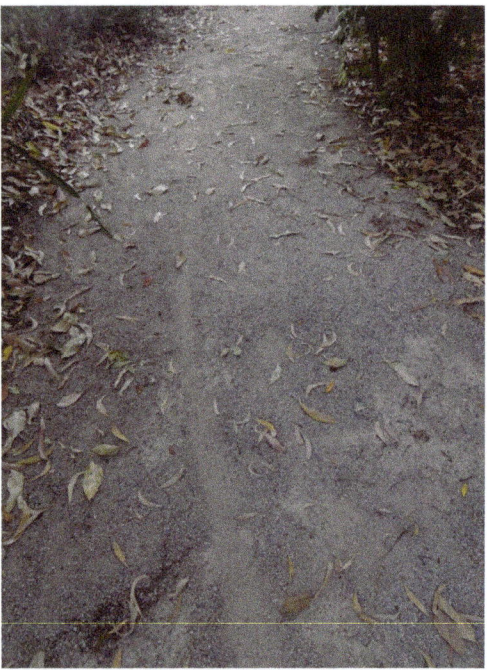

**Figure 5.** Loose gravel path.

Citizen scientist B recorded Figure 6 and was not alone (also citizen scientist H):

*"Damaged footpath could be a hazard for people tripping"*

This was a group consensus and citizen scientist advocates proposed a letter to be sent to the municipal council. In conversation with the CEO, it was further recommended that additional photographs be taken whereby the exact areas were precisely 'spot-marked' with paint. This data were then presented to the municipal Councillor. Preparatory repair work has started.

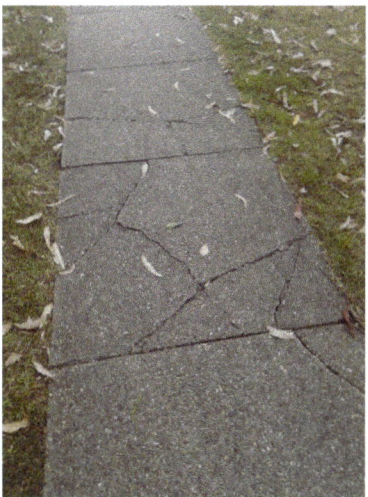

**Figure 6.** Damaged footpath.

*3.3. Traffic Related Safety/Parking*

Citizen scientist A expressed real safety concern related to Figure 7. Given other recorded images and narratives about the lack of parking ('car park always full'), the issue captured here takes on greater significance:

> *"On leaving the car park, it's very difficult when you're turning right with all the cars parked that you can't see cars coming down on the left-hand side and you need to take it out very carefully or you're likely to have an accident as all the cars on the left-hand side actually block your view"*

The citizen scientists' solution was to suggest the installation of a reverse mirror and/or to extend the yellow line road marking. This was a priority taken to municipal Councillor. The line marking has been completed.

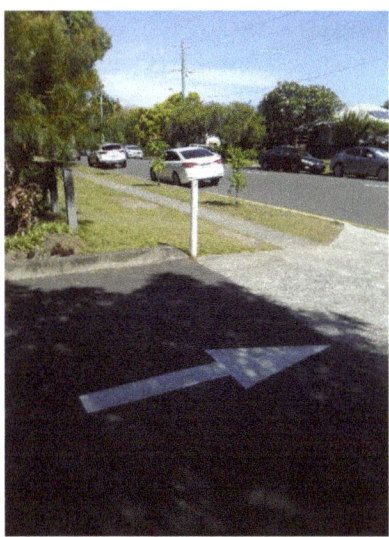

**Figure 7.** Likely to have an accident.

Citizen scientist E recognized that safely walking about the outside of the center relied on there being suitable line markings in the car park (Figure 8).

*"Carpark needs repainting for the lines in the carpark, it looks terrible"*

The Centre CEO accepted the citizen scientists' request that the line markings be redone.

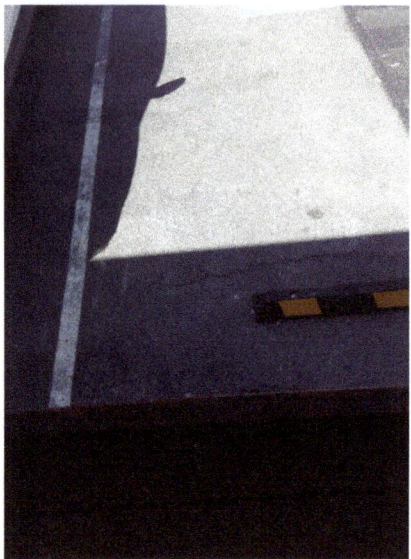

**Figure 8.** Carpark repainting.

Additional illustrative quotes for the hindrances to physical activity (walking) are included in Table 3.

## 4. Discussion

Our research allowed community dwelling older adults, as citizen scientists, to evaluate their physical environment around the Burnie Brae center for features that help or hinder their walking or access to it, respectively. These citizen scientists relied on smart technology in the form of the Discovery Tool to effectively capture digital geocoded images and record narratives about these features whilst undertaking a neighborhood walk. Collectively these citizen scientists analyzed their own data, allocating them to meaningful codes and from this they identified those hindrances to walking and access they wanted ameliorated. The group generated solutions which their nominated advocate pair presented to their center Chief Executive Officer, Chairman of the Board, Operating Manager; and the municipal Councillor at formal meetings. Adopting the *Our Voice* framework and the Discovery Tool for the first time in Australia, this study showed that it is possible for citizen scientists to enact changes in the neighborhood.

We have suggested [32] that the nature of the research reported here extends original forms of photo voice research [33–36]. Here we add smart technology in the form of the Discovery Tool application to underscore the critical opinions of older adults who not only identify their needs and assets but also offer real-world, real-time solutions to their identified problem(s) [37].

The *Our Voice* framework has been successfully tested in a number of lower-income neighborhoods in California's Bay Area (e.g., East Palo Alto, north San Mateo County, south Santa Clara County), and internationally in Mexico, Colombia, Chile and Israel [21]. These projects have addressed a range of challenges facing marginalized communities (e.g., walkability, food access, safe routes to school, park safety and land use) and have shown changes across multiple levels: individual, social, physical environment and policy [24,29–31,37]. An emerging Our Voice Citizen Science Global Research Network (CSGRN) (see http://med.stanford.edu/ourvoice.html) is advancing the paradigm in the USA-inspiring, for example, African-American woman to identify aspects of their local environments that if improved would support the daily habit of walking. In addition, the Our Voice CSGRN is targeting older adults (and adolescents) in Brazil, Chile, Manitoba (Canada), the UK and Taiwan as well as young adults and Maori communities in New Zealand.

We propose that there are a range of good reasons for the implementation of the *Our Voice* Citizen Scientist framework and community engagement process as an environmentally-focused intervention. Our proposals come with a caveat, namely the scope and reach of our findings must be set alongside our research limitations, which include a small sample size and reasonably short time frames in which impacts of the intervention have been evaluated. *Our Voice* projects are currently being conducted globally with larger numbers of citizen scientists (e.g., a hundred plus) and across longer time frames (e.g., two years).

The physical environment is a key to social participation which is vital to successful ageing [38,39]. The physical characteristics of the home, neighborhood and transport infrastructure all have a bearing on older adult's ability to maintain independence and engage socially [40] The latter is protective of older adult's physical, cognitive and mental health [41], and is facilitated through development of social capital (i.e., neighborhood trust, community belonging). The older adult as a citizen scientist, engaged in the way we have described, not only improves their immediate neighborhood to facilitate active living but also engages in a process that brings them together; sharing ideas, agreeing and disagreeing as they propose solutions that are meaningful to their immediate needs.

It is only by incorporating the perspectives and experiences of the citizens in our neighborhoods, communities and prefectures that we might expect to meet the UN 2030 Sustainable Development Goals of 'making cities and human settlements inclusive, safe, resilient and sustainable' [2]. Furthermore, the 2002 Madrid International Plan of Action on Ageing (MIPAA) recognizes that older adults ought to participate in and benefit equitably from the outcomes of development to advance their health and well-being and that societies should provide enabling environments for them to do so [42]. Increasingly, there is an expectation to create aged-friendly standards and environments to help prevent the onset or worsening of disabilities [42] and to design urban spaces free of barriers to mobility and access. Mindful of the earlier noted caveats, the citizen science we have described herein does all of these things.

Consistent with the 2002 MIPAA [42] our older adult as a citizen scientist is recognized as "participant(s) in development planning, emphasizing (they ought to be able to) participate in and benefit equitably from the (outcomes) of development to advance their health and well-being, and that societies should provide enabling environments for them to do so" [2] (p. 1). The participatory role of the public as citizen scientists in the *Our Voice* framework posits it as a perfect mechanism for decision making about the environment. *Our Voice* supports one of the core rights of the Aarhus Convention [43].

The WHO's *Global Age-Friendly Cities Project* and guide contains some eight (8) core age-friendly features as universal standards for an age-friendly city [44]. The WHO project identified, by listening to the voices of older adults, two urban living areas of specificity for the research being reported here, namely: age-friendly outdoor spaces and buildings and age-friendly respect and social inclusion [44]. The former means that the older adult expects well-maintained and safe green spaces, pedestrian friendly walkways, well-maintained pavements and well-designed roads. The latter means that the older adult is consulted on ways to serve them better; and that the older adult is included as a 'full partner in community decision-making affecting them' [45] (p. 50). Across the international literature, an age-friendly city takes as a starting point older adult's lives and experiences to identify desirable community services and support [46]. Mindful of our project's small size, we propose that older adults as citizen scientists engaging in the *Our Voice* processes are participating in the very assessments the WHO suggests a city can make about its age-friendly urban features [44].

Scaled-up, *Our Voice* can be enacted to address these big topics espoused by the 'big players'—we have named a few (e.g., UN 2030 Sustainable Development Goals; 2002 Madrid International Plan of Action on Ageing; UNECE Aarhus Convention). A planned future application for this work could also include persons with dementia (PWD), in the hope of driving change towards creating and maintaining dementia-friendly habitats [47].

*Limitations*

This project utilized a small purposive sample of motivated members of the Burnie Brae Centre as citizen scientists. Outcomes need to be weighed carefully against sample size. Whilst the relatively small sample generated a range of issues in the physical environment around the Centre and the project achieved its stated aim of consolidating feedback and solutions from the member base on ways to improve the walkability of their environment, caution must be taken about extrapolating outcomes. Equally, the sample was taken from a single Centre and caution should be paid when translating findings to other locales. Lastly, the small sample was predominantly female. Though this is reflective of the Center membership, it can be reasonably assumed that features of the physical environment that are identified by older women might not necessarily be the same as features identified by older men.

## 5. Conclusions

Older adults are often the recipients of services and solutions that are provided to them by an external other; by government, institution or organization. In this paper, we present a project were issues have been identified and solutions have been formulated by the older adult for the older adult. Further, the older adults have actively advocated for the implementation of these solutions to the benefit of their entire community. As outlined in the discussion, this has the potential to satisfy on many levels the objectives set by world-leading organizations who demand rights for older adults and for them to be to self-determining in all aspects of their lives.

**Author Contributions:** A.T., P.A.G. and A.K. designed the study; Citizen Scientists with the research team (A.F., S.H., A.T., P.A.G.) collected and analyzed the data; All authors contributed to the manuscript production.

**Funding:** This research received no external funding.

**Acknowledgments:** We must sincerely thank the Citizen Scientists for their commitment and enthusiasm: Hector Beveridge, Nancy Kerr, Christine Lamb, Sharon McNeil, Helleen Purdy, Diane Thornton, Patricia Vaughan, Di' Wheeler. We would also like to acknowledge the contribution of the staff of the Burnie Brae Centre. We also thank Ann Banchoff for her helpful comments on this manuscript.

**Conflicts of Interest:** The authors declare no conflicts of interest.

## References

1. Chen, W.-W.; Zhang, X.; Huang, W.-J. Role of physical exercise in Alzheimer's disease. *Biomed. Rep.* **2016**, *4*, 403–407. [CrossRef] [PubMed]
2. United Nations Department of Economic and Social Affairs Population Division. *World Population Ageing 2015*; United Nations: New York, NY, USA, 2015.
3. World Health Organisation National Institute on Ageing. *Global Health and Ageing*; National Institute of Health: Bethesda, MD, USA, 2011.
4. Balboa-Castillo, T.; Leon-Munoz, L.; Graciani, A.; Rodriguez-Artalejo, F.; Guallar-Castillon, P. Longitudinal association of physical activity and sedentary behaviour during leisure time with health-related quality of life in community-dwelling older adults. *Health Qual. Life Outcomes* **2011**, *9*. [CrossRef] [PubMed]
5. Fielding, R.; Vellas, B.; Evans, W.; Bhasin, S.; Morley, J.; Newman, A.; Zamboni, M. Sarcopenia: An undiagnosed condition in older adults. Current consensus definition: Prevalence, aetiology, and consequences. international working group on sarcopenia. *J. Am. Med. Dir. Assoc.* **2011**, *12*, 249–256. [CrossRef] [PubMed]

6.  Hamilton, M.; Hamilton, D.; Zderic, T. Exercise physiology versus inactivity physiology: An essential concept for understanding lipoprotein lipase regulation. *Exerc. Sport Sci. Rev.* **2004**, *32*, 161–166. [CrossRef] [PubMed]

7.  Santos, D.; Silva, A.; Baptista, F.; Santos, R.; Vale, S.; Mota, J. Sedentary behaviour and ohysical activity are independently related to functional fitness in older adults. *Exp. Gerontol.* **2012**, *47*, 908–912. [CrossRef] [PubMed]

8.  Darren, E.; Warburton, C.; Whitney, N.; Bredin, S. Health benefits of physical activity: The evidence. *Can. Med. Assoc. J.* **2006**, *174*, 801–809.

9.  Keogh, J.; Henwood, T.; Gardiner, P.; Tuckett, A.; Hodgkinson, B.; Rouse, K. Examining evidence based resistance plus balance training in community-dwelling older adults with complex health care needs: Trial protocol for the Muscling Up Against Disability project. *Arch. Gerontol. Geriatr.* **2016**, *68*, 97–105. [CrossRef] [PubMed]

10. Abbott, R.; White, L.; Webster Ross, G.; Masaki, K.; Curb, J.; Petrovitch, H. Walking and dementia in physically capable elderly men. *J. Am. Med. Assoc.* **2004**, *292*, 1447–1453. [CrossRef] [PubMed]

11. Cruwys, T.; Dingle, G.; Haslam, C.; Haslam, S.; Jetten, J.; Morton, T. Social group memberships protect against future depression, alleviate depression symptoms and prevent depression relapse. *Soc. Sci. Med.* **2013**, *98*. [CrossRef] [PubMed]

12. World Health Organisation. *Active Ageing: A Policy Framework*; World Health Organisation: Geneva, Switzerland, 2002.

13. Douglas, H.; Georgiou, A.; Westbrook, J. Social participation as an indicator of successful ageing: An overview of concepts and their associations with health. *Aust. Health Rev.* **2017**, *41*, 455–462. [CrossRef] [PubMed]

14. Haslam, C. Social connectedness and health in later life. *InPsych* **2016**, *38*, 1–3.

15. Cornwell, B.; Laumann, E.; Schumm, P. The social connectedness of older adults: A national profile. *Am. Sociol. Rev.* **2008**, *73*, 185–203. [CrossRef] [PubMed]

16. Umberson, D.; Karas Montez, J. Social relationships and health: A flashpoint for health policy. *J. Health Soc. Behav.* **2010**, *51*, 54S–66S. [CrossRef] [PubMed]

17. Freedman, V.; Grafova, I.; Schoeni, R.; Rogowski, J. Neighborhoods and disability in later life. *Soc. Sci. Med.* **2008**, *66*, 2253–2267. [CrossRef] [PubMed]

18. Kerr, J.; Rosenberg, D.; Frank, L. The role of the physical environment in healthy aging: Community design, physical activity and health among older adults. *J. Plan. Lit.* **2012**, *27*, 43–60. [CrossRef]

19. Carlson, J.; Sallis, J.; Conway, T.; Saelens, B.; Frank, L.; Kerr, J.; Cain, K.; King, A. Interactions between psychosocial and physical environment factors in explaining older adults' physical activity. *Prev. Med.* **2012**, *54*, 68–73. [CrossRef] [PubMed]

20. Li, F.; Harmer, P.; Cardinal, B.; Bosworth, M.; Johnson-Shelton, D.; Moore, J.; Acock, A.; Vongjaturapat, N. Physical environment and 1-year change in weight and waist circumference in middle-aged and older adults. *Am. J. Epidemiol.* **2009**, *169*, 1–12.

21. King, A.; Winter, S.; Sheats, J.; Rosas, L.; Buman, M.; Salvo, D.; Rodriguez, N.; Seguin, R.; Moran, M.; Garber, R.; et al. Leveraging Citizen Science and Information Technology for Population Physical Activity Promotion. *Transl. J. ACSM* **2016**, *1*, 30–44.

22. Winter, S.; Buman, M.; Sheats, J.; Hekler, E.; Otten, J.; Baker, C.; Cohen, D.; Butler, B.; King, A. Harnessing the potential of older adults to measure and modify their environments: Long-term success of the Neighborhood Eating and Activity Advocacy Team (NEAAT) Study. *Transl. Behav. Med.* **2014**, *4*, 226–227. [CrossRef] [PubMed]

23. Jansujwicz, J.; Calhoun, A.; Lilieholm, R. The Maine vernal pool mapping and assessment program: Engaing municipal officilas and private landowners in community-based citizen science. *Environ. Manag.* **2013**, *52*, 1369–1385. [CrossRef] [PubMed]

24. Buman, M.; Winter, S.; Baker, C.; Hekler, E.; Otten, J.; king, A. Neighborhood Eating and Activity Advocacy Teams (NEAAT): Engaging older adults in policy activities to improve food and physical environments. *Transl. Behav. Med.* **2012**, *2*, 249–253. [CrossRef] [PubMed]

25. Miller, A. The role of citizen scientists in nature resource decision-making: Lessons from the spruce budworm problem in Canada. *Environmentalist* **1993**, *13*, 47–59. [CrossRef]

26. Alaback, P. A true partnership. *Front. Ecol. Environ.* **2012**, *10*, 284. [CrossRef]

27. Vaughn, L.; Whetstone, C.; Boards, A.; Busch, M.; Magnusson, M.; Maatta, S. Partnering insiders: A review of peer models across community-engaged research, education and social care. *Health Soc. Care Community* **2018**, 1–18. [CrossRef] [PubMed]

28. Butsch Kovacic, M.; Stigler, S.; Smith, A.; Kidd, A.; Vaughn, L. Beginning a partnership with Photo Voice to explore environmental health and health inequities in minority communities. *Int. J. Environ. Res. Public Health* **2014**, *11*, 11132–11151. [CrossRef] [PubMed]

29. Buman, M.; Winter, S.; Sheats, J.; Hekler, E.; Otten, J.; Grieco, L.; king, A. The Stanford Healthy Neighborhood Discovery Tool: A computerised tool to assess active living environments. *Am. J. Prev. Med.* **2013**, *44*, e41–e47. [CrossRef] [PubMed]

30. Winter, S.; Goldman Rosas, L.; Padilla-Romero, P.; Sheats, J.; Buman, M.; Baker, C.; king, A. Using citizen scientists to gather, analyse and disseminate information about neighbourhood features that affect active living. *J. Immigr. Minor. Health* **2015**, 1–13. [CrossRef]

31. Sheats, J.; Winter, S.; Padilla-Romero, P.; Goldman Rosas, L.; Grieco, L.; King, A. Comparison of passive versus active photo capture of physical environment features by technology naïve Latinos using the SenseCam and Stanford Healthy Neighborhood Discovery Tool. *Assoc. Comput. Mach. Digit. Libr.* **2013**. [CrossRef]

32. Tuckett, A.; Banchroff, A.; Winter, S.; King, A. The physical environment and older adults: A literature review and an applied approach to engaging older adults in physical environment improvements for health. *Int. J. Older People Nurs.* **2018**, *13*. [CrossRef] [PubMed]

33. Catalani, C.; Minkler, M. Photovoice: A review of the literature in health and public health. *Health Educ. Behav.* **2010**, *37*, 424–451. [CrossRef] [PubMed]

34. Novek, S.; Menec, V. Older adults' perceptions of age-friendly communities in Canada: A photovoice study. *Ageing Soc.* **2014**, *34*, 1052–1072. [CrossRef]

35. Novek, S.; Morris-Oswald, T.; Macera, C. Using photovoice with older adults: Some methodological strenghts and issues. *Ageing Soc.* **2012**, *32*, 451–470. [CrossRef]

36. Roger, K.; Wetzel, M.; Penner, L. Living with Parkinson's disease—Perceptions of invisibility in a photovoice study. *Ageing Soc.* **2018**, *38*, 1041–1062. [CrossRef]

37. HelpAge International. *Ageing and the City: Making Urban Spaces Work for Older People*; HelpAge International: London, UK, 2016; pp. 3–26.

38. Bennett, K. Low level social engagement as a precursor of mortality among people in later life. *Age Ageing* **2002**, *31*, 165–168. [CrossRef] [PubMed]

39. Giles, L.; Anstey, K.; Walker, R.; Luszcz, M. Social networks and memory over 15 years of follow-up in a cohort of older Australians: Results from the Australian Longitudinal Study of Ageing. *J. Ageing Res.* **2012**, *2012*, 856048.

40. Judd, B. Housing solutions for older adults. In *Encyclopedia of Geropsychology*; Pachana, N., Ed.; Springer: New York, NY, USA, 2016.

41. Bennett, D.; Schneider, J.; Tang, Y.; Arnold, S.; Wilson, R. The effect of social networks on the relation between Alzheimer's disease pathology and level of cognitive function in old people: A longitudinal cohort study. *Lancet Neurol.* **2006**, *5*, 406–412. [CrossRef]

42. United Nations. *Political Declaration and Madrid International Plan of Action on Ageing*; United Nations: New York, NY, USA, 2002.

43. UNEC. Protecting your environment. In *The Power Is in Your Hands: Quick Guide to the Aarhus Convention*; UN: Geneva, Switzerland, 2014.

44. World Health Organisation. *WHO Global Age-Friendly Cities- A Guide*; WHO: Geneva, Switzerland, 2007.

45. McCormack, G.; Shiell, A. In search of causality: A systematic review of the relationship between the physical environment and physical activity among adults. *Int. J. Behav. Nutr. Phys. Act.* **2011**, *8*, 1–11. [CrossRef] [PubMed]

46. Lui, C.-W.; Everingham, J.-A.; Warburton, J.; Cuthill, M.; Bartlett, H. What makes a community age-friendly: A review of international literature. *Australas. J. Aging* **2009**, *28*, 116–121. [CrossRef] [PubMed]

47. Wisconsin Department of Health Services. A Toolkit for Building Dementia-Friendly Communities. Available online: https://www.dhs.wisconsin.gov/dementia/communities.htm (accessed on 29 September 2018).

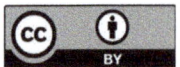

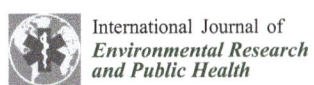

International Journal of
***Environmental Research***
***and Public Health***

*Article*

# Development of a Neighbourhood Walkability Index for Porto Metropolitan Area. How Strongly Is Walkability Associated with Walking for Transport?

**Ana Isabel Ribeiro [1,2,\*] and Elaine Hoffimann [1]**

[1]  EPIUnit—Instituto de Saúde Pública, Universidade do Porto, 4050-600 Porto, Portugal;
    elainehoffimann@gmail.com
[2]  Department of Public Health, Forensic Sciences and Medical Education, University of Porto Medical School,
    4200-319 Porto, Portugal
\*  Correspondence: ana.isabel.ribeiro@ispup.up.pt; Tel.: +351-22-206-1820

Received: 13 October 2018; Accepted: 5 December 2018; Published: 6 December 2018

**Abstract:** The creation of walkable communities constitutes a cost-effective health promotion strategy, as walking is an accessible and free intervention for increasing physical activity and health. In this cross-sectional ecological study, we developed a walkability index for the Porto Metropolitan Area and we validated it by assessing its association with walking for transportation. Neighborhood walkability was measured using a geographic information system and resulted from the weighted sum of residential density, street connectivity, and a destination-based entropy index. The index was categorized into quintiles of increasing walkability. Among the 1,112,555 individuals living in the study area, 28.1% resided in neighborhoods in the upper quintile of walkability and 15.8% resided in the least walkable neighborhoods. Adjusted regression models revealed that individuals residing in the most walkable neighborhoods are 81% more likely to report walking for transportation, compared with those from the least walkable neighborhoods (odds ratio: 1.81; 95% confidence intervals: 1.76–1.87). These results suggest that community design strategies to improve walkability may promote walking behavior.

**Keywords:** built environment; urban health; urban form; walking; physical activity; health promotion

---

## 1. Introduction

Despite the many benefits of physical activity (PA) [1], most people do not engage in regular PA. The Portuguese remain amongst the most physically inactive Europeans, as 68% of Portuguese adults were reported as never engaging in PA [2].

Walking is the most common form of PA. It is affordable, enjoyable, and versatile; it is recognized as a means of increasing levels of PA for the majority of the population [3]. Furthermore, walking can be easily incorporated into daily life routines, namely during trips from home to work/school, so-called "walking for transportation" (or active transportation).

Certain built environmental characteristics can act as facilitators or as barriers to walking. For instance, a well-connected street network shortens distances between origins and destinations, and the availability of a variety of destinations (recreation, services, and retail) within a walkable distance from residence reduces automobile trips and promotes walking [4].

To combine key built environmental features that encourage walking behavior—street network connectivity, land-use mix, and residential density—the walkability index was developed in the 2000s [5]. An increasing number of studies, mainly from the United States (US) and Australia, showed that neighborhood walkability is an important correlate of PA, i.e., walking behavior [3,6,7], suggesting that the creation of more walkable communities may constitute a powerful and cost-effective tool for promoting PA at population-level.

Despite the importance of addressing the built environmental correlates of PA, no validated measures of neighborhood walkability exist in Portugal. The walkability index was mostly applied in North America and Australia. Given the differences in urban form, extrapolation of findings to European cities such as Porto may not be appropriate [8]. Cities in America are more decentralized and sprawling, while cities in Europe are more central and compact [9]. Furthermore, the walkability index proposed by Frank and colleagues uses a set of well-established variables that were shown to be significantly associated with walking behavior [5]. Ideally, the same set of variables should be used in Porto (Portugal) to create a similar index. However, these variables were not available and alternate indexes must be computed. The creation of novel and modified walkability indexes requires validation to assess if they preserve the same explanatory power of the original index. In 2016, two indexes of walkability were developed for the Porto municipality [10,11], though these indexes were not validated by measuring their association with walking behavior. This is particularly relevant because the previously mentioned indexes used land-use data from a pan-European dataset—European Environment Agency Urban Atlas land-use map [12]—which has poor attribute accuracy. For instance, commercial, industrial, and military land-uses are collapsed in the same land-use category ("industrial, commercial, public, military, and private units"), which may not allow for the accurate quantification of the diversity of non-residential destinations, a key component of the walkability index.

Taking into account these research gaps, we aimed to develop a neighborhood walkability index for the Porto Metropolitan Area and to test if it is associated with walking for transportation.

## 2. Materials and Methods

### 2.1. Study Area

The Porto Metropolitan Area is the second largest metropolitan area of Portugal. It is located in the northern region of the country and has a population of 1.3 million [13].

For the development of the walkability index, we focused on the six core municipalities of the Metropolitan Area, which hold roughly 85% of its population ($N$ = 1,112,555 inhabitants): Porto, Matosinhos, Maia, Vila Nova de Gaia, Gondomar, and Valongo. These municipalities are divided into 10,444 census tracts. Census tracts are an operational unit for data collection and constitute the smallest geographical unit of census data dissemination (mean of 107 inhabitants/area, mean area of 53,852 m$^2$) [14]. Census tracts, from here onward simply referred to as neighborhoods, were used as the unit of analysis in the present study.

### 2.2. Walkability Index

Neighborhood walkability is generally composed of four elements [6]. Due to data unavailability, the ratio of retail building floor areas was not included; thus, our index incorporated the remaining three variables: residential density, street connectivity, and entropy index. Similarly to us, due to data unavailability, several other studies were also forced to remove this variable [7,8,10,15,16]. Despite this methodological modification, these studies were able to detect a significant association between the developed walkability index and walking for transport [7,8,15,16], which indicates that the explanatory power of the index may not be affected by this omission.

All the variables and procedures required to assess the components of neighborhood walkability are described in Table 1.

**Table 1.** Data sources and procedures used for assessing the characteristics of the built and socioeconomic environment of the neighborhoods.

| Variable | | Data Source | GIS and Statistical Procedure |
|---|---|---|---|
| Residential density | | 2011 Census available at Statistics Portugal (https://www.ine.pt/). | We computed the ratio of the dwellings per neighborhood area. |
| Street connectivity | | ESRI StreetMap for ArcPad Portugal TomTom (http://enterprise.arcgis.com/en/streetmap-premium/latest/get-started/dd-tomtom-data.htm). | Firstly, we removed the intersections of 2 streets or less, as well as intersections of motorways. Then, we computed the density of intersections (intersections per km$^2$) within 400 and 800 m of the neighborhood centroid. |
| Entropy index | Retail | Shopping centers, markets, and supermarkets obtained in 2018 from online business directories. | Whenever needed, destinations were georeferenced using Google Maps and ArcGIS Online Geocoding Service. Most destinations had a location represented by a single point; however, for green spaces, we used the entrances of these spaces. Then, using the ArcGIS Network Analysist tool, we determined the number of destinations of each type within 400 and 800 m of the neighborhood centroid. Finally, the index was obtained using the entropy index equation. |
| | Recreation | Restaurants, sport facilities, green spaces, libraries, zoos, art galleries, and museums obtained in 2018 from the TLA databases and online business directories. | |
| | Services | Banks, post-offices, pharmacies, hospitals, primary care centers, finance office, credit unions, courts, and notary, obtained in 2018 from the TLA databases, institutional websites, and online business directories. | |
| | Institutional | Schools, universities, kindergartens, churches, city halls, police stations, and fire stations, obtained in 2018 from the TLA databases, institutional websites, and online business directories. | |
| | Residential | Number of exclusively residential buildings obtained from the 2011 census available at Statistics Portugal (https://www.ine.pt/). | |

ESRI—Environmental Systems Research Institute; TLA—territorial local authorities.

### 2.2.1. Residential Density

Residential density was obtained by calculating the density of households (number of households per km$^2$) within each neighborhood. For that, data from the 2011 population and housing census, available at Statistics Portugal (https://www.ine.pt/), were used.

### 2.2.2. Street Connectivity

An updated street network dataset, provided courtesy of Environmental Systems Research Institute (ESRI), was used to compute the number of intersections ($\geq$3 intersecting streets) per km$^2$ within 800 m of the centroid of each neighborhood; only streets that allowed pedestrian circulation were included. For this assessment, we used the ArcGIS 10.4 Network Analyst tool (Environmental Systems Research Institute, ESRI, Redlands, CA, USA) and an 800-m (equivalent to a 10-min walk) threshold as employed in other studies focused on measuring pedestrian access to neighborhood facilities [17,18]. Additionally, to evaluate how sensitive our results were to the distance threshold, the 400-m distance was also employed. The 800-m and 400-m buffers contain approximately 2,011,000 and 503,000 square meters, respectively.

### 2.2.3. Entropy Index

To assess the variety of destinations available to each neighborhood, we computed an entropy index. Traditionally, the entropy index is based on the percentage area occupied by different types of land uses that promote PA, and reflects how varied the neighborhood is in terms of its land-use distribution [5,6]. However, no accurate polygon dataset of those land uses was openly available for the Porto Metropolitan Area. Thus, we computed an alternative, destination-based measure of entropy as described below.

(1) Step 1: Collection of the locations of commonly visited destinations in the study area. Based on previous studies [6,19], we considered the following types/groupings of destinations: retail, institutional, services, recreational, and residential. Several sources of data were used, fully detailed in Table 1. These data sources can be considered reliable and accurate, as details about most destinations were centralized in institutional and territorial local authority websites and datasets.

(2) Step 2: Assessment of the number of destinations of each type within 800 m of the centroid of each neighborhood, using the ArcGIS 10.4 Network Analyst tool and an updated street network. Again, for sensitivity analysis, the 400-m distance threshold was also employed.

(3) Step 3: After determining the number of destinations of each type at a walkable distance, we calculated the entropy index for each neighborhood, using the equation below.

$$Entropy\ index\ of\ j\ neighbourhood = \frac{-\sum p_{ij} \times \ln p_{ij}}{\ln N_i}, \tag{1}$$

where $p_{ij}$ is the fraction of destinations of type $i$ at a walkable distance from neighbourhood centroid $j$, and $N_i$ is the number of different destination types, i.e., five. Values may range from 0 (low diversity of destinations) to 1 (high diversity).

### 2.2.4. Walkability Index Calculation

Each of the previously described variables was standardized, and the walkability score was obtained by summing the three z-scores [10].

The walkability index was created to be used both as a continuous score and/or a categorical variable. As in the original version of the measure [5], the neighborhood walkability index was then categorized in quintiles of increasing value (Q1—least walkable to Q5—most walkable).

## 2.3. Walking for Transport

Data on the number of individuals that report walking from/to school/work were obtained from the 2011 population and housing census, available via Statistics Portugal (https://www.ine.pt/).

In the census survey, every inhabitant answered the following question: What is your main mode to travel to school/work? (1, walking; 2, car; 3, bus; 4, collective transport offered by school/work; 5, metro; 6, train; 7, motorcycle; 8, bike; 9, boat; 10, other). The person could select one option only. There were no missing data, as usual in universal population censuses.

In this study, we used the number of individuals (count) living in each neighborhood who reported walking to/from home/work and, as a denominator, we included the total number of individuals living in the same neighborhood.

## 2.4. Covariates

We also included data on potential confounders in the association between neighborhood walkability and walking for transport, identified in previous studies [5,20]: the population age and gender distribution (proportion of active-age population 15–64 years old, and proportion of women), the proportion of employed individuals, and the proportion of people working in other municipalities. These data were obtained from the 2011 population and housing census, available via Statistics Portugal (https://www.ine.pt/), Additionally, we considered the neighborhood socioeconomic deprivation index developed and fully described in previous publications [21,22]. In short, this index was calculated from the weighted sum of the following standardized variables: % overcrowded households, % households with no bath/shower, % households without indoor flushing, % households occupied by non-owners, % women aged 65 or more, % individuals with low education, % individuals in low-income occupation, and % unemployed individuals. The index was categorized into quintiles of increasing socioeconomic deprivation (Q1—least deprived to Q5—most deprived).

## 2.5. Associations with Transport Walking

Generalized additive models (GAM) were used to estimate the association between the proportion of individuals that reported walking from/to school/work and the walkability index score and quintiles.

GAM extends generalized linear models to include nonparametric smoothing. This approach, employed previously [23,24], allowed us to model the spatial distribution of the response variable, thus allowing for the control of spatial autocorrelation.

Firstly, we fitted a univariable model, which included the response variable, the walkability index, and a function (thin plate spline) applied on the coordinates of each neighborhood.

Then, the model was adjusted for potential confounders: the population age and gender distribution (proportion of active-age population 15–64 years, and proportion of women), the proportion of employed individuals, the proportion of people working in other municipalities, and the neighborhood socioeconomic deprivation index. Statistical analyses were conducted in the R software version 3.3.3. (R Foundation for Statistical Computing, Vienna, Austria) using the package "mgcv".

## 3. Results

The spatial distribution of the walkability index is shown in Figure 1. The average walkability index in the study area was 0.01, ranging from −2.81 to 15.05. Out of the 1,112,555 inhabitants living in the study area, 15.8% resided in neighborhoods in the first quintile of walkability (Q1—least walkable), 16.0% in Q2, 17.9% in Q3, 22.2% in Q4, and 28.1% in Q5 (the most walkable neighborhoods). For the geographical distribution of the index, we observed a clear radial decay in the walkability index of the Porto Metropolitan Area from the center (Porto municipality) to the periphery (municipalities of Matosinhos, Maia, Valongo, Gondomar, and Vila Nova de Gaia) (Figure 1).

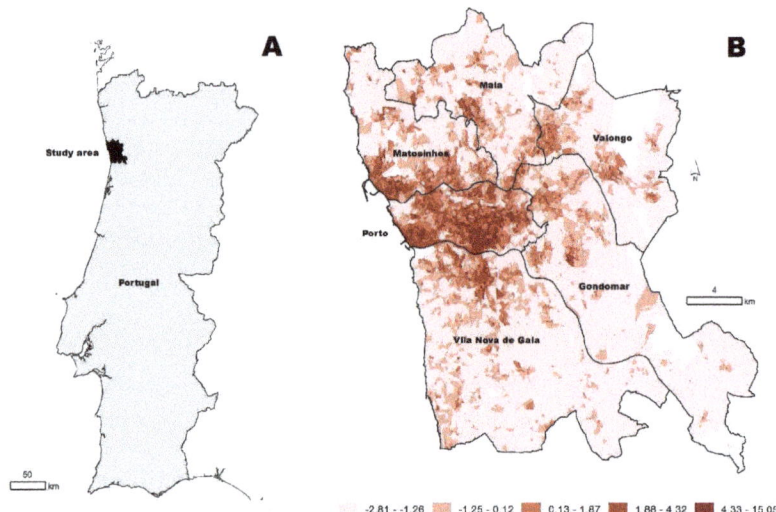

**Figure 1.** Location of the study area in Portugal (**A**). Spatial distribution of the walkability index at the neighborhood level (*n* = 10,444) (**B**).

Table 2 shows the population characteristics. Overall, 15.4% of the population reported walking to/from work/school. Table 3 depicts the association between the walkability index and the proportion of the population that walks to/from work/school. There is a graded and positive association between the walkability index and transport-related walking.

This association remained after adjustment for potential confounding variables. Compared with the least walkable neighborhoods, individuals residing in the most walkable neighborhoods were significantly more likely to walk to/from work/school (Q1 vs. Q5 odds ratio: 1.81; 95% confidence intervals: 1.76–1.87). When using the walkability index score, we observed that the odds of walking to/from work/school increased by 7% for every unit increase in the walkability index (odds ratio: 1.07; 95% confidence intervals: 1.07–1.08).

Similar results were obtained using the 400-m distance threshold, as shown in Table S1 (Supplementary Materials).

**Table 2.** Characteristics of the population residing in the study area (*N* = 1,112,555).

| Variables | % |
|---|---|
| Gender (men) | 47.4 |
| Active-age population 15–64 years | 68.5 |
| Employed individuals | 60.3 |
| Working in other municipalities | 24.1 |
| Walking from/to work/school | 15.4 |
| Neighborhood walkability index | |
| Q1—least walkable | 15.8 |
| Q2 | 16.0 |
| Q3 | 17.9 |
| Q4 | 22.2 |
| Q5—most walkable | 28.2 |
| Neighborhood socioeconomic deprivation | |
| Q1—least deprived | 15.5 |
| Q2 | 19.1 |
| Q3 | 22.4 |
| Q4 | 20.9 |
| Q5—most deprived | 22.2 |

**Table 3.** Crude and adjusted associations between the neighborhood walkability index and the proportion of residents walking from/to work/school.

|  | Walking from/to Work/School OR and 95% CIs [1] | Walking from/to Work/School AOR and 95% CIs [2] |
|---|---|---|
| Neighborhood walkability index |  |  |
| Q1—least walkable | 1.00 | 1.00 |
| Q2 | 1.08 (1.05–1.11) | 1.11 (1.08–1.15) |
| Q3 | 1.30 (1.27–1.34) | 1.37 (1.33–1.41) |
| Q4 | 1.44 (1.40–1.48) | 1.56 (1.51–1.60) |
| Q5—most walkable | 1.53 (1.48–1.57) | 1.81 (1.76–1.87) |
| Neighborhood walkability index (score) | 1.05 (1.04–1.05) | 1.07 (1.07–1.08) |

[1] Odds ratio (OR) and 95% confidence intervals. [2] Adjusted odds ratio (AOR) and 95% confidence intervals. Adjusted for the proportion of active-age population 15–64 years, proportion of men, proportion of employed people, proportion of people working in other municipalities, and neighborhood socioeconomic deprivation score.

## 4. Discussion

The present study was designed to measure of how well the Porto Metropolitan Area neighborhoods promote active forms of transportation, such as walking. This study fulfilled an important evidence gap in Portugal, where, despite the extremely low levels of PA, few investments were made in ascertaining how friendly urban environments are for pedestrian movement. To address this, we developed a walkability index at the neighborhood level by adapting an original methodological framework for walkability [5] to the data available in the study area.

Confirming findings from international investigations [3,6–8,15,16,25,26], we observed a positive and graded association between neighborhood walkability and walking. Residents in more walkable neighborhoods—areas with a variety of destinations within walking distance, a well-connected street network, and a high density of residences—presented 81% higher odds of walking for transportation (to/from work/school), as compared with those living in the least walkable areas. While our methods are not fully comparable with all those used in other studies on the topic, it is important to note that the effect sizes observed in the literature somehow match ours. For instance, Chudyk et al. reported that a 10-point increase in the walkability index score was associated with 45% greater odds of walking for transportation in a population of older adults from Canada [3]. In a sample of South Asians living in the US, for each 10-point increase in walk score, men engaged in 13 additional minutes per week of walking for transport [16]. Villanueva et al. collected data from a sample of Australian adults, and observed that a point increase in the walkability index score was associated with 6% greater odds of walking [7]. In Sweden, individuals living in highly walkable neighborhoods, compared to those living in less walkable neighborhoods, had 77% higher odds of walking for active transportation [15]. Studies using objective measures of walking, derived from accelerometry, also observed a positive association between neighborhood walkability and daily steps [25,26].

Regarding, the geographical distribution of the index, we observed a clear radial decay in the walkability index of the Porto Metropolitan Area from the center (Porto municipality) to the periphery, as expected. This is likely the case because the Porto municipality is the urban core, and the peripheral municipalities (Matosinhos, Valongo, Maia, Vila Nova de Gaia, and Gondomar) have lower land-use mix and street connectivity, two of the walkability index components. Similar radial decay patterns in the walkability index were observed in other urban areas [6,8,27].

This investigation has a number of limitations that should be discussed. Concerning the index development methodology, we could not include all possible destinations available in the study area (namely shops and small food outlets), due to difficulty in accessing high-quality and accurate datasets. This may affect the absolute walkability index value by underestimating it, but it is unlikely to influence the relative position of the neighborhoods, i.e., the quintiles. We were also unable to obtain information on a fourth variable commonly included (ratio of retail building floor areas). Concerning the measurement of associations, conclusions regarding causality and the directionality of the associations could not be made, given the study's cross-sectional design. We relied on a dichotomous (yes/no) self-reported variable to measure walking for transport, which might lead to recall and reporting bias. Previous studies found a low-to-moderate correlation between self-reported and objective measures of PA [28]. Thus, ideally, objective measures obtained using global position systems (GPS) and accelerometry, should be used to measure walking for transport [28]. Additionally, our variable on walking for transport did not capture the duration and intensity of walking, which are more relevant to health.

This study also has a number of strengths and implications. Firstly, we developed, for the first time, a validated walkability index for Porto area, which is critical for establishing priorities for the creation of more walkable and pedestrian-friendly communities. Secondly, we developed and tested an alternative measure of entropy, which may be useful in settings where no high-resolution land parcel maps are openly available. The methods employed in this study may be easily transposed and applied in other countries of high, medium, and low income, where accurate and updated land-use datasets may not be available, provided these new indexes are subject to proper validation. Moreover, we tested the impact of using different thresholds of geographical proximity to destinations (800 and 400 m); this is critical as there is no current consensual definition of what a walkable distance is. In sum, the validation of the index was based on census data, which have universal coverage in Portugal, and included data from 1.1 million citizens living in the second largest metro area of the country.

Demonstrating that the way the urban environment is built influences walking behavior provides important evidence for the development of area-based interventions for the creation of more PA-friendly communities. Moreover, the creation of walkable communities may lead to a series of co-benefits [29]: (1) significant health gains at population level, as physical inactivity is a leading risk factor for mortality and several non-communicable diseases [30]; (2) environmental sustainability, since it reduces car trips, which minimizes air pollution and noise [29]; (3) economic gains, by decreasing expenses related to car ownership and strengthening the local business environment [29].

## 5. Conclusions

In conclusion, this study showed that neighborhood walkability has a positive and graded association with walking for transportation. Although we cannot directly infer this from our study, our results suggest that implementing community design strategies to improve walkability might enhance PA among Portuguese urbanites, specifically by increasing walking for transportation. The study also demonstrated that, in the absence of land-use maps, an alternative and valid measure of the neighborhood entropy index could be developed based on the number and type of destinations within a certain area.

**Supplementary Materials:** The following are available online at http://www.mdpi.com/1660-4601/15/12/2767/s1: Table S1: Crude and adjusted associations between the neighborhood walkability index and the proportion of residents walking from/to work/school (threshold distance equal to 400 m).

**Author Contributions:** Conceptualization, A.I.R.; methodology, A.I.R.; formal analysis, A.I.R. and E.H.; writing—original draft preparation, A.I.R. and E.H.; writing—review and editing, A.I.R.

**Funding:** This study was supported by FEDER through the Operational Program Competitiveness and Internationalization and national funding from the Foundation for Science and Technology—FCT (Portuguese Ministry of Science, Technology and Higher Education) under the Unidade de Investigação em Epidemiologia—Instituto de Saúde Pública da Universidade do Porto (EPIUnit) (POCI-01-0145-FEDER-006862; Ref. UID/DTP/04750/2013). This study was also funded by the European Regional Development Fund (FEDER), through the Competitiveness and Internationalization Operational Program, and by national funding from the Foundation for Science and Technology (FCT) under the scope of the project PTDC/GES-AMB/30193/2017 (POCI-01-0145-FEDER-030193, 02/SAICT/2017-30193).

**Conflicts of Interest:** The authors declare no conflict of interest.

# References

1. Arem, H.; Moore, S.C.; Patel, A.; Hartge, P.; de Gonzalez, A.B.; Visvanathan, K.; Campbell, P.T.; Freedman, M.; Weiderpass, E.; Adami, H.O.; et al. Leisure Time Physical Activity and Mortality: A Detailed Pooled Analysis of the Dose-Response Relationship. *JAMA Intern. Med.* **2015**, *175*, 959–967. [CrossRef] [PubMed]

2. EU. Special Eurobarometer 472: Sport and physical activity. In *European Commission, Directorate-General for Education, Youth, Sport and Culture and Co-Ordinated by the Directorate-General for Communication*; European Union: Brussels, Belgium, 2018.

3. Chudyk, A.M.; McKay, H.A.; Winters, M.; Sims-Gould, J.; Ashe, M.C. Neighborhood walkability, physical activity, and walking for transportation: A cross-sectional study of older adults living on low income. *BMC Geriatr.* **2017**, *17*, 82. [CrossRef] [PubMed]

4. Jackson, L.E. The relationship of urban design to human health and condition. *Landsc. Urban Plan.* **2003**, *64*, 191–200. [CrossRef]

5. Frank, L.D.; Schmid, T.L.; Sallis, J.F.; Chapman, J.; Saelens, B.E. Linking objectively measured physical activity with objectively measured urban form: Findings from SMARTRAQ. *Am. J. Prev. Med.* **2005**, *28* (Suppl. 2), 117–125. [CrossRef] [PubMed]

6. Frank, L.D.; Sallis, J.F.; Saelens, B.E.; Leary, L.; Cain, K.; Conway, T.L.; Hess, P.M. The development of a walkability index: Application to the Neighborhood Quality of Life Study. *Br. J. Sports Med.* **2010**, *44*, 924. [CrossRef] [PubMed]

7. Villanueva, K.; Knuiman, M.; Nathan, A.; Giles-Corti, B.; Christian, H.; Foster, S.; Bull, F. The impact of neighborhood walkability on walking: Does it differ across adult life stage and does neighborhood buffer size matter? *Health Place* **2014**, *25*, 43–46. [CrossRef] [PubMed]

8. Stockton, J.C.; Duke-Williams, O.; Stamatakis, E.; Mindell, J.S.; Brunner, E.J.; Shelton, N.J. Development of a novel walkability index for London, United Kingdom: Cross-sectional application to the Whitehall II Study. *BMC Public Health* **2016**, *16*, 416. [CrossRef] [PubMed]

9. Huang, J.; Lu, X.X.; Sellers, J.M. A global comparative analysis of urban form: Applying spatial metrics and remote sensing. *Landsc. Urban Plan.* **2007**, *82*, 184–197. [CrossRef]

10. Ribeiro, A.I.; Krainski, E.T.; Autran, R.; Teixeira, H.; Carvalho, M.S.; de Pina, M.D.F. The influence of socioeconomic, biogeophysical and built environment on old-age survival in a Southern European city. *Health Place* **2016**, *41*, 100–109. [CrossRef] [PubMed]

11. Autran, R.G. Neighbourhood Environment and Physical Activity among Portuguese Adolescents. Ph.D. Thesis, University of Porto, Porto, Portugal, 2016.

12. EEA Urban Atlas 2012. Available online: https://land.copernicus.eu/local/urban-atlas (accessed on 10 September 2018).

13. INE Estimativas da população residente. Available online: https://www.ine.pt (accessed on 10 September 2018).

14. INE Censos. O que são? Available online: https://www.ine.pt/xportal/xmain?xpgid=censos21_sobre_censos&xpid=CENSOS21&xlang=pt (accessed on 4 October 2018).

15. Sundquist, K.; Eriksson, U.; Kawakami, N.; Skog, L.; Ohlsson, H.; Arvidsson, D. Neighborhood walkability, physical activity, and walking behavior: The Swedish Neighborhood and Physical Activity (SNAP) study. *Soc. Sci. Med.* **2011**, *72*, 1266–1273. [CrossRef] [PubMed]

16. Kelley, E.A.; Kandula, N.R.; Kanaya, A.M.; Yen, I.H. Neighborhood Walkability and Walking for Transport among South Asians in the MASALA Study. *J. Phys. Act. Health* **2016**, *13*, 514–519. [CrossRef] [PubMed]

17. Hoffimann, E.; Barros, H.; Ribeiro, I.A. Socioeconomic Inequalities in Green Space Quality and Accessibility—Evidence from a Southern European City. *Int. J. Environ. Res. Public Health* **2017**, *14*, 916. [CrossRef] [PubMed]

18. Witten, K.; Pearce, J.; Day, P. Neighbourhood Destination Accessibility Index: A GIS Tool for Measuring Infrastructure Support for Neighbourhood Physical Activity. *Environ. Plan. A Econ. Space* **2011**, *43*, 205–223. [CrossRef]

19. Brown, B.B.; Yamada, I.; Smith, K.R.; Zick, C.D.; Kowaleski-Jones, L.; Fan, J.X. Mixed land use and walkability: Variations in land use measures and relationships with BMI, overweight, and obesity. *Health Place* **2009**, *15*, 1130–1141. [CrossRef] [PubMed]

20. Frank, L.D.; Sallis, J.F.; Conway, T.L.; Chapman, J.E.; Saelens, B.E.; Bachman, W. Many Pathways from Land Use to Health: Associations between Neighborhood Walkability and Active Transportation, Body Mass Index, and Air Quality. *J. Am. Plan. Assoc.* **2006**, *72*, 75–87. [CrossRef]

21. Guillaume, E.; Pornet, C.; Dejardin, O.; Launay, L.; Lillini, R.; Vercelli, M.; Marí, D.; Olmo, M.; Fernández Fontelo, A.; Borrell, C.; et al. Development of a cross-cultural deprivation index in five European countries. *J. Epidemiol. Community Health* **2015**, *70*, 493–499. [CrossRef] [PubMed]

22. Ribeiro, A.I.; Mayer, A.; Miranda, A.; de Pina, M.D.F. The Portuguese Version of the European Deprivation Index: An Instrument to Study Health Inequalities. *Acta Méd. Port.* **2017**, *30*, 17–25. [CrossRef]

23. Ribeiro, A.I.; Mitchell, R.; Carvalho, M.S.; de Pina, M.D.F. Physical activity-friendly neighbourhood among older adults from a medium size urban setting in Southern Europe. *Prev. Med.* **2013**, *57*, 664–670. [CrossRef]

24. Ribeiro, A.I.; Pires, A.; Carvalho, M.S.; Pina, M.F. Distance to parks and non-residential destinations influences physical activity of older people, but crime doesn't: A cross-sectional study in a southern European city. *BMC Public Health* **2015**, *15*, 593. [CrossRef]

25. Van Dyck, D.; Deforche, B.; Cardon, G.; de Bourdeaudhuij, I. Neighbourhood walkability and its particular importance for adults with a preference for passive transport. *Health Place* **2009**, *15*, 496–504. [CrossRef]

26. Hajna, S.; Ross, N.A.; Joseph, L.; Harper, S.; Dasgupta, K. Neighbourhood walkability, daily steps and utilitarian walking in Canadian adults. *BMJ Open* **2015**, *5*, e008964. [CrossRef] [PubMed]

27. Xia, Z.; Li, H.; Chen, Y. Assessing neighborhood walkability based on usage characteristics of amenities under chinese metropolises context. *Sustainability* **2018**, 3879. [CrossRef]

28. Prince, S.A.; Adamo, K.B.; Hamel, M.E.; Hardt, J.; Connor Gorber, S.; Tremblay, M. A comparison of direct versus self-report measures for assessing physical activity in adults: A systematic review. *Int. J. Behav. Nutr. Phys. Act.* **2008**. [CrossRef] [PubMed]

29. Sallis, J.F.; Spoon, C.; Cavill, N.; Engelberg, J.K.; Gebel, K.; Parker, M.; Thornton, C.M.; Lou, D.; Wilson, A.L.; Cutter, C.L.; et al. Co-benefits of designing communities for active living: An exploration of literature. *Int. J. Behav. Nutr. Phys. Act.* **2015**, *12*, 30. [CrossRef] [PubMed]

30. Lee, I.M.; Shiroma, E.J.; Lobelo, F.; Puska, P.; Blair, S.N.; Katzmarzyk, P.T. Effect of physical inactivity on major non-communicable diseases worldwide: An analysis of burden of disease and life expectancy. *Lancet* **2012**, *380*, 219–229. [CrossRef]

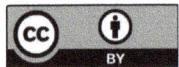

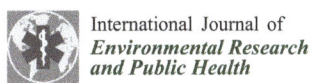

International Journal of
*Environmental Research and Public Health*

*Article*

# Walk Score® and Its Associations with Older Adults' Health Behaviors and Outcomes

**Yung Liao [1], Chien-Yu Lin [2], Ting-Fu Lai [1], Yen-Ju Chen [3], Bohyeon Kim [4] and Jong-Hwan Park [4,\*]**

[1]   Department of Health Promotion and Health Education, National Taiwan Normal University, 162, Heping East Road Section 1, Taipei 106, Taiwan; liaoyung@ntnu.edu.tw (Y.L.); ted971345@gmail.com (T.-F.L.)
[2]   Institute of Health Behaviors and Community Sciences, National Taiwan University, 17, Xuzhou Road, Taipei 100, Taiwan; chienyulin@ntu.edu.tw
[3]   Graduate Institute of Sport, Leisure and Hospitality Management, National Taiwan Normal University, 162, Heping East Road Section 1, Taipei 106, Taiwan; lulu0126@gmail.com
[4]   Health Behaviors & Disease Prevention Research Group, Institute of Convergence Bio-Health, Dong-A University, Busan 49201, Korea; gus8179@gmail.com
\*   Correspondence: jpark@dau.ac.kr; Tel.: +81-51-240-2763

Received: 4 December 2018; Accepted: 16 February 2019; Published: 20 February 2019

**Abstract:** This study aimed to investigate the associations between Walk Score® and lifestyle behaviors and health outcomes in older Taiwanese adults. A nationwide survey was conducted through telephone-based interviews with older adults (65 years and older) in Taiwan. Data on Walk Score®, lifestyle behaviors (physical activity, sedentary behavior, healthy eating behavior, alcohol use, and smoking status), health outcomes (overweight/obesity, hypertension, type 2 diabetes, and cardiovascular disease), and personal characteristics were obtained from 1052 respondents. A binary logistic regression adjusting for potential confounders was employed. None of the Walk Score® categories were related to the recommended levels of total physical activity. The categories "very walkable" and "walker's paradise" were positively related to total sedentary time and TV viewing among older adults. No significant associations were found between Walk Score® and other lifestyle health behaviors or health outcomes. While Walk Score® was not associated with recommended levels of physical activity, it was positively related to prolonged sedentary time in the context of a non-Western country. The different associations between the walk score and health lifestyle behaviors and health outcomes in different contexts should be noted.

**Keywords:** walkability; neighborhood; older adult; chronic diseases

## 1. Introduction

There is overwhelming evidence of the role of the neighborhood environment in individuals' lifestyle behaviors and health outcomes [1,2]. Compared to psychosocial intervention, manipulation of the built environment is expected to have long-term effects on various populations [3,4]. The neighborhood built environment is particularly important for older populations because they tend to spend most of their time in it as their mobility gradually declines with age [5]. Walkability, a key concept of the built environment, is the capacity of a neighborhood to support individuals' lifestyle behaviors such as walking and physical activity [6]. Previous studies have assessed neighborhood walkability using various measurements such as audits of streetscapes, residents' perceptions as well as indices of land use mix diversity, street connectivity, and residential density [7,8]. Research has associated an increased duration of physical activity with a decreased risk of negative health outcomes such as being overweight [9], symptoms of depression [10,11], and overall mortality [12,13]. A deeper understanding of neighborhood walkability and older adults' health is needed to develop initiatives and inform policymakers and urban designers on redesigning cities and suburbs to improve public health.

Walk Score® is a free, web-based, and publicly available estimate of neighborhood walkability that can minimize the limitations of observational, self-reported, and geographic information system (GIS) measures [14]. Although Walk Score® was initially developed as an indicator for housing prices and environment friendly neighborhoods (i.e. walkability and transportation), previous studies showed a positive association between walk score and walking behavior and overall physical activity [15–17] and a negative association with sedentary behaviors such as driving a car [18]. Moreover, the walk score is negatively related to health outcomes such as risk of obesity [19] and cardiovascular diseases (CVD) [20,21], and positively related to risks of type 2 diabetes [22]. However, studies using Walk Score® mostly reported data from Western countries, and the situation remains unclear in the context of non-Western countries. Thus, to our knowledge, only two studies have investigated the relationships between Walk Score® and physical activity, sedentary behavior, [18] and weight status [23] in Japan, an Asian country. Compared to Western countries, differences in the context of Asian countries include high population density, long working hours, transportation mode (i.e. motorcycles), and traditionally mixed land-use [24,25]. Based on different cultural, economic, and environmental contexts, the walk score may have different effects on public health in Asian countries. In addition, since neighborhood physical attributes influence lifestyle behaviors that contribute to chronic diseases [26], it remains unclear whether the walk score is linked with other lifestyle behaviors such as current smoking status, alcohol use, and healthy eating behavior (potentially influenced by access to amenities in the neighborhood), and other health outcomes (i.e., hypertension) in older adults. To fill this research gap, the present study aimed to explore the relationships between the walk score and lifestyle behaviors (total physical activity, sedentary time, smoking behavior, alcohol use, and eating behavior) and health outcomes (risks of overweight/ obesity, hypertension, type 2 diabetes, and CVD) of Taiwanese older adults.

## 2. Materials and Methods

### 2.1. Participants

A cross-sectional telephone-based survey was conducted across Taiwan in 2017. To ensure a representative sample, participants were randomly selected using a stratified two-stage sampling procedure. The four areas (i.e., northern, eastern, western, and southern) of Taiwan were first stratified according to geographic location. In the second stage, individuals were randomly selected based on gender and age group (aged 85+, 75–84, 65–74 years). Each interviewer underwent training and conducted a standardized questionnaire during each survey. Among 3,282 older adults asked to participate, 1,068 responded (response rate: 32.5%). After data cleaning, the data of 1052 participants was considered valid and included in our analysis (eligible rate: 32.1%). Before each telephone interview began, verbal informed consent was obtained. Furthermore, participants were not offered any rewards. The protocols of this study were assessed and approved by the Research Ethics Committee of the University (REC number: 201706HM020).

### 2.2. Outcome Variables

Seven lifestyle behaviors and four health outcomes were included in this study:

1. Lifestyle behaviors: (i) total physical activity, (ii) total sedentary behavior, (iii) TV viewing, (iv) driving time, (v) healthy eating behavior, (vi) alcohol use, and (vii) current smoking status
2. Health outcomes: (viii) overweight/obesity, (ix) hypertension, (x) diabetes, and (xi) CVD

### 2.2.1. Lifestyle Behaviors

Physical Activity

The total time spent doing physical activity was assessed using the Taiwanese version of the International Physical Activity Questionnaire (IPAQ), which is widely utilized in telephone interview surveys on older adults [27,28]. The Taiwanese version of the IPAQ has high test-retest reliability (r = 0.78) and content validity (intra-class correlation coefficient = 0.99) [29]. The self-reported time spent walking, on moderate-intensity physical activity excluding walking (e.g., dancing and table tennis), and vigorous-intensity physical activity (e.g., aerobic exercises and basketball) was summed as total physical activity. The total physical activity was then dichotomized into two categories according to the physical activity guidelines for older adults: sufficient ($\geq$150 min/week total physical activity) and insufficient (<150 min/week total physical activity) [30].

Sedentary Behavior

The total sedentary behavior, TV viewing time, and driving time were obtained using the Measure of Older Adults' Sedentary Time questionnaire. Total sedentary behavior in the past week was calculated as the sum of TV viewing (i.e., time spent watching TV or digital videos), screen time (i.e., time spent online via any medium such as a computer, cellphone, and tablet), reading, chatting with others while sitting, driving time, eating, sedentary hobbies (e.g., listening to music and playing cards), sitting for work or volunteering, and other sitting activities. The total sedentary behavior was then dichotomized as >8 h/d and $\leq$8 h/d [31]. Furthermore, two specific sedentary behaviors, namely TV viewing and driving time, were examined because they may be potentially related to environmental walkability [18,32]. The cutoffs of 2 h/d and 1 h/d were selected for TV viewing [33,34] and driving time, respectively [35].

Eating Behavior, Alcohol Use, Current Smoking Status

In addition to physical activity and sedentary behavior, eating behavior, alcohol use, and current smoking status were recorded. Based on the items used in previous studies [36], participants were asked about their healthy eating behavior (How many servings of fruits and vegetables do you consume on an average day?), total number of alcoholic drinks consumed (How many alcoholic drinks do you consume each week?), and current smoking status (Are you a current smoker?). We divided healthy eating behavior into "Yes (three servings of vegetables and two servings of fruit)" and "No" according to the Taiwanese dietary guidelines [37], and categorized "alcohol use" and "current smoking status" as "Yes" and "No."

### 2.2.2. Health Outcomes

Overweight/Obesity, Hypertension, Type 2 Diabetes, CVD

Health outcomes included self-reported body mass index (BMI), hypertension, type 2 diabetes, and CVD. BMI was calculated based on self-reported height and weight and classified as "normal weight, <24 kg/m$^2$" and "overweight/obesity, $\geq$24 kg/m$^2$" according to the criteria for Asian cutoff points [38]. According to the Taiwanese Chronic Disease Survey [39], the status of hypertension, type 2 diabetes, and CVD is determined by an affirmative response to a question (yes or no). The question is as follows: "Has a doctor, nurse, or other health professional ever told you that you have hypertension (type 2 diabetes, and CVD type 2 diabetes), or do you use medications for such conditions?"

### 2.3. Exposure Variable

The exposure variable was neighborhood walkability, which was measured using the Walk Score® website (Link: www.walkscore.com). Walk Score® was recently confirmed as a valid measure for assessing neighborhood walkability in the Asian context [40]. Our study also found significant positive correlations between Walk Score® and GIS-derived environmental attributes relevant to walking, namely residential density ($r$ = 0.64), intersection density ($r$ = 0.70), number of local destinations ($r$ = 0.70), sidewalk availability ($r$ = 0.38), and access to public transportation ($r$ = 0.53) in Taiwan. Walk Score® is first calculated by determining a raw score for each geographic location based on the network distance to nine amenity categories of walking destinations, namely grocery stores, restaurants, shopping, coffee shops, bank services, schools, entertainment, bookstores, and parks. These raw scores are then normalized from 0 to 100 adjusting for the "intersection density" and "block length" around each location [41,42]. To calculate the walk score of each respondent, each respondent's residential neighborhood was manually inputted into the Walk Score® website by one researcher and the validity checked by another researcher. Recent studies suggested that there may not be a linear association between the walk score and walking [16] and obesity [19]. Therefore, according to the methodology [42], the walk scores were classified into four categories: (1) "car-dependent" (walk score: 0–49), (2) "somewhat walkable" (walk score: 50–69), (3) "very walkable" (walk score: 70–89), and (4) "walker's paradise"(walk score: 90–100).

### 2.4. Covariates

The covariates were several demographic variables: gender, age groups (65–74, 75–84, 85+ years), education achievement (up to a high school degree or college degree or more), occupational status (full-time job or no full-time job), marital status (married or not married), and living status (living alone or living with others).

### 2.5. Data Analysis

Data from 1052 Taiwanese older adults who completed the survey on the study variables were analyzed. Since the outcome variables were skewed (i.e., health behaviors) or categorical (i.e., health outcomes) and the walk score category was provided, an adjusted binary logistic regression was performed to investigate the relationship between the four walk score categories and seven lifestyle behaviors and four health outcome variables. For the association between walk score and each lifestyle behavior, socio-demographic covariates including gender, age group, education level, occupational status, marital status, and living status were adjusted. For the association between the walk score and each health outcome, all health lifestyle behaviors (excluding TV viewing and driving) and the abovementioned socio-demographic variables were further adjusted. We considered the total sedentary behavior; therefore, we excluded these two types of sedentary behavior to avoid issues of multicollinearity. The odds ratio and 95% confidence interval (CIs) were calculated for each variable. Inferential statistics were performed using IBM SPSS 22.0 and the level of significance was set at $P < 0.05$.

### 3. Results

#### 3.1. Participants' Demographic Characteristics

Table 1 presents the demographic characteristics of the sample. Among the participants, the mean age was 73.0 years (standard deviation (SD) = 6.10), 50.1% were male, 64.5% were aged 65–74 years, 69.7% had a high school degree and lower, 90% did not have a full-time job, 75.6% were married, and 85.7% lived with others. Older adults who lived in car-dependent neighborhoods tended to be male, had up to a high school degree, and did not have a full-time job.

We demonstrate the association between 11 health-related characteristics and 4 walk score categories in Table 2. Older adults living in a "walker's paradise" were more likely to have a total sedentary behavior time of more than 8 h per day (41.8%) and TV viewing time of more than 2 h per day (58.5%). No proportional differences were observed for total physical activity, driving time, healthy eating behavior, alcohol use, current smoking status, BMI, hypertension, type 2 diabetes, and CVD across the walk score categories.

Table 1. Demographic characteristics of participants by walk score category (*n* = 1052).

| Demographic Characteristics | Total | | Walk Score Category | | | | | | | | P-Value |
|---|---|---|---|---|---|---|---|---|---|---|---|
| | | | Car-Dependent | | Somewhat Walkable | | Very Walkable | | Walker's Paradise | | |
| | *n* | % | *n* | % | *n* | % | *n* | % | *n* | % | |
| | 1052 | 100% | 396 | 37.6% | 136 | 12.9% | 197 | 18.7% | 323 | 30.7% | |
| **Gender** | | | | | | | | | | | <0.001 |
| Male | 527 | 50.1% | 232 | 58.6% | 76 | 55.9% | 85 | 43.1% | 134 | 41.5% | |
| Female | 525 | 49.9% | 164 | 41.4% | 60 | 44.1% | 112 | 56.9% | 189 | 58.5% | |
| **Age group** | | | | | | | | | | | 0.363 |
| 65–74 years | 679 | 64.5% | 267 | 67.4% | 88 | 64.7% | 120 | 60.9% | 204 | 63.2% | |
| 75–84 years | 311 | 29.6% | 104 | 26.3% | 37 | 27.2% | 67 | 34.0% | 103 | 31.9% | |
| 85+ years | 62 | 5.9% | 25 | 6.3% | 11 | 8.1% | 10 | 5.1% | 16 | 5.0% | |
| **Education achievement** | | | | | | | | | | | <0.001 |
| Up to a high school degree | 733 | 69.7% | 319 | 80.6% | 92 | 67.6% | 140 | 71.1% | 182 | 56.3% | |
| College degree or more | 319 | 30.3% | 77 | 19.4% | 44 | 32.4% | 57 | 28.9% | 141 | 43.7% | |
| **Occupational status** | | | | | | | | | | | 0.005 |
| Full-time job | 105 | 10.0% | 56 | 14.1% | 12 | 8.8% | 15 | 7.6% | 22 | 6.8% | |
| No full-time job | 947 | 90.0% | 340 | 85.9% | 124 | 91.2% | 182 | 92.4% | 301 | 93.2% | |
| **Marital status** | | | | | | | | | | | 0.381 |
| Married | 795 | 75.6% | 307 | 77.5% | 104 | 76.5% | 151 | 76.6% | 233 | 72.1% | |
| Not married | 257 | 24.4% | 89 | 22.5% | 32 | 23.5% | 46 | 23.4% | 90 | 27.9% | |
| **Living status** | | | | | | | | | | | 0.554 |
| Living alone | 150 | 14.3% | 50 | 12.6% | 23 | 16.9% | 27 | 13.7% | 50 | 15.5% | |
| Living with others | 902 | 85.7% | 346 | 87.4% | 113 | 83.1% | 170 | 86.3% | 273 | 84.5% | |

Table 2. Participants' health lifestyle behaviors and outcomes by walk score category (n = 1052).

| Health-Related Characteristics | Total | | Walk Score Category | | | | | | | | p-Value |
|---|---|---|---|---|---|---|---|---|---|---|---|
| | | | Car-Dependent | | Somewhat Walkable | | Very Walkable | | Walker's Paradise | | |
| | n | % | n | % | n | % | n | % | n | % | |
| **Lifestyle behaviors** | | | | | | | | | | | |
| Total PA * | | | | | | | | | | | 0.251 |
| Sufficient | 834 | 79.3% | 317 | 80.1% | 99 | 72.8% | 156 | 79.2% | 262 | 81.1% | |
| Insufficient | 218 | 20.7% | 79 | 19.9% | 37 | 27.2% | 41 | 20.8% | 61 | 18.9% | |
| Total SB † | | | | | | | | | | | <0.001 |
| >8h/day | 326 | 31.0% | 89 | 22.5% | 38 | 27.9% | 64 | 32.5% | 135 | 41.8% | |
| ≤8h/day | 726 | 69.0% | 307 | 77.5% | 98 | 72.1% | 133 | 67.5% | 188 | 58.2% | |
| TV viewing | | | | | | | | | | | 0.010 |
| >2h/day | 560 | 53.2% | 191 | 48.2% | 65 | 47.8% | 115 | 58.4% | 189 | 58.5% | |
| ≤2h/day | 492 | 46.8% | 205 | 51.8% | 71 | 52.2% | 82 | 41.6% | 134 | 41.5% | |
| Driving time | | | | | | | | | | | 0.154 |
| >1h/day | 195 | 18.5% | 82 | 20.7% | 31 | 22.8% | 32 | 16.2% | 50 | 15.5% | |
| ≤1h/day | 857 | 81.5% | 314 | 79.3% | 105 | 77.2% | 165 | 83.8% | 273 | 84.5% | |
| Healthy eating behavior | | | | | | | | | | | 0.399 |
| Yes | 864 | 82.1% | 315 | 79.5% | 113 | 83.1% | 164 | 83.2% | 272 | 84.2% | |
| No | 188 | 17.9% | 81 | 20.5% | 23 | 16.9% | 33 | 16.8% | 51 | 15.8% | |
| Alcohol use | | | | | | | | | | | 0.701 |
| Yes | 102 | 9.7% | 36 | 9.1% | 17 | 12.5% | 19 | 9.6% | 30 | 9.3% | |
| No | 950 | 90.3% | 360 | 90.9% | 119 | 87.5% | 178 | 90.4% | 293 | 90.7% | |
| Current smoking status | | | | | | | | | | | 0.359 |
| Yes | 71 | 6.7% | 33 | 8.3% | 9 | 6.6% | 13 | 6.6% | 16 | 5.0% | |
| No | 981 | 93.3% | 363 | 91.7% | 127 | 93.4% | 184 | 93.4% | 307 | 95.0% | |
| **Health outcomes** | | | | | | | | | | | |
| BMI ‡ | | | | | | | | | | | 0.511 |
| Normal | 557 | 52.9% | 200 | 50.5% | 78 | 57.4% | 108 | 54.8% | 171 | 52.9% | |
| Underweight/Overweight | 495 | 47.1% | 196 | 49.5% | 58 | 42.6% | 89 | 45.2% | 152 | 47.1% | |
| Hypertension | | | | | | | | | | | 0.489 |
| Yes | 502 | 47.7% | 178 | 44.9% | 64 | 47.1% | 96 | 48.7% | 164 | 50.8% | |
| No | 550 | 52.3% | 218 | 55.1% | 72 | 52.9% | 101 | 51.3% | 159 | 49.2% | |
| Diabetes | | | | | | | | | | | 0.300 |
| Yes | 201 | 19.1% | 83 | 21.0% | 28 | 20.6% | 40 | 20.3% | 50 | 15.5% | |
| No | 851 | 80.9% | 313 | 79.0% | 108 | 79.4% | 157 | 79.7% | 273 | 84.5% | |
| CVD § | | | | | | | | | | | 0.903 |
| Yes | 198 | 18.8% | 78 | 19.7% | 27 | 19.9% | 38 | 19.3% | 55 | 17.0% | |
| No | 854 | 81.2% | 318 | 80.3% | 109 | 80.1% | 159 | 80.7% | 268 | 83.0% | |

* PA = physical activity; † SB = sedentary behavior; ‡ BMI = body mass index; § CVD = cardiovascular disease.

## 3.2. Association Between Walk Score and Lifestyle Behaviors and Health Outcomes

The adjusted logistic regression models showed the associations between 11 health-related characteristics and 4 walk score categories (Table 3). In the unadjusted model, some covariates (i.e., gender, education achievement, and occupational status) and two sedentary behaviors (i.e., total sedentary behavior and TV viewing) were associated with the walk score category (data are not shown). After adjusting for potential covariates, the associations of the walk score categories with the two studied sedentary behaviors were slightly attenuated. Participants living in very walkable neighborhoods and walker's paradises were more likely to have a total sedentary behavior time > 8 h/day (very walkable: OR = 1.68, 95% CI = 1.13–2.48; walker's paradise: OR = 2.28, 95% CI = 1.62–3.21) and more TV viewing time (>2 h/day) (very walkable: OR = 1.47, 95% CI = 1.03–2.09; walker's paradise: OR = 1.50, 95% CI = 1.10–2.05). No significant relationships were found between walk score category and total physical activity, driving time, healthy eating behavior, alcohol use, and current smoking status. Furthermore, walk score category was not related to health outcome variables including BMI, hypertension, type 2 diabetes, and CVD.

**Table 3.** Adjusted odds ratios (ORs) for the association of walk score category with lifestyle behaviors and health outcomes.

| Health-Related Characteristics | Walk Score Category | | | | | | |
|---|---|---|---|---|---|---|---|
| | Car-Dependent | Somewhat Walkable | | Very Walkable | | Walker's Paradise | |
| | OR * (95% CI †) | OR * (95% CI †) | | OR * (95% CI †) | | OR * (95% CI †) | |
| Lifestyle behaviors | | | | | | | |
| Total PA ‡ (ref. Insufficient) | | | | | | | |
| Sufficient | 1.00 | 0.65 | (0.41, 1.03) | 0.93 | (0.60, 1.43) | 1.01 | (0.68, 1.49) |
| Total SB § (ref. ≤ 8h/day) | | | | | | | |
| > 8h/day | 1.00 | 1.28 | (0.81, 2.01) | **1.68** | **(1.13, 2.48)** | **2.28** | **(1.62, 3.21)** |
| TV viewing (ref. ≤ 2h/day) | | | | | | | |
| > 2h/day | 1.00 | 0.97 | (0.65, 1.44) | **1.47** | **(1.03, 2.09)** | **1.50** | **(1.10, 2.05)** |
| Driving time (ref. ≤ 1h/day) | | | | | | | |
| > 1h/day | 1.00 | 1.18 | (0.73, 1.90) | 0.83 | (0.52, 1.32) | 0.75 | (0.50, 1.14) |
| Healthy eating behavior (ref. Yes) | | | | | | | |
| No | 1.00 | 0.81 | (0.48, 1.36) | 0.86 | (0.54, 1.36) | 0.82 | (0.54, 1.23) |
| Alcohol use (ref. Yes) | | | | | | | |
| No | 1.00 | 0.57 | (0.29, 1.09) | 0.59 | (0.32, 1.11) | 0.66 | (0.38, 1.17) |
| Current smoking status (ref. Yes) | | | | | | | |
| No | 1.00 | 1.08 | (0.48, 2.39) | 0.79 | (0.39, 1.61) | 1.12 | (0.57, 2.19) |
| Health outcomes | | | | | | | |
| BMI ‖ (ref. Overweight/obesity) | | | | | | | |
| Normal | 1.00 | 1.18 | (0.79, 1.77) | 1.13 | (0.79, 1.61) | 1.07 | (0.78, 1.48) |
| Hypertension (ref. Yes) | | | | | | | |
| No | 1.00 | 0.96 | (0.64, 1.44) | 0.90 | (0.63, 1.28) | 0.76 | (0.55, 1.04) |
| Diabetes (ref. Yes) | | | | | | | |
| No | 1.00 | 1.02 | (0.63, 1.67) | 1.05 | (0.68, 1.61) | 1.41 | (0.94, 2.12) |
| CVD ** (ref. Yes) | | | | | | | |
| No | 1.00 | 0.97 | (0.59, 1.59) | 1.06 | (0.68, 1.65) | 1.18 | (0.79, 1.77) |

* ORs = odds ratios; † CI = confidence interval; ‡ PA = physical activity; § SB = sedentary behavior; ‖ BMI = body mass index; ** CVD = cardiovascular disease; Lifestyle behaviors adjusted for gender, age group, education achievement, occupational status, marital status, and living status; Health outcomes adjusted for gender, age group, education achievement, occupational status, marital status, and living status, total PA, total SB, healthy eating behavior, alcohol use, and current smoking status.

## 4. Discussion

The present research is one of the limited number of studies that explore the relationships of the walk score with seven lifestyle behaviors and four health outcomes among older adults in an Asian country. The findings revealed that the walk score is not associated with physical activity recommendations, but positively related to prolonged sedentary time and TV viewing among older adults in the context of Taiwan. These findings are inconsistent with previous findings on physical activity [16,17,43] and sedentary behavior [19,44] conducted in Western countries. The present findings may have significant implications for the inconsistency in the associations of the walk score with physical activity and sedentary behavior between Western countries and other contexts.

Contrary to our expectations, none of the walk score categories were related to physical activity, although the categories "very walkable" and "walker's paradise" were positively related to total sedentary time and TV viewing. Previous studies provided conflicting findings regarding the association between walkability and physical activity. Many associated a higher walk score with higher physical activity [45,46], although several others demonstrated no association between walkability and physical activity [46] or walking [47]. The lack of association between Walk Score® and physical activity may reflect the nature of the participants, because regardless of the walk score, around 70–80% of older adults engage in sufficient physical activity. Consistent with previous studies using GIS-derived environmental measures, a highly walkable environment and total sedentary time [48] and screen time [49] were positively associated. To our knowledge, the previous literature does not provide much evidence of the potential mechanisms regarding the different relationships between the walk score and physical activity and sedentary time in older adults. Possibly, as highly walkable neighborhood environments in Taiwan are usually crowded and accompanied by more traffic (i.e., motorcycles) [50], older adults may tend to not go outdoors and spend more time engaging in sedentary behavior and watching TV at home. In addition, total physical activity, not context-specific walking behavior was used in the present study, which may partly explain why no significant relationships were found between walk score and physical activity. These results are important in terms of informing public health policymakers and urban designers that more highly walkable neighborhoods may not necessarily facilitate older adults' physical activity, but could prolong their sedentary time, at least in Taiwan.

Although previous studies associated the walk score with several health outcomes such as lowered obesity [19], type 2 diabetes [22], and CVD [20,21], no significant relationship was found in our study. Our results were consistent with those of previous studies that found no associations between the walk score and overweight [51] or excessive body weight [52]. These results could also be attributed to key lifestyle behaviors such as physical activity, driving, eating, drinking, and smoking, which are strongly associated with health outcomes [53–55], not with the walk score in the present study. This suggests that walkability, as measured by the walk score, may not play a direct role in older adults' health outcomes in the context of Taiwan. Future research in different contexts should be conducted to confirm these results.

There are several limitations in the present study that must be considered. First, because of the cross-sectional design, we were unable to determine the causality between variables. Second, we used self-reported lifestyle behaviors and health outcome measures that may be subject to recall bias. Third, self-selection (older adults' preference to live in highly walkable neighborhoods), a potential confounder, was not accounted for in this study. Fourth, previous studies suggested that the Walk Score® algorithm did not account for micro-scale characteristics that may impact walking behavior, such as sufficient light and traffic volume [56,57]. Fifth, although gender differences in the associations between neighborhood walkability and health behavior have been found [58,59], the present study has not further examined this issue. Future studies examining the gender difference in the association between walk score and health behaviors/outcomes are warranted. Furthermore, in this study, the walk score was obtained using participants' residential neighborhood, not address, because residential address is a private and sensitive question for Taiwanese older adults. In our pilot survey, a large number of older adults refused to provide their complete address. However, Walk Score® has been shown to provide a visualized and valid measurement of walkability in neighborhoods [56]. In this study, the neighborhood analyzed was a relatively small area in Taiwan (mean population is nearly 3,000) [60]. Future studies using participants' residential address to confirm our results are needed. Finally, we were unable to obtain a representative sample because a telephone survey was conducted. It is impossible to reach older adults without a household telephone in Taiwan (estimated to be around 7.3% of households) [61]. Thus, our findings may be less germane and relevant to the general population.

In conclusion, Walk Score®, an indicator of neighborhood walkability, was not related to the recommended levels of physical activity in this study, but positively associated with prolonged sedentary time in Taiwan, a non-Western country. Thus, the different relationships between Walk Score® and lifestyle behaviors and health outcomes in different contexts should be noted.

**Author Contributions:** Conceptualization: Y.L. and J.-H.P.; Methodology: C.-Y.L., T.-F.L., Y.-J.C., B.K., and Y.L.; Software, C.-Y.L. and T.-F.L.; Formal Analysis: C.-Y.L. and T.-F.L.; Writing—Original Draft Preparation: Y.L., C.-Y.L., T.-F.L., and J.-H.P.; Writing—Review & Editing: Y.L., B.K., and Y.-J.C.; Supervision: Y.L. and J.-H.P.; Project Administration: Y.-J.C. and B.K.; Funding Acquisition: Y.L. and J.-H.P.

**Acknowledgments:** Liao received a personal grant from the Ministry of Science and Technology of Taiwan (MOST 107-2410-H-003-117-MY2). The Ministry of Science and Technology of Taiwan was not involved in the study design, data collection, analysis, interpretation, and writing of the manuscript. This work was supported by a Global Research Network program through the Ministry of Education of the Republic of Korea and National Research Foundation of Korea (NRF-Project number: NRF-2017S1A2A2038558).

**Conflicts of Interest:** The authors declare that they have no conflicts of interest. None of the authors have any financial interest in walkscore.com.

## References

1. Berke, E.M.; Vernez-Moudon, A. Built environment change: A framework to support health-enhancing behaviour through environmental policy and health research. *J. Epidemiol. Community Health* **2014**, *68*, 586–590. [CrossRef] [PubMed]

2. Sallis, J.F.; Owen, N.; Fisher, E. Ecological models of health behavior. *Health Behav. Theory Res. Pract.* **2015**, *5*, 43–64.

3. Glanz, K.; Rimer, B.K.; Viswanath, K. *Health Behavior and Health Education: Theory, Research, and Practice*, 4th ed.; Jossey-Bass: San Francisco, CA, USA, 2008.

4. Chokshi, D.A.; Farley, T.A. Changing behaviors to prevent noncommunicable diseases. *Science* **2014**, *345*, 1243–1244. [CrossRef] [PubMed]

5. World Health Organization Active Ageing: A Policy Framework. Available online: http://apps.who.int/iris/bitstream/10665/67215/1/WHO_NMH_NPH_02.8.pdf (accessed on 20 February 2019).

6. Carr, L.J.; Dunsiger, S.I.; Marcus, B.H. Validation of Walk Score for estimating access to walkable amenities. *Br. J. Sports Med.* **2011**, *45*, 1144–1148. [CrossRef] [PubMed]

7. Villanueva, K.; Knuiman, M.; Nathan, A.; Giles-Corti, B.; Christian, H.; Foster, S.; Bull, F. The impact of neighborhood walkability on walking: Does it differ across adult life stage and does neighborhood buffer size matter? *Health Place* **2014**, *25*, 43–46. [CrossRef]

8. Van Dyck, D.; Cerin, E.; Conway, T.L.; De Bourdeaudhuij, I.; Owen, N.; Kerr, J.; Cardon, G.; Frank, L.D.; Saelens, B.E.; Sallis, J.F. Associations between perceived neighborhood environmental attributes and adults' sedentary behavior: Findings from the U.S.A., Australia and Belgium. *Soc. Sci. Med.* **2012**, *74*, 1375–1384. [CrossRef]

9. Mushtaq, M.U.; Gull, S.; Mushtaq, K.; Shahid, U.; Shad, M.A.; Akram, J. Dietary behaviors, physical activity and sedentary lifestyle associated with overweight and obesity, and their socio-demographic correlates, among Pakistani primary school children. *Int. J. Behav. Nutr. Phys. Act.* **2011**, *8*, 130. [CrossRef]

10. Liao, Y.; Shibata, A.; Ishii, K.; Oka, K. Independent and Combined Associations of Physical Activity and Sedentary Behavior with Depressive Symptoms Among Japanese Adults. *Int. J. Behav. Med.* **2016**, *23*, 402–409. [CrossRef]

11. Strawbridge, W.J.; Deleger, S.; Roberts, R.E.; Kaplan, G.A. Physical activity reduces the risk of subsequent depression for older adults. *Am. J. Epidemiol.* **2002**, *156*, 328–334. [CrossRef]

12. Richardson, C.R.; Kriska, A.M.; Lantz, P.M.; Hayward, R.A. Physical activity and mortality across cardiovascular disease risk groups. *Med. Sci. Sports Exerc.* **2004**, *36*, 1923–1929. [CrossRef]

13. O'Donovan, G.; Lee, I.; Hamer, M.; Stamatakis, E. Association of "weekend warrior" and other leisure time physical activity patterns with risks for all-cause, cardiovascular disease, and cancer mortality. *JAMA Internal Med.* **2017**, *177*, 335–342. [CrossRef] [PubMed]

14. Carr, L.J.; Dunsiger, S.I.; Marcus, B.H. Walk score as a global estimate of neighborhood walkability. *Am. J. Prev. Med.* **2010**, *39*, 460–463. [CrossRef] [PubMed]
15. Chudyk, A.M.; McKay, H.A.; Winters, M.; Sims-Gould, J.; Ashe, M.C. Neighborhood walkability, physical activity, and walking for transportation: A cross-sectional study of older adults living on low income. *BMC Geriatr.* **2017**, *17*, 82. [CrossRef] [PubMed]
16. Cole, R.; Dunn, P.; Hunter, I.; Owen, N.; Sugiyama, T. Walk Score and Australian adults' home-based walking for transport. *Health Place* **2015**, *35*, 60–65. [CrossRef] [PubMed]
17. Winters, M.; Barnes, R.; Venners, S.; Ste-Marie, N.; McKay, H.; Sims-Gould, J.; Ashe, M.C. Older adults' outdoor walking and the built environment: Does income matter? *BMC Public Health* **2015**, *15*, 876. [CrossRef] [PubMed] .
18. Koohsari, M.J.; Sugiyama, T.; Shibata, A.; Ishii, K.; Hanibuchi, T.; Liao, Y.; Owen, N.; Oka, K. Walk Score® and Japanese adults' physically-active and sedentary behaviors. *Cities* **2018**, *74*, 151–155. [CrossRef]
19. Chiu, M.; Shah, B.R.; Maclagan, L.C.; Rezai, M.R.; Austin, P.C.; Tu, J.V. Walk Score® and the prevalence of utilitarian walking and obesity among Ontario adults: A cross-sectional study. *Health Rep.* **2015**, *26*, 3–10.
20. Chiu, M.; Rezai, M.R.; Maclagan, L.C.; Austin, P.C.; Shah, B.R.; Redelmeier, D.A.; Tu, J.V. Moving to a Highly Walkable Neighborhood and Incidence of Hypertension: A Propensity-Score Matched Cohort Study. *Environ. Health Perspect.* **2016**, *124*, 754–760. [CrossRef]
21. Meline, J.; Chaix, B.; Pannier, B.; Ogedegbe, G.; Trasande, L.; Athens, J.; Duncan, D.T. Neighborhood walk score and selected Cardiometabolic factors in the French RECORD cohort study. *BMC Public Health* **2017**, *17*, 960. [CrossRef]
22. Herrick, C.J.; Yount, B.W.; Eyler, A.A. Implications of supermarket access, neighbourhood walkability and poverty rates for diabetes risk in an employee population. *Public Health Nutr.* **2016**, *19*, 2040–2048. [CrossRef]
23. Koohsari, M.J.; Kaczynski, A.T.; Hanibuchi, T.; Shibata, A.; Ishii, K.; Yasunaga, A.; Nakaya, T.; Oka, K. Physical Activity Environment and Japanese Adults' Body Mass Index. *Int. J. Environ. Res. Public Health* **2018**, *15*, 596. [CrossRef]
24. Sugiyama, T.; Inoue, S.; Cerin, E.; Shimomitsu, T.; Owen, N. Walkable area within which destinations matter: Differences between Australian and Japanese cities. *Asia Pac. J. Public Health* **2015**, *27*, NP2757–NP2763. [CrossRef]
25. Leather, J.; Fabian, H.; Gota, S.; Mejia, A. *Walkability and Pedestrian Facilities in Asian Cities State and Issues*; Asian Development Bank (ADB): Mandaluyong City, Phillippines, 2011.
26. Perdue, W.C.; Stone, L.A.; Gostin, L.O. The built environment and its relationship to the public's health: The legal framework. *Am. J. Public Health* **2003**, *93*, 1390–1394. [CrossRef]
27. Hsueh, M.C.; Liao, Y.; Chang, S.H. Associations of Total and Domain-Specific Sedentary Time with Type 2 Diabetes in Taiwanese Older Adults. *J. Epidemiol.* **2016**, *26*, 348–354. [CrossRef]
28. Liao, Y.; Wang, I.T.; Hsu, H.H.; Chang, S.H. Perceived environmental and personal factors associated with walking and cycling for transportation in Taiwanese adults. *Int. J. Environ. Res. Public Health* **2015**, *12*, 2105–2119. [CrossRef] [PubMed]
29. Liou, Y.M.; Jwo, C.J.; Yao, K.G.; Chiang, L.C.; Huang, L.H. Selection of appropriate Chinese terms to represent intensity and types of physical activity terms for use in the Taiwan version of IPAQ. *J. Nurs. Res.* **2008**, *16*, 252–263. [CrossRef] [PubMed]
30. Nelson, M.E.; Rejeski, W.J.; Blair, S.N.; Duncan, P.W.; Judge, J.O.; King, A.C.; Macera, C.A.; Castaneda-Sceppa, C. Physical activity and public health in older adults: Recommendation from the American College of Sports Medicine and the American Heart Association. *Med. Sci. Sports Exerc.* **2007**, *39*, 1435–1445. [CrossRef]
31. van der Ploeg, H.P.; Chey, T.; Korda, R.J.; Banks, E.; Bauman, A. Sitting time and all-cause mortality risk in 222,497 Australian adults. *Arch. Intern. Med.* **2012**, *172*, 494–500. [CrossRef]
32. Ding, D.; Sugiyama, T.; Winkler, E.; Cerin, E.; Wijndaele, K.; Owen, N. Correlates of change in adults' television viewing time: A four-year follow-up study. *Med. Sci. Sports Exerc.* **2012**, *44*, 1287–1292. [CrossRef] [PubMed]
33. Bowman, S.A. Television-viewing characteristics of adults: Correlations to eating practices and overweight and health status. *Prev. Chronic Dis.* **2006**, *3*, A38. [PubMed]
34. Dunstan, D.W.; Salmon, J.; Owen, N.; Armstrong, T.; Zimmet, P.Z.; Welborn, T.A.; Cameron, A.J.; Dwyer, T.; Jolley, D.; Shaw, J.E.; et al. Associations of TV viewing and physical activity with the metabolic syndrome in Australian adults. *Diabetologia* **2005**, *48*, 2254–2261. [CrossRef] [PubMed]

35. Sugiyama, T.; Wijndaele, K.; Koohsari, M.J.; Tanamas, S.K.; Dunstan, D.W.; Owen, N. Adverse associations of car time with markers of cardio-metabolic risk. *Prev. Med.* **2016**, *83*, 26–30. [CrossRef] [PubMed]

36. Lin, C.Y.; Liao, Y.; Park, J.H. Association of Motorcycle Use with Risk of Overweight in Taiwanese Urban Adults. *Int. J. Environ. Res. Public Health* **2017**, *14*, 410. [CrossRef] [PubMed]

37. Health Promotion Administration, Ministry of Health and Welfare Daily Dietary Guideline Manual. Available online: https://www.hpa.gov.tw/Pages/EBook.aspx?nodeid=1208 (accessed on 20 February 2019).

38. Health Promotion Administration, Ministry of Health and Welfare Body Mass Index Test. Available online: http://health99.hpa.gov.tw/OnlinkHealth/Onlink_BMI.aspx (accessed on 20 February 2019).

39. Health Promotion Administration, Ministry of Health and Welfare the Behavioral Risk Factor Surveillance System (BRFSS). Available online: https://www.hpa.gov.tw/EngPages/Index.aspx (accessed on 20 February 2019).

40. Koohsari, M.J.; Sugiyama, T.; Hanibuchi, T.; Shibata, A.; Ishii, K.; Liao, Y.; Oka, K. Validity of Walk Score(R) as a measure of neighborhood walkability in Japan. *Prev. Med. Rep.* **2018**, *9*, 114–117. [CrossRef] [PubMed]

41. Nykiforuk, C.I.; McGetrick, J.A.; Crick, K.; Johnson, J.A. Check the score: Field validation of Street Smart Walk Score in Alberta, Canada. *Prev. Med. Rep.* **2016**, *4*, 532–539. [CrossRef] [PubMed]

42. Walk Score® Walk Score Methodology. Available online: http://www.walkscore.com/methodology.shtml (accessed on 20 February 2019).

43. Chudyk, A.M.; Winters, M.; Moniruzzaman, M.; Ashe, M.C.; Gould, J.S.; McKay, H. Destinations matter: The association between where older adults live and their travel behavior. *J. Transp. Health* **2015**, *2*, 50–57. [CrossRef] [PubMed]

44. Thielman, J.; Manson, H.; Chiu, M.; Copes, R.; Rosella, L.C. Residents of highly walkable neighbourhoods in Canadian urban areas do substantially more physical activity: A cross-sectional analysis. *CMAJ Open* **2016**, *4*, E720–E728. [CrossRef] [PubMed]

45. Hirsch, J.A.; Moore, K.A.; Evenson, K.R.; Rodriguez, D.A.; Diez Roux, A.V. Walk Score(R) and Transit Score(R) and walking in the multi-ethnic study of atherosclerosis. *Am. J. Prev. Med.* **2013**, *45*, 158–166. [CrossRef]

46. Riley, D.L.; Mark, A.E.; Kristjansson, E.; Sawada, M.C.; Reid, R.D. Neighbourhood walkability and physical activity among family members of people with heart disease who participated in a randomized controlled trial of a behavioural risk reduction intervention. *Health Place* **2013**, *21*, 148–155. [CrossRef]

47. Takahashi, P.Y.; Baker, M.A.; Cha, S.; Targonski, P.V. A cross-sectional survey of the relationship between walking, biking, and the built environment for adults aged over 70 years. *Risk Manag. Healthc. Policy* **2012**, *5*, 35–41. [CrossRef]

48. Van Dyck, D.; Cardon, G.; Deforche, B.; Owen, N.; Sallis, J.F.; De Bourdeaudhuij, I. Neighborhood walkability and sedentary time in Belgian adults. *Am. J. Prev. Med.* **2010**, *39*, 25–32. [CrossRef] [PubMed]

49. Liao, Y.; Shibata, A.; Ishii, K.; Koohsari, M.J.; Oka, K. Cross-sectional and prospective associations of neighbourhood environmental attributes with screen time in Japanese middle-aged and older adults. *BMJ Open* **2018**, *8*, e019608. [CrossRef] [PubMed]

50. Ministry of Transportation and Communication (Ed.) *2013 Daily Transportation Report*; Ministry of Transportation and Communication: Taipei, Taiwan, 2014.

51. Sriram, U.; LaCroix, A.Z.; Barrington, W.E.; Corbie-Smith, G.; Garcia, L.; Going, S.B.; LaMonte, M.J.; Manson, J.E.; Sealy-Jefferson, S.; Stefanick, M.L.; et al. Neighborhood Walkability and Adiposity in the Women's Health Initiative Cohort. *Am. J. Prev. Med.* **2016**, *51*, 722–730. [CrossRef] [PubMed]

52. Xu, Y.; Wen, M.; Wang, F. Multilevel built environment features and individual odds of overweight and obesity in Utah. *Appl. Geogr.* **2015**, *60*, 197–203. [CrossRef] [PubMed]

53. Byrne, D.W.; Rolando, L.A.; Aliyu, M.H.; McGown, P.W.; Connor, L.R.; Awalt, B.M.; Holmes, M.C.; Wang, L.; Yarbrough, M.I. Modifiable Healthy Lifestyle Behaviors: 10-Year Health Outcomes from a Health Promotion Program. *Am. J. Prev. Med.* **2016**, *51*, 1027–1037. [CrossRef]

54. Meyers, D.G.; Neuberger, J.S.; He, J. Cardiovascular effect of bans on smoking in public places: A systematic review and meta-analysis. *J. Am. Coll. Cardiol.* **2009**, *54*, 1249–1255. [CrossRef]

55. Thorp, A.A.; Owen, N.; Neuhaus, M.; Dunstan, D.W. Sedentary behaviors and subsequent health outcomes in adults a systematic review of longitudinal studies, 1996–2011. *Am. J. Prev. Med.* **2011**, *41*, 207–215. [CrossRef]

56. Bereitschaft, B. Walk Score® versus residents' perceptions of walkability in Omaha, N.E. *J. Urban.* **2018**, *11*, 412–435.

57. Harvey, C.; Aultman-Hall, L. Measuring Urban Streetscapes for Livability: A Review of Approaches. *Prof. Geogr.* **2015**, *68*, 149–158. [CrossRef]

58. Kelley, E.A.; Kandula, N.R.; Kanaya, A.M.; Yen, I.H. Neighborhood Walkability and Walking for Transport Among South Asians in the MASALA Study. *J. Phys. Act. Health* **2016**, *13*, 514–519. [CrossRef]

59. Wasfi, R.A.; Dasgupta, K.; Eluru, N.; Ross, N.A. Exposure to walkable neighbourhoods in urban areas increases utilitarian walking: Longitudinal study of Canadians. *J. Transp. Health* **2016**, *3*, 440–447. [CrossRef]

60. Ministry of the Interior Number of Villages, Neighborhoods, Households and Resident Population. Available online: https://www.moi.gov.tw/files/site_stuff/321/1/month/month_en.html (accessed on 20 February 2019).

61. Directorate General of Budget, Accounting and Statistics Report on the Survey of Family Income and Expendture. Available online: http://win.dgbas.gov.tw/fies/e11.asp?year=105 (accessed on 20 February 2019).

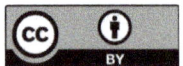

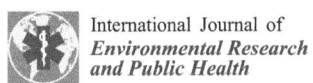

International Journal of
*Environmental Research and Public Health*

*Article*

# Area-Level Walkability and the Geographic Distribution of High Body Mass in Sydney, Australia: A Spatial Analysis Using the 45 and Up Study

**Darren J. Mayne** [1,2,3,4,*], **Geoffrey G. Morgan** [1,5], **Bin B. Jalaludin** [6,7] and **Adrian E. Bauman** [1]

[1]   The University of Sydney, School of Public Health, Sydney, NSW 2006, Australia;
     geoffrey.morgan@sydney.edu.au (G.G.M.); adrian.bauman@sydney.edu.au (A.E.B.)
[2]   Illawarra Shoalhaven Local Health District, Public Health Unit, Warrawong, NSW 2502, Australia
[3]   University of Wollongong, School of Medicine, Wollongong, NSW 2522, Australia
[4]   Illawarra Health and Medical Research Institute, University of Wollongong,
     Wollongong, NSW 2522, Australia
[5]   The University of Sydney, University Centre for Rural Health, Rural Clinical School—Northern Rivers,
     Sydney, NSW 2006, Australia
[6]   Ingham Institute, University of New South Wales, Sydney, NSW 2052, Australia; b.jalaludin@unsw.edu.au
[7]   Epidemiology, Healthy People and Places Unit, Population Health,
     South Western Sydney Local Health District, Liverpool, NSW 1871, Australia
*   Correspondence: dmay8519@uni.sydney.edu.au; Tel.: +61-2-4221-6733

Received: 16 December 2018; Accepted: 19 February 2019; Published: 24 February 2019

**Abstract:** Improving the walkability of built environments to promote healthy lifestyles and reduce high body mass is increasingly considered in regional development plans. Walkability indexes have the potential to inform, benchmark and monitor these plans if they are associated with variation in body mass outcomes at spatial scales used for health and urban planning. We assessed relationships between area-level walkability and prevalence and geographic variation in overweight and obesity using an Australian population-based cohort comprising 92,157 Sydney respondents to the 45 and Up Study baseline survey between January 2006 and April 2009. Individual-level data on overweight and obesity were aggregated to 2006 Australian postal areas and analysed as a function of area-level Sydney Walkability Index quartiles using conditional auto regression spatial models adjusted for demographic, social, economic, health and socioeconomic factors. Both overweight and obesity were highly clustered with higher-than-expected prevalence concentrated in the urban sprawl region of western Sydney, and lower-than-expected prevalence in central and eastern Sydney. In fully adjusted spatial models, prevalence of overweight and obesity was 6% and 11% lower in medium-high versus low, and 10% and 15% lower in high versus low walkability postcodes, respectively. Postal area walkability explained approximately 20% and 9% of the excess spatial variation in overweight and obesity that remained after accounting for other individual- and area-level factors. These findings provide support for the potential of area-level walkability indexes to inform, benchmark and monitor regional plans aimed at targeted approaches to reducing population-levels of high body mass through environmental interventions. Future research should consider potential confounding due to neighbourhood self-selection on area-level walkability relations.

**Keywords:** body mass; disease mapping; geographic variation; obese; overweight; spatial analysis; walkability

## 1. Introduction

The increasing prevalence of overweight and obesity is a universal and urgent public health problem [1]. High body mass index $\geq 25$ kg/m$^2$ (overweight or obese) contributed 5.7% of total disability adjusted life years (DALY) to the global burden of disease in 2016, making it the fifth leading risk factor—up from 2.7% of total DALYs and a ranking of 12 in 1990 [2]. High body mass is a risk factor for cardiovascular disease, cancer, type 2 diabetes mellitus, and musculoskeletal conditions [3,4], while its economic costs to health care systems and communities grow with increasing levels of overweight and obesity [5]. The physiological energy imbalance that underlies high body mass is influenced by genetic, behavioural, social, economic, and environmental factors operating within multiple complex systems [6–8]. Reducing the health and economic burdens of overweight and obesity will require shifts in these population-level systems [7]. For example, environmental interventions that typically produce small individual-level effects may aggregate into large population-level benefits because exposure is ubiquitous [8,9] and relatively persistent [10,11].

The built environment refers to that "part of the physical environment...Constructed by human activity" ( [12] p. S550), and is hypothesised to contribute to high body mass by influencing lifestyle behaviours that underlie its development [8]. The emerging consensus from the extensive literature is that the built environment evidence base is sufficiently developed to incorporate into planning, policy and interventions aimed at reducing high body mass [7,13], although uncertainties remain (see reviews by [14–18]). "Walkability" describes the capacity of the built environment to promote walking for multiple purposes [19], and may contribute to reducing overweight and obesity by promoting participation in total daily moderate-intensity physical activity [8,9,17,20–22]. To this end, it is increasingly considered in development plans aimed at enhancing physical and social infrastructure to promote healthy lifestyles and reduce the burden of chronic conditions like high body mass on populations (e.g., [23–26]).

Walkability indexes have been identified as potentially useful tools for planning, benchmarking and monitoring environmental policies and interventions to improve walkability, and translating the outcomes of walkability research from rhetoric to action [27,28]. While numerous indexes exist (e.g., [29–37]), the Neighborhood Quality of Life Study (NQLS) [38] and Physical Activity in Localities and Community Environments (PLACE) Study [19] indexes remain the most influential [39]; underpin a majority of research linking walkability to health behaviours and outcomes, including high body mass [17]; and are applicable in planning, policy and practice settings [28], which is facilitated by their capacity to be constructed at multiple spatial resolutions [38,40]. These indexes operationalise walkability using residential density, street connectivity, land use mix and, if available, retail floor area ratio, destinations or density within a geographic information system [19,38,40]. Index variables serve as proxy measures for built environment attributes associated with walking. Land use mix measures the diversity and concentration of land uses in an area, while intersection density measures the directness of paths [38]. Compact areas with diverse land uses that are highly connected promote walking by reducing the distance between origins and destinations [9,19,40]. Similarly, high population densities provide critical masses that concentrate diverse destinations within compact areas [12,38,40], and is measured by residential density. The ratio of retail floor area to retail land use is a measure of pedestrian access, with larger values indicating greater area given to pedestrian uses and less area to car parking [41].

The extent to which walkability indexes are associated with health outcomes at population scales is a key consideration in their utility to benchmark and guide planning and policy aimed at reducing population-levels of overweight and obesity [27,42]. This is because health and urban planning that influences environmental walkability occurs at local, urban and regional scales [43,44]; that is, for communities and populations. These meso (neighbourhoods/communities) and macro (cities) geographic scales are much coarser than typically used in studies to derive built environment exposure-response evidence [42,45], which mostly focus on individual (micro) level risk (see reviews by [14–17,22,46]). Measured at the micro-scale, walkability is typically derived within a radial or street-based network buffer of 200–1600 metres around a residential address; reflects the immediate built environment to which an individual is exposed [47,48]; and is preferred for individual-level research.

In contrast, when measured at meso- and macro-scales, walkability (or sprawl) is usually calculated within an administrative boundary; represents a contextual variable describing the shared built environment to which groups, communities and populations are exposed; and is especially useful for area-level (ecological) research and planning applications [42]. Using individual-level walkability evidence to inform activity at coarser planning scales has raised concern in the literature for its potential to result in flawed public health action [49]. This is a concern about atomistic [50] or individualistic [51] fallacy, which is the area-level corollary of the ecological fallacy and refers to the erroneous use of data on individuals to make inferences about groups [52].

Analysis at the geographic scale of planning addresses concern about erroneous cross-level inference [42], and has been identified as highly relevant to "local area" walkability planning because it produces evidence at the level where decisions are made [43]. Rydin and colleagues have also identified the need for "urban scale" data to inform planning and policy interventions that maintain the urban advantage in health outcomes [44]. However, studies that match walkability exposures and body mass outcomes at these planning scales are uncommon [16,17,46], despite calls from planners and policy makers for evidence at this level [45,53–55]. What evidence is available at these planning scales comes largely from ecological analyses in the United States, which have consistently found higher body mass and prevalence of obesity in sprawling versus compact counties (e.g., [30,53,56–58]). Compactness at this scale is generally considered synonymous with more walkable environments. However, sprawl indexes have been criticized for conflating multiple built environment concepts, and not providing a coherent, unitary measure of walkability [38,40].

Geographic variation in overweight and obesity has been reported within many countries [59], and needs to be considered in health programming and planning. In addition to identifying areas at increased risk of adverse health outcomes [59,60], geographic variation in excess of that due to known factors can indicate place-based influences on health that are distinct to the contextual effects arising from differences in the demographic, social and economic composition of populations between areas [61,62]. Spatial analysis is particularly useful in identifying these place-based effects because it quantifies the contribution of both observed and unobserved factors to geographic variation in outcomes while accounting for spatial autocorrelation that can lead to biased statistical inference [62]. In this context, geographic variation encompasses more than just differences between areas, which is well addressed in the body mass literature (e.g., [63–72]). It is also the spatial expression or distribution of this variation [73]. Spatial analysis is concerned with location [74]. It leverages the underlying process giving rise to the geographic variation rather than reducing it to a naïve dummy-coded comparison of areas in the case of fixed-effects analysis, or focusing on reductions in intraclass correlation coefficients that conflate spatial and non-spatial sources of variation through a common random effect term as in multilevel analysis [42].

Spatial analysis has the potential to provide unique information on relations between walkability and high body mass. For example, we have previously reported that physical activity is geographically structured in Sydney, and that area-level walkability accounts for some of this spatial patterning [42]. The "disease mapping" approach [75] used in this study also produces smoothed maps that can be used to communicate spatially varying risks to planners, policy-makers and other interested stakeholders [42]. Identifying spatial disparities in contextual factors that contribute to adverse health outcomes at appropriate intervention scales has been identified as essential for informing place-based interventions aimed at improving population health [76]. Spatial analysis is uniquely placed to assist in addressing these disparities and environmental inequalities through its capacity to identify and target geographic areas where environment-related health risks are disproportionately higher and potentially amenable to intervention [42,77]. However, despite an increasing use of geographic information systems in the high body mass literature, the application of spatial analysis at any scale is rare [78]. For example, only a few area-level studies have used an explicitly spatial approach to address geographic variation in overweight and obesity [56,59,62,72,79–89]; an even smaller number have considered built environment influences on this geographic variation [62,81,82,89]; and only one appears to have evaluated the contribution of walkability to this geographic variation directly [81].

The objective of this study was to build on our previous work in the Sydney statistical district [39,42] and assess relations between area-level walkability and population-levels of overweight and obesity using an explicitly spatial approach, and at a geographic scale representative of those used for "local area" [43] and "urban scale" [44] planning. The specific aims of the study were to (i) assess area-level associations between walkability and prevalence of overweight and obesity in Sydney; (ii) assess geographic variation in area-level prevalence of overweight and obesity in Sydney; and (iii) assess the extent to which area-level walkability accounts for geographic variation in overweight and obesity in Sydney beyond that due to individual-level demographic, social, economic and health factors, and area-level socioeconomic disadvantage.

## 2. Materials and Methods

### 2.1. Study Design and Area

We investigated associations between area-level walkability and prevalence of overweight and obesity in the Sydney statistical division of New South Wales, Australia [90], using a cross-sectional ecological study design, which is appropriate and valid for area-level inference [52]. Sydney has a land area of 12,142 km$^2$, and was Australia's most populous city at the 2006 Australian Census with an estimated resident population of 4.1 million people living in 1.6 million dwellings [91]. We used Census postal areas as our units of analysis to coincide with the smallest spatial unit at which individual-level data were geographically identified by the data custodian. In 2006 there were 260 conterminous postal areas across the Sydney statistical division [92] with median and inter quartile range (IQR) values for land area of 7.6 (IQR = 3.7–19.4) km$^2$, 5304 (IQR = 2694–8426) residential dwellings, and 13,090 (IQR = 6529–22,092) residents [91]. The median land area of postal areas corresponds to a radial buffer of 1550 m, which is within the range of buffer sizes for which consistent environment-behaviour associations have been reported in individual-level studies of walkability [47,48], and is likely a reasonable analogue of the "local areas" and "urban scales" at which health and urban planning decisions occur [43,44].

### 2.2. Participants

Individual-level data used in this study were obtained from participants of The Sax Institute 45 and Up Study [93] approved and monitored by the University of New South Wales Human Research Ethics Committee (ref no. HREC 05035/HREC 10186). This population-based cohort study was established to investigate healthy ageing in the New South Wales population aged 45 years and over [93]. Study recruitment occurred between January 2006 and December 2009 [94] for a final cohort size of 267,153 participants or approximately 10% of the total New South Wales target population [95]. Eligible persons were randomly sampled from the the Department of Human Services (formerly Medicare Australia) enrolment database. Selected individuals were mailed an invitation letter, and asked to return a signed, written consent form with their baseline survey via reply-paid mail if they consented to participating in the study [93]. We were provided access to the April 2009 data release, which the data custodian had geocoded to 2006 Census statistical divisions and postal areas. We limited our analysis to 115,153 respondents living in the Sydney statistical division to coincide with the spatial extent of our exposure variable. Our research comprised a sub-study of the Social, Environmental, and Economic Factors Study approved and monitored by the University of Sydney Human Research Ethics Committee (ref No. 10-2009/12187). Details on accessing 45 and Up Study data are available on The Sax Institute website (www.saxinstitute.org.au/our-work/45-up-study).

## 2.3. Data

Individual-level data included self-reported responses to the baseline survey of 45 and Up Study collected between January 2006 and April 2009 [93], which we used to calculate and adjust area-level outcome variables. Postal area contextual variables comprised the Sydney Walkability Index (SWI) [40] and 2006 Index of Relative Socioeconomic Disadvantage [96], which we included as study and covariate factors, respectively.

## 2.4. Outcome Variable

The primary outcome measures used in our study were self-reported overweight and obesity, which we defined using the standard body mass index (BMI) formula of weight in kilograms (kg) over height in metres (m) squared (kg/m²) and World Health Organisation (WHO) cut-points of 25.0–<30.0 kg/m² for overweight and ≥30.0 kg/m² for obesity [97]. Self-reported BMI has been validated against measured BMI as a generally appropriate method for quantifying body size in the 45 and Up Study cohort, although it is known to underestimate prevalence of obesity when classified using standard BMI categories [98]. Overweight and obesity status were represented as dichotomous (yes/no) variables for individual-level analyses, and as counts of overweight and obese respondents within postcodes in area-level analyses.

## 2.5. Exposure Variable

The exposure variable used for all analyses was postal area walkability, which we measured using the Sydney Walkability Index [40]. This three-factor index is derived using methods and data comparable to the PLACE and NQLS walkability index [19,38]. The Sydney Walkability Index is calculated within a geographical information system using three built environment variables: residential dwelling density (the number of residential dwellings per square kilometre of residential land use); intersection density (the number of intersections with three or more roads per square kilometre of total land area); and land use mix (the entropy of residential, commercial, industrial, recreational and other land uses). The Sydney Walkability Index was derived at the 2006 postal area level using 2007 spatial data to temporally align it with the midpoint of the of the 45 and Up Study baseline data collection.

Environmental variable values are divided into deciles, scored from 1 (lowest) to 10 (highest), summed to give a total score between 3–30, and then divided into quartiles corresponding to low, low-medium, medium-high and high walkability [40]. Environmental values increase monotonically within strata and have median values of 2.3, 13.4, 19.8 and 46 dwellings per hectare for residential density; 3.4, 46.1, 79.5 and 162.5 intersections per square kilometre for street network connectivity; and entropies of 0.005, 0.033, 0.056, and 0.134 for land use mix (see [42]). The Sydney Walkability Index has predictive validity for utilitarian walking, is comparable to four-variable indexes in the research literature, and is associated with population-levels of moderate and vigorous physical activity [40,42].

Walkability was entered as an index in our analysis for consistency with the interest expressed in the literature on using "walkability indexes" to benchmark, inform and monitor regional development plans [27,28], and because the non-parametric functions used in other studies [99–101] to model index components separately would have made our already computationally-intensive spatial analyses intractable.

## 2.6. Covariates

Individual- and area-level factors from the 45 and Up Study and substantive literature likely to contribute to, or confound, associations between walkability and body mass were included as covariates in our analysis (see [102–113]). Individual-level covariates included self-reported sex; five-year age group at baseline interview; language spoken at home; educational level; relationship status; employment status; health insurance type; level of psychosocial distress measured using the

Kessler Psychological Distress Scale [114] (minor, moderate, high, very high [115–117]); smoking status; number of chronic conditions ever diagnosed and treated in the previous four weeks; and functional capacity, which was measured using the Medical Outcomes Study (MOS) 36-Item Short-Form Health Survey (SF-36) physical functioning scale [118,119] and classified as none (0 to <60), minor (60 to <90), moderate (90 to <100), and severe (100) [120]. Postal area socioeconomic disadvantage was measured using the Index of Relative Socio-economic Disadvantage from the 2006 Australian Census [96]. We did not include physical activity in our analysis because it likely mediates relations between the built environment and high body mass [8,14–17].

### 2.7. Statistical Analysis

The objective of our analysis was to assess relations between walkability and the prevalence and geographic distribution of overweight and obesity in the Sydney statistical district at a scale analogous to those at which health and urban planning decisions are made. This objective is appropriately addressed by an ecological (spatial) analysis because the targets of inference are areas, not individuals [52]. We have previously identified high levels of spatial autocorrelation in 45 and Up Study data that have both research and planning utility, and the potential to bias inference if not addressed in the analysis [42]. Multilevel models can account for spatial autocorrelation but typically conflate spatial and non-spatial variation through a common variance component [42]. We therefore explicitly modelled the underlying spatial and non-spatial sources of variation in our data using a relative risk implementation of the ecological Besag, York and Mollié (BYM) conditional auto regressive model.

The BYM is a fully Bayesian ecological spatial model fit to aggregate data, which is commonly used in epidemiology for "disease mapping" applications [75]. The goal of disease mapping is to recover a map displaying variation in the geographic distribution of risks for spatial units within a study area that is "smoothed" of extreme and unreliable estimates that can arise from differences between units in the sizes of their underlying populations [75]. This is achieved in the BYM model by decomposing map variation into an unstructured variance component that smooths risk estimates towards the global mean of the study area, and a spatially structured (geographic) variance component that smooths risk estimates towards the local mean of contiguous spatial units [75,121]. These components also indicate the extent to which map variation is due to structured (spatial) and unstructured (non-spatial) factors.

The BYM model can be extended to ecological regression problems by incorporating area-level covariates into its specification [75], but it cannot parsimoniously control for individual-level factors that may confound area-level effect estimates. We therefore used a two stage modelling strategy adopted by other researchers in the epidemiological literature whereby individual-level regression models are used to estimate expected cases for each outcome, which are then used as offset terms in area-level spatial analyses to adjust for the varying size and composition of populations between spatial units (see [39,42,122–124]).

In the first step, we estimated the predicted log odds ($l_{ij}$) of overweight and obesity for individuals using conditional fixed-effects logistic regression models:

$$\hat{l}_{ij} = \alpha + x_i \beta \tag{1}$$

where $\hat{l}_{ij}$ is the predicted log odds of being either overweight or obese for the $i^{th}$ person in the $j^{th}$ postal area, $\alpha$ is the model intercept, and $x_i\beta$ is an optional vector of individual-level covariates. We fit two models for each outcome: (1) an unadjusted null model with no covariates; and (2) an adjusted model including all individual-level covariates described previously. The log odds for individuals from each model were converted to a predicted probability using the inverse link function:

$$\hat{Y}_{ij} = \frac{e^{l_{ij}}}{1 + e^{l_{ij}}} \tag{2}$$

We then summed these probabilities within each postal area to obtain the expected number of cases for each outcome based on (1) the prevalence in the study area from unadjusted logistic regression estimates; and (2) the underlying respondent structure of our sample from adjusted logistic regression estimates (see [39,42,122–124]). These expected case counts were used as offsets in the spatial Poisson regressions described in step 2, and are referred to as unadjusted and adjusted offsets, respectively.

In the second step, we used relative risk implementations of the BYM model with Poisson likelihoods to estimate prevalence ratios for postal areas relative to the study area [125]. The BYM model is a fully Bayesian spatial model fit to aggregate data that decomposes total variation into observed and unobserved sources [75,121] using:

$$log(\theta_j) = \alpha + x_j\beta + s_j + u_j + log(e_j) \tag{3}$$

where $\theta_j$ is the prevalence ratio for the $j^{th}$ postal area; $\alpha$ is the prevalence ratio for the study area; $x_j$ and $\beta$ are vectors of observed area-level explanatory variables and associated regression parameters estimates; $s_j$ and $u_j$ are unobserved spatially structured and unstructured random effects; and $e_j$ is an offset term representing the expected number cases in the $j^{th}$ area. The unstructured variance ($u_j$) is a normal independent and identically distributed residual, while the spatial variance ($s_j$) is conditionally normally distributed on the mean prevalence of the surrounding $k$ contiguous postal areas [75]. Model offsets ($e_j$) corresponded to those derived for postal areas in step one, and were either unadjusted or adjusted for individual-level factors.

The total count of overweight and obese respondents ($o_j$) in each postal area served as the dependent variable in each model. We fit six BYM spatial regressions for each outcome: (1) a null model with unadjusted offsets; (2) a null model with adjusted offsets; (3) a covariate model with adjusted offsets and postal area walkability; (4) a covariate model with adjusted offsets and postal area socioeconomic disadvantage; (5) a covariate model with adjusted offsets and postal area walkability and socioeconomic disadvantage, and (6) an effect modification model with adjusted offsets, postal area walkability and socioeconomic disadvantage, and their interaction. A total of 10,000 draws from the posterior distributions of two Monte Carlo Markov Chains sampled every 250th iteration were used to obtain medians and 95% credible intervals for each model. Chain convergence was assessed using autocorrelation plots and the Gelman-Rubin diagnostic [126]. We chose between alternate models using the *Deviance Information Criterion* (DIC) [127], and mapped exponentiated linear predictors and variance estimates using quintiles to visualise geographic variation in risk of high body mass. The spatial fraction ($\rho$) for each model was calculated from the marginal variances of the random effects, and used to index the proportion of residual variation due to unobserved spatial factors (i.e., $\sigma_s^2/[\sigma_s^2 + \sigma_u^2]$) (see [128,129]). Models were fit in WinBUGS 1.4.3 using R 3.3.2 and unweighted survey data, which produce unbiased, representative and generalisable relative effect estimates for individual- and area-level analyses in this cohort [42,130,131].

## 3. Results

Complete data were available for 92,157 of 115,153 (80.0%) Sydney respondents residing in 254 of 260 (97.7%) study postal areas. The median number of respondents per postal area was 212, and ranged from 0 to 2532 with an inter-quartile range of 110–363. Individual-level attributes for respondents included in analyses are shown in the *Characteristics* section of Table 1. Consistent with the larger 45 and Up Study cohort [132], our sample had a similar gender and employment profile to the study area but was otherwise younger, more highly educated, less likely to speak a language other than English at home, and more likely to be living with a partner than the general Sydney population aged 45 years and over [91].

**Table 1.** Sample characteristics and prevalence of overweight and obesity among study participants.

| Variable | Characteristics | | Prevalence | | | |
| | | | Overweight | | Obesity | |
| | N | % | n | % | n | % |
|---|---|---|---|---|---|---|
| **AREA-LEVEL VARIABLES** | | | | | | |
| *Walkability* | | | | | | |
| Low | 25,454 | 27.6 | 10,150 | 52.9 | 6251 | 40.8 |
| Low-medium | 31,404 | 34.1 | 12,380 | 50.0 | 6655 | 35.0 |
| Medium-high | 19,449 | 21.1 | 7543 | 47.2 | 3454 | 29.0 |
| High | 15,850 | 17.2 | 5861 | 44.0 | 2516 | 25.2 |
| *Socioeconomic disadvantage* | | | | | | |
| Q1 - Most | 17,425 | 18.9 | 6697 | 52.1 | 4559 | 42.5 |
| Q2 | 19,517 | 21.2 | 7579 | 51.7 | 4847 | 40.6 |
| Q3 - Middling | 14,984 | 16.3 | 5877 | 49.4 | 3082 | 33.8 |
| Q4 | 19,982 | 21.7 | 7938 | 47.8 | 3392 | 28.2 |
| Q5 - Least | 20,249 | 22.0 | 7843 | 45.5 | 2996 | 24.1 |
| **INDIVIDUAL-LEVEL VARIABLES** | | | | | | |
| *Sex* | | | | | | |
| Male | 44,690 | 48.5 | 20,802 | 58.1 | 8912 | 37.3 |
| Female | 47,467 | 51.5 | 15,132 | 40.3 | 9964 | 30.8 |
| *Age* | | | | | | |
| 45–49 | 13,550 | 14.7 | 4871 | 45.1 | 2761 | 31.8 |
| 50–54 | 16,723 | 18.1 | 6188 | 47.4 | 3665 | 34.8 |
| 55–59 | 16,717 | 18.1 | 6568 | 51.2 | 3885 | 38.3 |
| 60–64 | 13,742 | 14.9 | 5696 | 53.7 | 3136 | 39.0 |
| 65–69 | 10,188 | 11.1 | 4297 | 54.0 | 2227 | 37.8 |
| 70–74 | 6910 | 7.5 | 2969 | 53.3 | 1341 | 34.0 |
| 75–79 | 4999 | 5.4 | 2047 | 49.0 | 820 | 27.8 |
| 80–84 | 6614 | 7.2 | 2513 | 43.2 | 801 | 19.5 |
| 85+ | 2714 | 2.9 | 785 | 31.7 | 240 | 12.4 |
| *Language spoken at home* | | | | | | |
| English | 78,028 | 84.7 | 30,768 | 49.9 | 16,330 | 34.6 |
| Other | 14,129 | 15.3 | 5166 | 44.6 | 2546 | 28.4 |
| *Education level* | | | | | | |
| Less than secondary school | 7434 | 8.1 | 2704 | 50.6 | 2086 | 44.1 |
| Secondary school graduation | 26,741 | 29.0 | 10,171 | 49.2 | 6052 | 36.5 |
| Trade, certificate or diploma | 28,932 | 31.4 | 11,814 | 51.8 | 6143 | 35.9 |
| University degree | 29,050 | 31.5 | 11,245 | 46.0 | 4595 | 25.8 |
| *Relationship status* | | | | | | |
| Partner | 68,759 | 74.6 | 27,826 | 50.7 | 13,863 | 33.9 |
| No partner | 23,398 | 25.4 | 8108 | 44.1 | 5013 | 32.8 |
| *Employment status* | | | | | | |
| Full-time work | 32,716 | 35.5 | 13,622 | 53.5 | 7246 | 37.9 |
| Part-time work | 13,177 | 14.3 | 4418 | 41.0 | 2408 | 27.5 |
| Other work | 1358 | 1.5 | 426 | 39.6 | 281 | 30.2 |
| Not working | 44,906 | 48.7 | 17,468 | 48.6 | 8941 | 32.6 |
| *Health insurance type* | | | | | | |
| Private with extras | 54,218 | 58.8 | 21,751 | 50.1 | 10,830 | 33.4 |
| Private without extras | 12,961 | 14.1 | 5058 | 47.2 | 2255 | 28.5 |
| Government health care card | 11,993 | 13.0 | 4351 | 47.8 | 2881 | 37.7 |
| None | 12,985 | 14.1 | 4774 | 47.4 | 2910 | 35.4 |
| *Smoking status* | | | | | | |
| Never smoked | 54,117 | 58.7 | 20,518 | 46.6 | 10,072 | 30.0 |
| Past smoker | 31,639 | 34.3 | 13,145 | 54.2 | 7397 | 40.0 |
| Current smoker | 6401 | 6.9 | 2271 | 45.5 | 1407 | 34.1 |

Table 1. *Cont.*

| Variable | Characteristics | | Prevalence | | | |
|---|---|---|---|---|---|---|
| | | | Overweight | | Obesity | |
| | N | % | n | % | n | % |
| *Psychosocial distress* | | | | | | |
| Low | 70,218 | 76.2 | 27,960 | 49.1 | 13,318 | 31.5 |
| Moderate | 14,573 | 15.8 | 5433 | 49.0 | 3475 | 38.0 |
| High | 5152 | 5.6 | 1828 | 48.4 | 1375 | 41.4 |
| Very high | 2214 | 2.4 | 713 | 47.3 | 708 | 47.2 |
| *Diagnosed chronic conditions* | | | | | | |
| 0 | 31,297 | 34.0 | 11,955 | 44.1 | 4218 | 21.8 |
| 1 | 36,917 | 40.1 | 14,726 | 50.2 | 7560 | 34.1 |
| 2 | 18,186 | 19.7 | 7145 | 54.4 | 5040 | 45.6 |
| 3 or more | 5757 | 6.2 | 2108 | 57.0 | 2058 | 56.4 |
| *Treated chronic conditions* | | | | | | |
| 0 | 41,580 | 45.1 | 15,904 | 45.5 | 6590 | 25.7 |
| 1 | 30,121 | 32.7 | 12,141 | 51.3 | 6448 | 35.9 |
| 2 | 14,524 | 15.8 | 5721 | 53.5 | 3835 | 43.6 |
| 3 or more | 5932 | 6.4 | 2168 | 55.2 | 2003 | 53.2 |
| *Limited physical functioning* | | | | | | |
| None | 32,392 | 35.1 | 12,656 | 44.4 | 3908 | 19.8 |
| Minor | 25,125 | 27.3 | 10,628 | 52.4 | 4838 | 33.4 |
| Moderate | 20,316 | 22.0 | 7801 | 52.8 | 5555 | 44.4 |
| Severe | 14,324 | 15.5 | 4849 | 49.7 | 4575 | 48.3 |
| SENSITIVITY VARIABLES | | | | | | |
| *Total physical activity* | | | | | | |
| 0 min | 5478 | 5.9 | 1868 | 50.9 | 1807 | 50.1 |
| 1–149 min | 15,365 | 16.7 | 5895 | 52.1 | 4053 | 42.8 |
| 150–299 min | 15,833 | 17.2 | 6241 | 50.5 | 3468 | 36.2 |
| ≥300 min | 55,481 | 60.2 | 21,930 | 47.7 | 9548 | 28.5 |

N—Stratum total, n—Stratum outcome frequency, %—Stratum outcome per cent.

## 3.1. Prevalence Overweight and Obesity

The within-cohort prevalence of overweight and obesity were 49.0% (48.7–49.4%) and 33.6% (33.2–34.0%), respectively. Table 1 reports prevalence by area- and individual-level characteristics. Prevalence of both overweight and obesity were highest in postal areas with low walkability, lowest in postal areas with high walkability, and displayed a exposure-response gradient. Likewise, overweight and obesity reduced with reducing levels of postal area socioeconomic disadvantage. For individual-level factors, overweight and obesity were more prevalent in males, persons speaking English at home or living with a partner, less educated individuals and full-time workers, persons without private health insurance, and past smokers; and increased with age to 65–69 years, psychosocial distress, number of diagnosed and treated chronic health conditions, and reduced functional capacity.

## 3.2. Individual-Level Factors

Table 2 shows adjusted fixed-effects estimates for overweight and obesity used to derive adjusted offsets for postal area spatial models. All effects were significantly associated with body mass outcomes and mostly consistent with the prevalence patterns reported in Table 1. The stand-out exception was a reversal in gradient between obesity and psychosocial distress from positive to negative after adjustment. This was due to confounding by functional capacity, which was both an independent risk factor for obesity (see Table 2) and strongly associated with psychosocial distress ($\chi_9^2 = 4072.4$, $p < 0.0001$). Other notable differences following adjustment were relationship status, which was unrelated to either overweight or obesity; age, which became associated with monotonically decreasing odds of obesity across the lifespan; and smoking status, which became associated with reduced odds of obesity for current compared to non smokers.

**Table 2.** Adjusted odds ratios for individual-level analyses of overweight and obesity.

|  | Overweight | | Obese | |
|---|---|---|---|---|
|  | **OR** | **95% CI** | **OR** | **95% CI** |
| *Sex* | *p* < 0.0001 | | *p* < 0.0001 | |
| Male | 1.00 | | 1.00 | |
| Female | 0.47 | 0.46–0.49 | 0.62 | 0.59–0.64 |
| *Age* | *p* < 0.0001 | | *p* < 0.0001 | |
| 45–49 | 1.00 | | 1.00 | |
| 50–54 | 1.00 | 0.95–1.05 | 0.94 | 0.88–1.00 |
| 55–59 | 1.07 | 1.01–1.13 | 0.90 | 0.84–0.97 |
| 60–64 | 1.08 | 1.02–1.15 | 0.76 | 0.70–0.82 |
| 65–69 | 1.00 | 0.93–1.07 | 0.59 | 0.54–0.65 |
| 70–74 | 0.87 | 0.81–0.94 | 0.39 | 0.35–0.43 |
| 75–79 | 0.66 | 0.60–0.72 | 0.23 | 0.21–0.26 |
| 80–84 | 0.50 | 0.46–0.54 | 0.12 | 0.11–0.14 |
| 85+ | 0.31 | 0.28–0.35 | 0.06 | 0.05–0.07 |
| *Language spoken at home* | *p* < 0.0001 | | *p* < 0.0001 | |
| English | 1.00 | | 1.00 | |
| Other | 0.81 | 0.78–0.84 | 0.72 | 0.68–0.77 |
| *Education level* | *p* < 0.0001 | | *p* < 0.0001 | |
| Less than secondary school | 1.53 | 1.43–1.63 | 2.47 | 2.28–2.67 |
| Secondary school graduation | 1.35 | 1.29–1.40 | 1.77 | 1.67–1.86 |
| Trade, certificate or diploma | 1.27 | 1.22–1.32 | 1.54 | 1.46–1.62 |
| University degree | 1.00 | | 1.00 | |
| *Relationship status* | *p* < 0.0001 | | *p* = 0.1285 | |
| Partner | 1.00 | | 1.00 | |
| No partner | 0.89 | 0.86–0.92 | 0.96 | 0.92–1.01 |
| *Employment status* | *p* < 0.0001 | | *p* < 0.0001 | |
| Full-time work | 1.00 | | 1.00 | |
| Part-time work | 0.75 | 0.71–0.79 | 0.61 | 0.57–0.65 |
| Other work | 0.72 | 0.64–0.82 | 0.61 | 0.52–0.71 |
| Not working | 0.78 | 0.75–0.82 | 0.66 | 0.62–0.70 |
| *Health insurance type* | *p* < 0.0001 | | *p* < 0.0001 | |
| Private with extras | 1.00 | | 1.00 | |
| Private without extras | 0.90 | 0.86–0.94 | 0.83 | 0.78–0.88 |
| Government health care card | 0.94 | 0.89–0.99 | 1.02 | 0.96–1.09 |
| None | 0.91 | 0.87–0.95 | 0.99 | 0.93–1.05 |
| *Smoking status* | *p* < 0.0001 | | *p* < 0.0001 | |
| Never smoked | 1.00 | | 1.00 | |
| Past smoker | 1.17 | 1.13–1.21 | 1.28 | 1.23–1.34 |
| Current smoker | 0.78 | 0.74–0.84 | 0.73 | 0.68–0.79 |
| *Psychosocial distress* | *p* < 0.0001 | | *p* < 0.0001 | |
| Low | 1.00 | | 1.00 | |
| Moderate | 0.94 | 0.90–0.98 | 0.91 | 0.86–0.96 |
| High | 0.88 | 0.82–0.95 | 0.82 | 0.76–0.89 |
| Very high | 0.83 | 0.74–0.92 | 0.88 | 0.78–1.00 |
| *Diagnosed chronic conditions* | *p* < 0.0001 | | *p* < 0.0001 | |
| 0 | 1.00 | | 1.00 | |
| 1 | 1.19 | 1.15–1.24 | 1.58 | 1.51–1.66 |
| 2 | 1.35 | 1.29–1.42 | 2.13 | 2.01–2.27 |
| 3 or more | 1.48 | 1.37–1.60 | 2.69 | 2.46–2.93 |

**Table 2.** *Cont.*

| | Overweight | | Obese | |
|---|---|---|---|---|
| | **OR** | **95% CI** | **OR** | **95% CI** |
| *Treated chronic conditions* | $p < 0.0001$ | | $p < 0.0001$ | |
| 0 | 1.00 | | 1.00 | |
| 1 | 1.22 | 1.18–1.27 | 1.47 | 1.40–1.54 |
| 2 | 1.38 | 1.31–1.45 | 1.89 | 1.77–2.01 |
| 3 or more | 1.57 | 1.45–1.69 | 2.48 | 2.27–2.71 |
| *Limited physical functioning* | $p < 0.0001$ | | $p < 0.0001$ | |
| None | 1.00 | | 1.00 | |
| Minor | 1.36 | 1.30–1.41 | 2.10 | 1.99–2.21 |
| Moderate | 1.58 | 1.51–1.65 | 3.77 | 3.56–4.00 |
| Severe | 1.61 | 1.52–1.70 | 5.31 | 4.96–5.68 |

OR—Odds ratio, CI—Confidence interval.

### 3.3. Spatial Analysis

Tables 3 and 4 report parameter estimates and diagnostics for spatial regressions fit to overweight and obesity data. Smoothed prevalance ratios for postal areas from unadjusted null models ranged from 0.83–1.16 for overweight and 0.46–1.68 for obesity. Variation in risks between postal areas was principally due to unobserved spatial factors, with >96% of residual variation attributed to the spatial variance component for both overweigtht and obesity (see spatial fractions for Model 1 in Tables 3 and 4). Adjusting for individual-level factors (Model 2) attenuated the ranges of smoothed prevalence ratios to 0.88–1.08 for overweight and 0.63–1.23 for obesity, but had little effect on the proportions of residual variation from spatial sources, which remained high at >93% for both outcomes. Univariable parameter estimates for area-level associations including walkability and socioeconomic disadvantage are shown in the Model 3 and 4 columns of Tables 3 and 4. Risk ratios for walkability indicated consistent exposure gradients for both outcomes, with prevalence of overweight reduced by 4% and 9% and obesity by 8% and 11% in medium-high and high versus low walkability postal areas. Likewise, high body mass reduced monotonically with decreasing socioeconomic disadvantage. Overweight was 6% lower in the least versus most disadvantaged postal areas, and obesity was 11% and 9% lower in the least and second-to-least versus most disadvantaged postal areas. Fully-adjusted spatial regressions including individual- and area-level factors (Model 5) had the lowest DIC values and were the best fitting models for both outcomes (see DIC row in Tables 3 and 4). Prevalence ratios for socioeconomic disadvantage in these models were largely unaffected; however, gradients for area-level walkability strengthened with overweight 6% and 10% lower and obesity 11% and 15% lower in medium-high and high versus low walkability postcodes. These fully-adjusted spatial models also had the smallest amounts of residual spatial variation, with 67% of unexplained model variation attributed to unobserved spatial factors for overweight and 90% for obesity. Interaction analyses (Models 6) provided no evidence that the observed associations between walkability and overweight ($DIC_{M6} - DIC_{M5} = 18.21$) or obesity ($DIC_{M6} - DIC_{M5} = 12.12$) were modified by postal area socioeconomic disadvantage.

**Table 3.** Spatial regression summaries for postal area analyses of associations between overweight, walkability and relative socioeconomic disadvantage.

| | Model 1 | Model 2 | Model 3 | Model 4 | Model 5 |
|---|---|---|---|---|---|
| Individual-level adjustment | No | Yes | Yes | Yes | Yes |
| *Prevalence ratios (95% CrI)* | | | | | |
| Constant | 0.99 (0.98–1.00) | 1.00 (0.98–1.01) | 1.03 (1.00–1.06) | 1.01 (0.99–1.04) | 1.07 (1.02–1.11) |
| Walkability | | | | | |
| Low | – | – | 1.00 | – | 1.00 |
| Low–medium | – | – | 0.98 (0.95–1.01) | – | 0.98 (0.95–1.01) |
| Medium–high | – | – | 0.96 (0.92–1.00) | – | 0.94 (0.91–0.98) |
| High | – | – | 0.91 (0.87–0.97) | – | 0.90 (0.86–0.94) |
| Socioeconomic disadvantage | | | | | |
| Q1 - Most | – | – | – | 1.00 | 1.00 |
| Q2 | – | – | – | 1.01 (0.97–1.05) | 1.01 (0.97–1.04) |
| Q3 - Middling | – | – | – | 0.99 (0.95–1.03) | 0.99 (0.95–1.03) |
| Q4 | – | – | – | 0.97 (0.93–1.01) | 0.97 (0.93–1.00) |
| Q5 - Least | – | – | – | 0.94 (0.90–0.99) | 0.93 (0.89–0.97) |
| *Model diagnostics* | | | | | |
| pD | 55.73 | 37.48 | 33.64 | 35.05 | 27.01 |
| DIC | 1832.77 | 1787.67 | 1787.12 | 1787.85 | 1782.70 |
| Spatial fraction | 0.965 | 0.932 | 0.882 | 0.900 | 0.673 |

CrI—credible interval, pD—effective parameters, DIC—Deviance Information Criterion. Model 1—null model with expected cases proportional to the overall prevalence. Model 2—null model with expected cases adjusted for individual-level factors. Model 3—Model 2 + Sydney Walkability Index. Model 4—Model 2 + Index of Relative Socioeconomic Disadvantage. Model 5—Model 3 + Index of Relative Socioeconomic Disadvantage.

**Table 4.** Spatial regression summaries for postal area analyses of associations between obesity, walkability and relative socioeconomic disadvantage.

| | Model 1 | Model 2 | Model 3 | Model 4 | Model 5 |
|---|---|---|---|---|---|
| Individual-level adjustment | No | Yes | Yes | Yes | Yes |
| *Prevalence ratios (95% CrI)* | | | | | |
| Constant | 0.95 (0.93–0.97) | 0.96 (0.95–0.98) | 1.02 (0.97–1.08) | 1.01 (0.96–1.05) | 1.10 (1.02–1.17) |
| Walkability | | | | | |
| Low | – | – | 1.00 | – | 1.00 |
| Low-medium | – | – | 0.97 (0.91–1.02) | – | 0.96 (0.91–1.01) |
| Medium-high | – | – | 0.92 (0.85–0.99) | – | 0.89 (0.83–0.96) |
| High | – | – | 0.89 (0.80–0.99) | – | 0.85 (0.78–0.94) |
| Socioeconomic disadvantage | | | | | |
| Q1 - Most | – | – | – | 1.00 | 1.00 |
| Q2 | – | – | – | 1.03 (0.98–1.09) | 1.02 (0.97–1.08) |
| Q3 - Middling | – | – | – | 0.97 (0.92–1.03) | 0.97 (0.91–1.03) |
| Q4 | – | – | – | 0.91 (0.85–0.97) | 0.90 (0.85–0.96) |
| Q5 - Least | – | – | – | 0.88 (0.82–0.95) | 0.85 (0.79–0.92) |
| *Model diagnostics* | | | | | |
| pD | 128.60 | 72.36 | 70.99 | 63.02 | 56.79 |
| DIC | 1794.88 | 1711.26 | 1712.90 | 1705.26 | 1703.00 |
| Spatial fraction | 0.992 | 0.985 | 0.981 | 0.978 | 0.961 |

CrI—credible interval, pD—effective parameters, DIC—Deviance Information Criterion. Model 1—null model with expected cases proportional to the overall prevalence. Model 1—null model with expected cases proportional to the overall prevalence. Model 3—Model 2 + Sydney Walkability Index. Model 4—Model 2 + Index of Relative Socioeconomic Disadvantage. Model 5—Model 3 + Index of Relative Socioeconomic Disadvantage.

*3.4. Prevalence Maps*

Figures 1 and 2 graphically display smoothed prevalence ratios for overweight and obesity obtained from spatial models 1 (unadjusted null model), 2 (adjusted null model) and 5 (adjusted model with walkability and socioeconomic disadvantage). Total excess prevalence is shown in Maps A, D and G, and decomposed into excess risk due to spatial factors in maps B, E and H, and unstructured factors in maps C, F and I. Two features stand-out in each set of maps. First, residual prevalence is principally due to unobserved place-based factors, with higher ratios in spatial (B, E and H) versus unstructured (C, F and I) maps; and second, this geographic variation in risk reduces as individual- (Model 2) and area-level (Model 5) factors are added to spatial models. In unadjusted (Model 1) and adjusted (Model 2) null models, higher-than-expected prevalence was concentrated in western Sydney, and lower-than-expected prevalence in central and eastern Sydney. Including area-level walkability and relative socioeconomic disadvantage (Model 5) substantially attenuated excess prevalence by reducing excess risk attributable to unobserved spatial factors (see maps G and H of Figures 1 and 2). Final excess prevalence estimates were reduced in western Sydney and the peri-urban fringe for both overweight and obesity; and remained higher-than-expected for obesity through south-central Sydney, and lower-than-expected for both outcomes on the eastern seaboard north of the Sydney central business district.

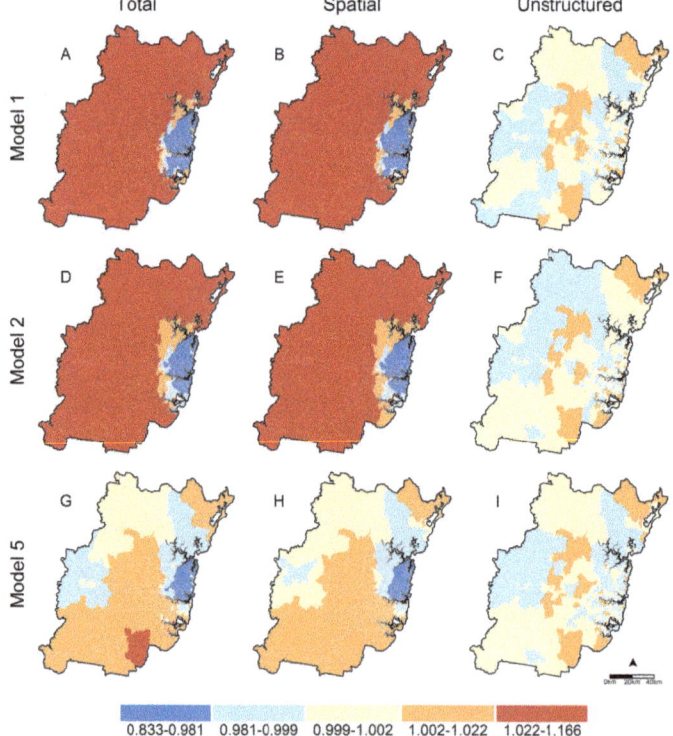

**Figure 1.** Total, Spatial and Unstructured prevalence ratios for overweight body mass in Sydney postal areas. Total prevalence ratios are derived by exponentiating the sum of spatial (*s*) and unstructured (*u*) random effects; Spatial and Unstructured prevalence ratios are obtained by exponentiating individual *s* and *u* components, respectively. Total, Spatial, and Unstructured prevalence ratio estimates are reported in maps (**A–C**) for Model 1, maps (**D–F**) for Model 2, and maps (**G–I**) for Model 5.

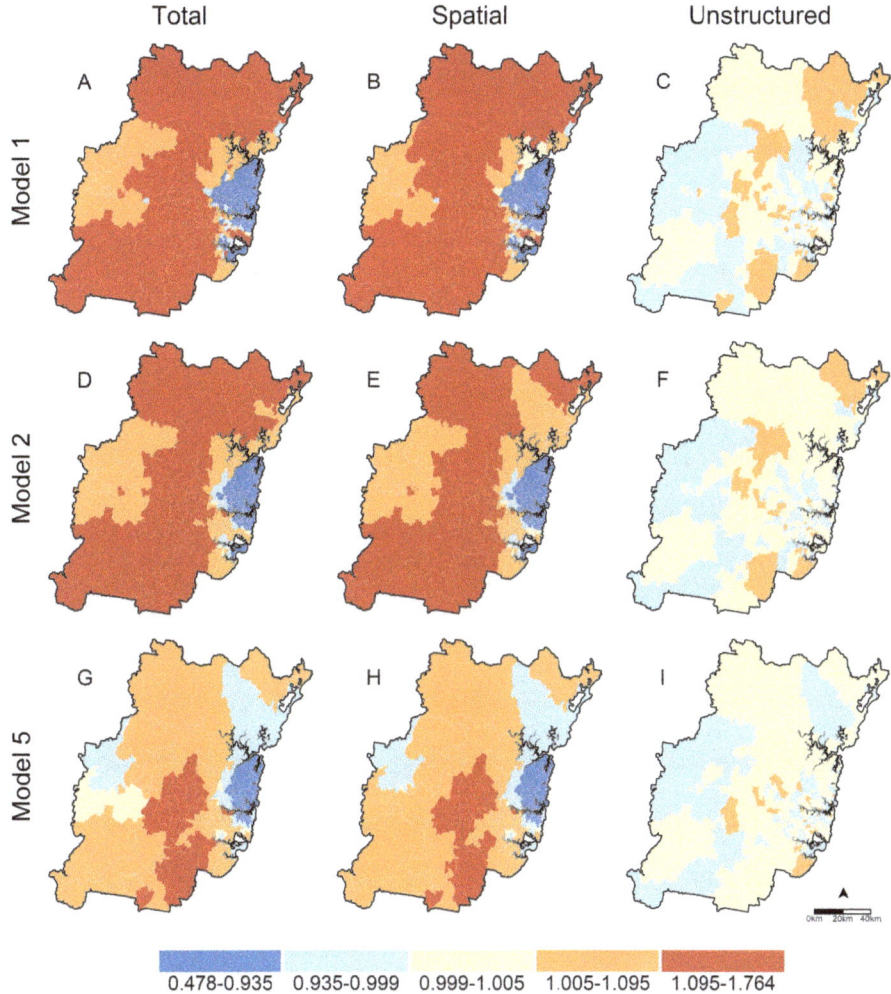

**Figure 2.** Total, Spatial and Unstructured prevalence ratios for obese body mass in Sydney postal areas. Total prevalence ratios are derived by exponentiating the sum of spatial (*s*) and unstructured (*u*) random effects; Spatial and Unstructured prevalence ratios are obtained by exponentiating individual *s* and *u* components, respectively. Total, Spatial, and Unstructured prevalence ratio estimates are reported in maps (**A–C**) for Model 1, maps (**D–F**) for Model 2, and maps (**G–I**) for Model 5.

## 4. Discussion

This is one of only a small number of studies to examine geographic variation in high body mass and its association with environmental walkability using a large population-derived cohort and spatial analytic framework. We find strong support for associations between postal area walkability and area-levels of overweight and obesity among persons aged 45 years and over living in Sydney, Australia. Prevalence in postal areas with medium-high and high walkability is reduced by 6% and 10% for overweight and 11% and 15% for obesity compared to postal areas with low walkability, and are independent of individual-level social, economic and health status factors, and area-level socioeconomic disadvantage. We also find that both overweight and obesity are geographically clustered at the postal area level with lowest prevalence in and to the north of the central business district, and highest prevalence in western Sydney. Postal area walkability explains approximately 20% and 9% of this geographic variation in overweight and obesity, respectively, that is not attributable to individual-level factors and area-level socioeconomic disadvantage. Our findings confirm associations between high body mass and walkability at spatial scales typical of those used for public health planning; highlight the potential for spatial analysis to better integrate "place" into walkability research; and provide novel methods and data for New South Wales Government initiatives aimed at creating built environments that support active transportation and promote healthy lifestyles, and monitoring these initiatives.

Despite some limitations, the existing built environment evidence base appears sufficiently developed to inform interventions aimed at addressing high body mass at individual and population levels [13]. A recent review concluded that the strongest evidence is for meso- and macro-level correlates, and identifies urban sprawl, land use mix, street connectivity, population density, and proximity to services and destinations as the important environmental characteristics at these levels [17]. Walkability indexes combine many of these key environmental variables into summary metrics that can be easily implemented at multiple spatial scales for planning purposes [19,27,28,40]. Our study is novel because it directly addresses exposure-outcome relations at a geographic scale more proximal to those typically used by government agencies for population-level health and urban planning [43–45]. We observed that higher levels of postal area walkability measured by our index were associated with lower prevalence of overweight and obesity in postal area populations aged ≥45 years, even after adjusting for other individual- and area-level characteristics related to body mass. These findings coincide with the small but consistent body of area-level findings that increased body mass and prevalence of obesity are associated with greater urban sprawl (see review by [17]), and extend recent individual-level associations between walkability and body mass [133–137] to populations and the spatial scales at which health and urban planning decisions are made. Our study also provides new evidence on the potential of tools like the Sydney Walkability Index [40] to benchmark, inform and monitor health and urban planning activities aimed at reducing population-levels of overweight and obesity. This will have relevance in the Australian context where open-access tools have been developed that allow researchers and planners to calculate NQLS-PLACE index values at mutiple spatial scales (see [28,138]).

Action to address overweight and obesity should target populations of greatest need [59,60]. However, it is unlikely that at-risk groups will be uniformly distributed across an area such as the Sydney statistical district [88]. Spatial analysis is especially useful in this regard with its ability to identify geographic locations with higher (or lower) than expected rates of overweight and obesity, and whether this variation is explained by, or in addition to, factors known to influence the distribution of health, such as demographic and socioeconomic characteristics [61]. We observed very strong clustering of overweight and obesity through central Sydney that was due to unobserved and spatially structured factors, and which contributed the majority of excess risk. Including individual-level demographic, social, economic and health status factors in our analysis attenuated excess prevalence of high body mass and reduced spatial variance but had little effect on outcome clustering across the study region. This is consistent with Canadian findings that individual-level variables were important correlates of within-region variation but explained little between-area geographic variation [85]. In contrast, adding postal-area walkability and socioeconomic disadvantage to our models reduced area-level clustering of overweight and, to a lesser extent, obesity. However, our final maps remained weakly clustered. This residual variation could suggest the presence of other unobserved spatial factors structuring the residual prevalence of high body mass in our study area. Identifying these additional factors was beyond the aims of our study but may include greenspace, access to shops and services, aesthetics, the food environment, and proximity to public transport [7,8,13,62]. It is also possible that some of this residual variation is due to residual confounding of associations between walkability and high body mass by sociodemographic factors. For example, Frank and colleagues have reported that features of walkable neighbourhoods are associated with lower overweight in males but greater overweight in females without a degree, and with lower obesity in men with a degree but higher obesity in unemployed non-white men without a degree and white women without a degree [139]. Likewise, there is some evidence that higher body mass is negatively associated with features of walkable neighbourhoods in high socioeconomic communities, and positively associated in low socioeconomic minority communities [140]. Future spatial studies employing our approach should consider alternate adjustment techniques to account for this possibility; for example, by calculating offsets using a logistic machine learning classifier.

Our findings are consistent with a growing evidence base indicating geographic variation at multiple spatial scales in the distribution of overweight and obesity that have relevance for health, urban and transport planning [56,59,62,79–89], although only a few studies have investigated built environment correlates of this variation within a geospatial context [62,81,82]. While Shuurman and colleagues were unable to assess whether population density—included in most walkability indexes—patterned obesity in Metro Vancouver because obesity itself did not cluster in their study area [82], Congdon has reported that not only are obesity rates 13–20% higher in sprawling versus compact US counties—an effect size similar to that obtained for physical inactivity, but that adding environmental measures to spatial models of county-level obesity prevalence reduced unexplained spatial variation by 22%. Lathey et al. have also examined associations between obesity rates and sprawl factors, including walkability, for census blocks in Maricopa County, Arizona [81]. They defined walkability as accessibility to places of social interaction, and found it was the strongest model predictor of being in a "high disease" obesity cluster with odds halved for the most versus least walkable census blocks [81]. Cluster membership was also associated with residential and commercial land use, and street connectivity, although effect sizes were very small [81]. Unfortunately, the focus on correlates of cluster membership reduces the analysis to a consideration of between-group differences, which is not especially informative geographically. Our study adds to the evidence base by its explicit focus on walkability and its contribution to geographical variation in high body mass at the spatial scales where health and urban planning decisions are made. We found effect sizes for walkability that were meaningful at population-scales [10], and sizable reductions in unexplained spatial variation comparable to other area-level spatial analyses [62].

Despite substantial reductions in unexplained variation due to spatially structured factors of 93.6% for overweight and 89.1% for obese, we observed little impact on spatial fractions except for overweight model 5, which reduced from ≥88.2% (models 1–4) to 67.3%. This is not surprising given the unstructured variance reduced by just 12.9% for overweight and 46.1% for obesity over the range of models fitted; with most of this decrease occurring between models 1 and 2 when we first adjusted for individual-level factors. Lunn et al. have noted that either the spatial ($s$) or unstructured ($u$) variance component will typically dominate the other in practical implementations of the Besag, York and Mollié model but will only be apparent once the posterior distributions of the components are examined [141]. A key strength of the Besag, York and Mollié model is its robustness to spatial and non spatial variation, and will produce unbiased parameter and variance estimates in the absence of either [142]. The large residual spatial fractions from our analyses also suggests the likely existence of additional geographically distributed factors related to overweight and obesity within in the Sydney Statistical Division.

The geographic variation observed in our data and reported in the substantive literature highlight the importance of appropriately controlling for spatial autocorrelation at analysis [39,42,61]. Spatial autocorrelation is problematic for standard regression methods that assume model residuals are independently and identically distributed (IDD), and its violation may result in biased inference [143]. Clustering is most typically handled by multilevel models that conflate unexplained spatial and non-spatial variation into a single random effect error term [42]. This approach addresses the issue of spatial autocorrelation; however, the potential value of the spatial variation for informing health planning is lost in the process. We have consistently identified variation in health risk-factors and outcomes in the Sydney region using 45 and Up Study data that indicate geographic areas with excess risk attributable to unobserved and spatially structured factors [39,42]. For example, we have reported variation in physical activity [42] and psychosocial distress [39] that indicates excess risk due to unobserved and spatially structured factors in addition to that attributable to observed individual-level factors, and postal area walkability and relative socioeconomic disadvantage. Pattenden and colleagues contend that outcome variation in excess of socioeconomic factors may indicate opportunities to address disparities in health status [61], while Fitzpatrick et al highlight its potential role in suggesting causal pathways [144]. We believe our approach is helpful because it not only locates inequalities in the geographic distribution of risk but also quantifies that attributable to known factors that may, or may not, be amenable to intervention, and to unknown factors requiring further investigation.

We observed statistically significant associations between most individual-level covariates and body mass outcomes in all fixed-effects models used to derive offset terms in spatial models. Consistent with our previous work on physical activity [42] and psychosocial distress [39] in this cohort, we observed strong positive associations between prevalence of high body mass and numbers of chronic care conditions ever diagnosed and recently treated, and even stronger associations with reduced functional capacity. These findings agree with previous reports on this cohort [103,120] and in the broader literature [145–147]. High body mass is considered a "gateway" into non-communicable diseases [148], and possibly multi-morbidity [149–152] and reduced physical functioning [145,153,154], although reverse causality is plausible with multi-morbidity and reduced physical functioning leading to lower levels of physical activity and poorer dietary choices [155]. We also observed an inverse association between high body mass and lower levels of psychosocial distress after adjusting for functional capacity. This is consistent with previous findings of increased risk of psychosocial distress with greater functional limitations in this cohort [39,156,157], and a strong contemporaneous effect of physical disability on depressive symptoms [158]. Depression and anxiety disorders are also known causes of weight loss in community-dwelling older adults [159], and may be influential on our findings as the Kessler Psychological Distress Scale [114] is specific for current anxiety and affective disorders in Australian community populations at the cut-points used in our study [160].

A major strength of our study is the large sample size drawn from the 45 and Up Study [93]. This high-quality, population-based cohort comprises approximately 10% of the Sydney statistical district aged 45 and over. While we make no claims to the external validity of our point-estimates beyond our sample, it is well established in the epidemiological literature that relative measures of effect are generalisable irrespective of representativeness and non response [161,162]. Methodological investigations of the 45 and Up Study cohort support this likelihood. Mealing et al. [130] have reported that odds ratios derived from the full cohort correspond to those from the population-representative New South Wales Adult Population Health Survey [163], while we have reported high correlations between postal area relative risks and disease maps estimated from unweighted and post-stratification weighted data [42,131]. These observations support the generalisability of our risk estimators and their geographical distribution to postal area populations within the Sydney Statistical Division area. We also used the Sydney Walkability Index as our exposure metric, which is derived using high-quality government agency spatial data [40]. The strengths of this index include its demonstrated predictive validity for moderate-intensity walking at multiple spatial scales, a cohesive latent variable structure, and comparability to other indexes (e.g., NQLS [38] and PLACE [19]) frequently used in walkability research [40,42]. The spatial data used in its construction are routinely updated to support NSW Government business, and are accessible via the *NSW Open Data Policy* [164]. This allows the Sydney Walkability Index to be re-calculated annually to monitor changes in the spatial distribution of walkability across the Sydney statistical district. There is also an ongoing effort to develop a national walkability index using similar methods to our index that would benchmark and monitor changes in walkability across Australia [28]. Finally, our study employed an explicitly spatial approach that controlled for individual-level factors to investigate geographic variation in high body mass and its association with environmental walkability at the postal area level. The substantial levels of clustering in our data indicate the importance of accounting for spatial autocorrelation in analyses where it is expected or observed, and highlights the potentially informative nature of this variation for health and urban planning that is ignored when spatial and non-spatial sources of variation are conflated [42].

Our study reported on associations between postal area walkability and high body mass outcomes, which are not necessarily causal. An important limitation of our study is that we were unable to control for potential bias due to participant self-selection into postal areas, which raises the potential for reverse causation. Self-selection bias occurs when individuals choose to live in neighbourhoods that support their physical activity and travel behaviour preferences [8,17]. Systematic reviews indicate that neighbourhood self-selection may account for up to 50% of the built environment's effect on physical activity [17]. Its contribution to built environment associations with high body mass is less clear. Some studies have reported that self-selection fully accounts for these associations [165,166], while others have reported more modest attenuation effects [167–169]. There is also some evidence that it may selectively attenuate associations for continuous but not categorical body mass outcomes [170,171]. The 45 and Up Study does not collect information on respondents' preferences for the neighbourhoods in which they reside, and so we are unable to discount this as contributing to some portion of the estimated effect of walkability in our study.

We used self-reported BMI to classify overweight and obesity, which is generally appropriate for quantifying body size in the 45 and Up Study cohort but known to underestimate prevalence of obesity using standard BMI classifications by 6% [98]. In the context of our study, this means both overweight and obesity are likely to have been systematically misclassified. Monte Carlo simulation studies have found that systematic misclassification of binary dependent variables on the order of 2–5% can bias relative effects estimates by 12–25% in either direction [172,173]. This has the potential to weaken the magnitude of our observed associations for both overweight and obesity, but would still result in meaningful effect sizes at the population-level [8,10]. Another limitation of our analysis is that it was conducted at a single geographic scale, and so our findings may differ if conducted at a finer or coarser scale. This is the Modifiable Areal Unit Problem [174,175], which is germane to all analyses using areal units or zones [175]. We were only provided with access to postal area identifiers by the data custodian, and so were unable to assess the sensitivity of our results to different spatial scales. We have previously examined associations between walkability and health-enhancing physical activity at different spatial scales and found similar relations [40,42], which provides some reassurance on the robustness of our findings to spatial scale. However, the influence of scale on matched exposure-response relations in the walkability literature remains opens and warrants further investigation.

The Sydney Walkability Index [40] is comparable to other indexes used in the substantive literature [19] and so is subject to the same limitation that walkability quartiles may be data-dependent as they are derived using population-specific cut-points [176,177]. We therefore encourage planners, policy makers and researchers to review the quartile cut-points used in constructing the Sydney Walkability Index to evaluate their appropriateness and the applicability of our findings to their geographic context. Further, modelling walkability as an index means we are unable to identify which built environment components in the index contribute to the observed associations with prevalence and geographic distribution of overweight and obesity, which would be useful for framing policy interventions. This was partly a choice for consistency with the expressed interest in the literature about the potential for "walkability indexes" to benchmark, inform and monitor development plans, but also because the added complexity would have made our models intractable. Our analysis used a two stage approach in which individual-level conditional probabilities of overweight and obesity were modelled first and then used as offset terms to adjust spatial models. While this approach is not uncommon in the epidemiological literature (see [39,42,122–124]), ideally we would have modelled individual and area-level effects simultaneously in a single, parsimonious model. However, despite the relative ease with which Besag, York and Mollié models can be fit in available software [75,178], they remain computationally prohibitive to implement outside of high performance computing environments when extended to multi-level problems comprising samples of the size used in our study [179]. Our units of analysis comprised Australian postal areas, which correspond in spatial extent to the upper limit of buffers sizes used in individual-level research linking walkability to high body mass but may not be representative of all spatial extents at which health and urban planning decisions occur. Finally, our study precludes causal inference due to its cross-sectional design.

## 5. Conclusions

Walkability indexes have been identified as potentially useful tools for planning and monitoring the built environment to improve health [27]. Our results provide support for their potential application to body mass outcomes by demonstrating that: (1) rates of overweight and obesity are negatively associated walkability at the postcode level for Sydney residents aged ≥45 years; and (2) that area-level walkability makes a small but meaningful contribution to the geographic clustering of high body mass in the Sydney metropolitan region. Our results also suggest the presence of other unobserved and spatially structured factors contributing to this clustering. *The Greater Sydney Region Plan* aims to create healthy, resilient and socially connected communities over the next 40 years by creating fine scaled urban form, mixed land use and amenity within walkable urban centres [25]. The methods and outcomes described here may assist in the geographical targeting of strategies and monitoring their progress towards achieving its liveability objectives.

**Author Contributions:** Conceptualization, D.J.M., G.G.M., B.B.J. and A.E.B.; Data curation, D.J.M.; Formal analysis, D.J.M.; Methodology, D.J.M., G.G.M. and A.E.B.; Supervision, G.G.M. and A.E.B.; Writing—original draft, D.J.M., G.G.M., B.B.J. and A.E.B.; Writing—review & editing, D.J.M., G.G.M., B.B.J. and A.E.B.

**Acknowledgments:** This research was completed using data collected through the 45 and Up Study (www.saxinstitute.org.au). The 45 and Up Study is managed by the Sax Institute in collaboration with major partner Cancer Council NSW; and partners: the National Heart Foundation of Australia (NSW Division); NSW Ministry of Health; NSW Government Family & Community Services—Ageing, Carers and the Disability Council NSW; and the Australian Red Cross Blood Service. We thank the many thousands of people participating in the 45 and Up Study. Details on accessing 45 and Up Study data are available on the The Sax Institute website (www.saxinstitute.org.au/our-work/45-up-study). We wish to acknowledge Associate Professor Philayrath Phongsavan for her tireless and effective coordination of this project. DJM is grateful to Hevan Corrimal and WHC Sutherland for their ongoing support and providing office space. This study is part of the "Understanding the impact of the social, economic and environmental factors on the health of Australians in mid - later life; where are the opportunities for prevention?" study (National Health & Medical Research Council (NHMRC) Grant 402810).

**Conflicts of Interest:** The authors declare no conflict of interest. This manuscript was reviewed for technical accuracy by The 45 and Up Study coordinating centre prior to its submission for peer review. Neither the 45 and Up Study coordinating centre nor the NHMRC had a role in the design of the study; the collection, analysis, or interpretation of data; the writing of the manuscript; or in the decision to publish the results.

## References

1.  Gregg, E.W.; Shaw, J.E. Global Health Effects of Overweight and Obesity. *N. Engl. J. Med.* **2017**, *377*, 80–81. [CrossRef] [PubMed]
2.  Gakidou, E.; Afshin, A.; Abajobir, A.A.; Abate, K.H.; Abbafati, C.; Abbas, K.M.; Abd-Allah, F.; Abdulle, A.M.; Abera, S.F.; Aboyans, V.; et al. Global, regional, and national comparative risk assessment of 84 behavioural, environmental and occupational, and metabolic risks or clusters of risks, 1990–2016: A systematic analysis for the Global Burden of Disease Study 2016. *Lancet* **2017**, *390*, 1345–1422. [CrossRef]
3.  Must, A.; Spadano, J.; Coakley, E.H.; Field, A.E.; Colditz, G.; Dietz, W.H. The disease burden associated with overweight and obesity. *JAMA* **1999**, *282*, 1523–1529. [CrossRef] [PubMed]
4.  The GBD Obesity Collaborators. Health Effects of Overweight and Obesity in 195 Countries over 25 Years. *N. Engl. J. Med.* **2017**, *377*, 13–27. [CrossRef]
5.  Lehnert, T.; Sonntag, D.; Konnopka, A.; Riedel-Heller, S.; König, H.H. Economic costs of overweight and obesity. *Best Pract. Res. Clin. Endocrinol. Metab.* **2013**, *27*, 105–115. [CrossRef] [PubMed]
6.  Speakman, J.R. Obesity: The Integrated Roles of Environment and Genetics. *J. Nutr.* **2004**, *134*, 2090S–2105S. [CrossRef] [PubMed]
7.  Rutter, H.; Savona, N.; Glonti, K.; Bibby, J.; Cummins, S.; Finegood, D.T.; Greaves, F.; Harper, L.; Hawe, P.; Moore, L.; et al. The need for a complex systems model of evidence for public health. *Lancet* **2017**, *390*, 2602–2604. [CrossRef]

8.  Lakerveld, J.; Mackenbach, J.D.; Rutter, H.; Brug, J. Obesogenic environment and obesogenic behaviours. In *Advanced Nutrition and Dietetics in Obesity*; Hankey, C., Ed.; John Wiley & Sons, Incorporated: Newark, NJ, USA, 2017; Chapter 3.7, pp. 132–137.
9.  Saelens, B.E.; Sallis, J.F.; Frank, L.D. Environmental correlates of walking and cycling: Findings from the transportation, urban design, and planning literatures. *Ann. Behav. Med.* **2003**, *25*, 80–91. [CrossRef] [PubMed]
10. Rose, G. Sick individuals and sick populations. *Int. J. Epidemiol.* **2001**, *30*, 427–432. [CrossRef] [PubMed]
11. Giles-Corti, B.; Timperio, A.; Bull, F.; Pikora, T. Understanding physical activity environmental correlates: Increased specificity for ecological models. *Exerc. Sport Sci. Rev.* **2005**, *33*, 175–181. [CrossRef] [PubMed]
12. Saelens, B.E.; Handy, S.L. Built environment correlates of walking: A review. *Med. Sci. Sports Exerc.* **2008**, *40*, S550–S566. [CrossRef] [PubMed]
13. Townshend, T.; Lake, A. Obesogenic environments: Current evidence of the built and food environments. *Perspect. Public Health* **2017**, *137*, 38–44. [CrossRef] [PubMed]
14. Feng, J.; Glass, T.A.; Curriero, F.C.; Stewart, W.F.; Schwartz, B.S. The built environment and obesity: A systematic review of the epidemiologic evidence. *Health Place* **2010**, *16*, 175–190. [CrossRef] [PubMed]
15. Durand, C.P.; Andalib, M.; Dunton, G.F.; Wolch, J.; Pentz, M.A. A systematic review of built environment factors related to physical activity and obesity risk: Implications for smart growth urban planning. *Obes. Rev.* **2011**, *12*, e173–e182. [CrossRef] [PubMed]
16. Mackenbach, J.D.; Rutter, H.; Compernolle, S.; Glonti, K.; Oppert, J.M.; Charreire, H.; De Bourdeaudhuij, I.; Brug, J.; Nijpels, G.; Lakerveld, J. Obesogenic environments: A systematic review of the association between the physical environment and adult weight status, the SPOTLIGHT project. *BMC Public Health* **2014**, *14*, 233. [CrossRef] [PubMed]
17. Garfinkel-Castro, A.; Kim, K.; Hamidi, S.; Ewing, R. Obesity and the built environment at different urban scales: Examining the literature. *Nutr. Rev.* **2017**, *75*, 51–61. [CrossRef] [PubMed]
18. Ding, D.; Gebel, K. Built environment, physical activity, and obesity: What have we learned from reviewing the literature? *Health Place* **2012**, *18*, 100–105. [CrossRef] [PubMed]
19. Leslie, E.; Coffee, N.; Frank, L.; Owen, N.; Bauman, A.; Hugo, G. Walkability of local communities: Using geographic information systems to objectively assess relevant environmental attributes. *Health Place* **2007**, *13*, 111–122. [CrossRef] [PubMed]
20. Sallis, J.F.; Frank, L.D.; Saelens, B.E.; Kraft, M. Active transportation and physical activity: Opportunities for collaboration on transportation and public health research. *Transp. Res. Part A Policy Pract.* **2004**, *38*, 249–268. [CrossRef]
21. Hamer, M.; Chida, Y. Active commuting and cardiovascular risk: A meta-analytic review. *Prev. Med.* **2008**, *46*, 9–13, [CrossRef] [PubMed]
22. Bird, E.L.; Ige, J.O.; Pilkington, P.; Pinto, A.; Petrokofsky, C.; Burgess-Allen, J. Built and natural environment planning principles for promoting health: An umbrella review. *BMC Public Health* **2018**, *18*, 930. [CrossRef] [PubMed]
23. City Planning Department of Helsinki. Helsinki City Plan: Urban Plan—The New Helsinki City Plan, Vision 2050. Available online: https://www.hel.fi/hel2/ksv/julkaisut/yos_2013-23_en.pdf (accessed on 2 February 2019).
24. Salt Lake City Council. Pedestrian & Bicycle Master Plan. Available online: https://www.slc.gov/transportation/bike/pbmp/ (accessed on 2 February 2019).
25. GreaterSydneyCommission. Greater Sydney Region Plan: A Metropolis of Three Cities—Connecting People. Available online: https://www.planning.nsw.gov.au/plans-for-your-area/a-metropolis-of-three-cities/a-metropolis-of-three-cities (accessed on 17 September 2018).
26. Transport for London. Walking Action Plan: Making London the World'S Most Walkable City. Available online: http://content.tfl.gov.uk/mts-walking-action-plan.pdf (accessed on 2 February 2019).
27. Grasser, G.; Van Dyck, D.; Titze, S.; Stronegger, W. Objectively measured walkability and active transport and weight-related outcomes in adults: A systematic review. *Int. J. Public Health* **2013**, *58*, 615–625. [CrossRef] [PubMed]
28. Giles-Corti, B.; Macaulay, G.; Middleton, N.; Boruff, B.; Bull, F.; Butterworth, I.; Badland, H.; Mavoa, S.; Roberts, R.; Christian, H. Developing a research and practice tool to measure walkability: A demonstration project. *Health Promot. J. Aust.* **2014**, *25*, 160–166. [CrossRef] [PubMed]

29. Cervero, R.; Kockelman, K. Travel demand and the 3Ds: Density, diversity, and design. *Transp. Res. D Transp. Environ.* **1997**, *2*, 199–219. [CrossRef]

30. Ewing, R.; Schmid, T.; Killingsworth, R.; Zlot, A.; Raudenbush, S. Relationship between urban sprawl and physical activity, obesity, and morbidity. *Am. J. Health Promot.* **2003**, *18*, 47–57, [CrossRef] [PubMed]

31. Krizek, K.J. Operationalizing Neighborhood Accessibility for Land Use-Travel Behavior Research and Regional Modeling. *J. Plan. Educ. Res.* **2003**, *22*, 270–287. [CrossRef]

32. Lopez, R. Urban sprawl and risk for being overweight or obese. *Am. J. Public Health* **2004**, *94*, 1574–1579. [CrossRef] [PubMed]

33. Levine, J.; Inam, A.; Torng, G.W. A Choice-Based Rationale for Land Use and Transportation Alternatives: Evidence from Boston and Atlanta. *J. Plan. Educ. Res.* **2005**, *24*, 317–330. [CrossRef]

34. Lee, C.; Moudon, A.V. The 3Ds + R: Quantifying land use and urban form correlates of walking. *Transp. Res. Transp Environ.* **2006**, *11*, 204–215. [CrossRef]

35. Ross, N.A.; Tremblay, S.; Khan, S.; Crouse, D.; Tremblay, M.; Berthelot, J.M. Body mass index in urban Canada: Neighborhood and metropolitan area effects. *Am. J. Public Health* **2007**, *97*, 500–508. [CrossRef] [PubMed]

36. Carr, L.J.; Dunsiger, S.I.; Marcus, B.H. Validation of Walk Score for estimating access to walkable amenities. *Br. J. Sports Med.* **2011**, *45*, 1144–1148, doi:10.1136/bjsm.2009.069609. [CrossRef] [PubMed]

37. Zick, C.D.; Hanson, H.; Fan, J.X.; Smith, K.R.; Kowaleski-Jones, L.; Brown, B.B.; Yamada, I. Re-visiting the relationship between neighbourhood environment and BMI: An instrumental variables approach to correcting for residential selection bias. *Int. J. Behav. Nutr. Phys. Act.* **2013**, *10*, 27. [CrossRef] [PubMed]

38. Frank, L.D.; Sallis, J.F.; Saelens, B.E.; Leary, L.; Cain, K.; Conway, T.L.; Hess, P.M. The development of a walkability index: Application to the Neighborhood Quality of Life Study. *Br. J. Sports Med.* **2010**, *44*, 924–933. [CrossRef] [PubMed]

39. Mayne, D.J.; Morgan, G.G.; Jalaludin, B.B.; Bauman, A.E. Does Walkability Contribute to Geographic Variation in Psychosocial Distress? A Spatial Analysis of 91,142 Members of the 45 and Up Study in Sydney, Australia. *Int. J. Environ. Res. Public Health* **2018**, *15*, 275. [CrossRef] [PubMed]

40. Mayne, D.; Morgan, G.; Willmore, A.; Rose, N.; Jalaludin, B.; Bambrick, H.; Bauman, A. An objective index of walkability for research and planning in the Sydney metropolitan region of New South Wales, Australia: An ecological study. *Int. J. Health Geogr.* **2013**, *12*, 61. [CrossRef] [PubMed]

41. Frank, L.D.; Andresen, M.A.; Schmid, T.L. Obesity relationships with community design, physical activity, and time spent in cars. *Am. J. Prev. Med.* **2004**, *27*, 87–96. [CrossRef] [PubMed]

42. Mayne, D.J.; Morgan, G.G.; Jalaludin, B.B.; Bauman, A.E. The contribution of area-level walkability to geographic variation in physical activity: A spatial analysis of 95,837 participants from the 45 and Up Study living in Sydney, Australia. *Popul. Health Metr.* **2017**, *15*, 38. [CrossRef] [PubMed]

43. Sugiyama, T.; Cole, R.; Koohsari, M.J.; Kynn, M.; Sallis, J.F.; Owen, N. Associations of local-area walkability with disparities in residents' walking and car use. *Prev. Med.* **2019**, *120*, 126–130. [CrossRef] [PubMed]

44. Rydin, Y.; Bleahu, A.; Davies, M.; Dávila, J.D.; Friel, S.; De Grandis, G.; Groce, N.; Hallal, P.C.; Hamilton, I.; Howden-Chapman, P.; et al. Shaping cities for health: Complexity and the planning of urban environments in the 21st century. *Lancet* **2012**, *379*, 2079–2108. [CrossRef]

45. Merom, D.; Ding, D.; Corpuz, G.; Bauman, A. Walking in Sydney: Trends in prevalence by geographic areas using information from transport and health surveillance systems. *J. Transp. Health* **2015**, *2*, 350–359. [CrossRef]

46. Papas, M.A.; Alberg, A.J.; Ewing, R.; Helzlsouer, K.J.; Gary, T.L.; Klassen, A.C. The built environment and obesity. *Epidemiol. Rev.* **2007**, *29*, 129–143. [CrossRef] [PubMed]

47. James, P.; Berrigan, D.; Hart, J.E.; Aaron Hipp, J.; Hoehner, C.M.; Kerr, J.; Major, J.M.; Oka, M.; Laden, F. Effects of buffer size and shape on associations between the built environment and energy balance. *Health Place* **2014**, *27*, 162–170. [CrossRef] [PubMed]

48. Villanueva, K.; Knuiman, M.; Nathan, A.; Giles-Corti, B.; Christian, H.; Foster, S.; Bull, F. The impact of neighborhood walkability on walking: Does it differ across adult life stage and does neighborhood buffer size matter? *Health Place* **2014**, *25*, 43–46. [CrossRef] [PubMed]

49. Sato, M.; Du, J.; Inoue, Y. Rate of Physical Activity and Community Health: Evidence From U.S. Counties. *J. Phys. Act. Health* **2016**, *13*, 640–648. [CrossRef] [PubMed]

50. Riley, M.W. Special Problems of Sociological Analysis. In *Sociological Research: A Case Approach*; Riley, M.W., Merton, R.K., Eds.; Harcourt, Brace, and World: New York, NY, USA, 1963; Volume 1, pp. 700–725.

51. Alker H.A.J. A Typology of Ecological Fallacies. In *Quantitative Ecological Analysis*; Dogan, M., Rokkan, S., Eds.; Massachusetts Institute of Technology Press: Cambridge, MA, USA, 1969; pp. 69–86.

52. Schwartz, S. The fallacy of the ecological fallacy: The potential misuse of a concept and the consequences. *Am. J. Public Health* **1994**, *84*, 819–824. [CrossRef] [PubMed]

53. Ewing, R.; Hamidi, S. *Measuring Sprawl 2014*; Smart Growth America: Washington, DC, USA, 2014.

54. Hooper, P.; Knuiman, M.; Foster, S.; Giles-Corti, B. The building blocks of a 'Liveable Neighbourhood': Identifying the key performance indicators for walking of an operational planning policy in Perth, Western Australia. *Health Place* **2015**, *36*, 173–183. [CrossRef] [PubMed]

55. Fazli, G.S.; Creatore, M.I.; Matheson, F.I.; Guilcher, S.; Kaufman-Shriqui, V.; Manson, H.; Johns, A.; Booth, G.L. Identifying mechanisms for facilitating knowledge to action strategies targeting the built environment. *BMC Public Health* **2017**, *17*, 1. [CrossRef] [PubMed]

56. Cho, S.H.; Chen, Z.; Eastwood, D.B.; Yen, S.T. The effects of urban sprawl on body mass index: Where people live does matter? *Consum. Interest Ann.* **2006**, *52*, 159–169.

57. Ewing, R.; Hamidi, S. *Measuring Urban Sprawl and Validating Sprawl Measures*; Metropolitan Research Centre: Salt Lake City, UT, USA, 2010.

58. Hamidi, S.; Ewing, R.; Preuss, I.; Dodds, A. Measuring Sprawl and Its Impacts: An Update. *J. Plan. Educ. Res.* **2015**, *35*, 35–50. [CrossRef]

59. Kinge, J.M.; Steingrímsdóttir, O.A.; Strand, B.H.; Kravdal, Ø. Can socioeconomic factors explain geographic variation in overweight in Norway? *SSM Popul. Health* **2016**, *2*, 333–340. [CrossRef] [PubMed]

60. Gehlert, S.; Sohmer, D.; Sacks, T.; Mininger, C.; McClintock, M.; Olopade, O. Targeting Health Disparities: A Model Linking Upstream Determinants To Downstream Interventions. *Health Aff. (Millwood)* **2008**, *27*, 339–349. [CrossRef] [PubMed]

61. Pattenden, S.; Casson, K.; Cook, S.; Dolk, H. Geographical variation in infant mortality, stillbirth and low birth weight in Northern Ireland, 1992–2002. *J. Epidemiol. Commun. Health* **2011**, *65*, 1159–1165. [CrossRef] [PubMed]

62. Congdon, P. Variations in obesity rates between US counties: Impacts of activity access, food environments, and settlement patterns. *Int. J. Environ. Res. Public Health* **2017**, *14*, 1023. [CrossRef] [PubMed]

63. Sichieri, R.; Coitinho, D.C.; Leão, M.M.; Recine, E.; Everhart, J.E. High temporal, geographic, and income variation in body mass index among adults in Brazil. *Am. J. Public Health* **1994**, *84*, 793–798. [CrossRef] [PubMed]

64. Willms, J.D.; Tremblay, M.S.; Katzmarzyk, P.T. Geographic and Demographic Variation in the Prevalence of Overweight Canadian Children. *Obesity* **2003**, *11*, 668–673. [CrossRef] [PubMed]

65. Ackerson, L.K.; Kawachi, I.; Barbeau, E.M.; Subramanian, S.V. Geography of underweight and overweight among women in India: A multilevel analysis of 3204 neighborhoods in 26 states. *Econ. Hum. Biol.* **2008**, *6*, 264–280. [CrossRef] [PubMed]

66. Lebel, A.; Pampalon, R.; Hamel, D.; Thériault, M. The geography of overweight in Québec: A multilevel perspective. *Can. J. Public Health* **2009**, *100*, 18–23. [PubMed]

67. Simen-Kapeu, A.; Khule, S.; Veugelers, P.J. Geographic Differences in Childhood Overweight, Physical Activity, Nutrition and Neighbourhood Facilities: Implications for Prevention. *Can. J. Public Health* **2010**, *101*, 128–132. [PubMed]

68. El Mouzan, M.; Al Herbish, A.; Al Salloum, A.; Al Omar, A.; Qurachi, M. Regional variation in prevalence of overweight and obesity in Saudi children and adolescents. *Saudi J. Gastroenterol.* **2012**, *18*, 129–132. [CrossRef] [PubMed]

69. Toft, U.; Vinding, A.L.; Larsen, F.B.; Hvidberg, M.F.; Robinson, K.M.; Glümer, C. The development in body mass index, overweight and obesity in three regions in Denmark. *Eur. J. Public Health* **2015**, *25*, 273–278. [CrossRef] [PubMed]

70. Ajayi, I.O.; Adebamowo, C.; Adami, H.O.; Dalal, S.; Diamond, M.B.; Bajunirwe, F.; Guwatudde, D.; Njelekela, M.; Nankya-Mutyoba, J.; Chiwanga, F.S.; et al. Urban–rural and geographic differences in overweight and obesity in four sub-Saharan African adult populations: A multi-country cross-sectional study. *BMC Public Health* **2016**, *16*, 1126. [CrossRef] [PubMed]

71. Adachi-Mejia, A.M.; Lee, C.; Lee, C.; Carlos, H.A.; Saelens, B.E.; Berke, E.M.; Doescher, M.P. Geographic variation in the relationship between body mass index and the built environment. *Prev. Med.* **2017**, *100*, 33–40. [CrossRef] [PubMed]

72. Torres-Roman, J.S.; Urrunaga-Pastor, D.; Avilez, J.L.; Helguero-Santin, L.M.; Malaga, G. Geographic differences in overweight and obesity prevalence in Peruvian children, 2010–2015. *BMC Public Health* **2018**, *18*, 353. [CrossRef] [PubMed]

73. Mayhew, S. *A Dictionary of Geography*; Oxford University Press: Oxford, UK, 2015.

74. Fischer, M.M.; Getis, A. Introduction. In *Handbook of Applied Spatial Analysis: Software Tools, Methods and Applications*; Fischer, M.M., Getis, A., Eds.; Springer: Berlin/Heidelberg, Germany, 2010; Chapters 1–24.

75. Lawson, A.; Browne, W.J.; Vidal Rodeiro, C.L. *Disease Mapping with WinBUGS and MLwiN*; Statistics in Practice; Wiley: Hoboken, NJ, USA, 2003.

76. Smedley, B.; Amaro, H. Advancing the Science and Practice of Place-Based Intervention. *Am. J. Public Health* **2016**, *106*, 197–197. [CrossRef]

77. Miranda, M.L.; Edwards, S.E.; Keating, M.H.; Paul, C.J. Making the Environmental Justice Grade: The Relative Burden of Air Pollution Exposure in the United States. *Int. J. Environ. Res. Public Health* **2011**, *8*, 1755. [CrossRef] [PubMed]

78. Jia, P.; Cheng, X.; Xue, H.; Wang, Y. Applications of geographic information systems (GIS) data and methods in obesity-related research. *Obes. Rev.* **2017**, *18*, 400–411. [CrossRef] [PubMed]

79. Gutiérrez-Fisac, J.L.; Rodríguez Artalejo, F.; Guallar-Castillon, P.; Banegas Banegas, J.R.; del Rey Calero, J. Determinants of geographical variations in body mass index (BMI) and obesity in Spain. *Int. J. Obes.* **1999**, *23*, 342–347. [CrossRef]

80. Ford, E.S.; Mokdad, A.H.; Giles, W.H.; Galuska, D.A.; Serdula, M.K. Geographic Variation in the Prevalence of Obesity, Diabetes, and Obesity-Related Behaviors. *Obes. Res.* **2005**, *13*, 118–122. [CrossRef] [PubMed]

81. Lathey, V.; Guhathakurta, S.; Aggarwal, R.M. The Impact of Subregional Variations in Urban Sprawl on the Prevalence of Obesity and Related Morbidity. *J. Plan. Educ. Res.* **2009**, *29*, 127–141. [CrossRef]

82. Schuurman, N.; Peters, P.A.; Oliver, L.N. Are Obesity and Physical Activity Clustered? A Spatial Analysis Linked to Residential Density. *Obesity* **2009**, *17*, 2202–2209. [CrossRef] [PubMed]

83. Þórisdóttir, I.E.; Kristjansson, A.L.; Sigfusdottir, I.D.; Allegrante, J.P. The landscape of overweight and obesity in Icelandic adolescents: Geographic variation in body-mass index between 2000 and 2009. *J. Commun. Health* **2012**, *37*, 234–241. [CrossRef] [PubMed]

84. Myers, C.A.; Slack, T.; Martin, C.K.; Broyles, S.T.; Heymsfield, S.B. Regional disparities in obesity prevalence in the United States: A spatial regime analysis. *Obesity* **2015**, *23*, 481–487. [CrossRef] [PubMed]

85. Dutton, D.J.; McLaren, L. How important are determinants of obesity measured at the individual level for explaining geographic variation in body mass index distributions? Observational evidence from Canada using Quantile Regression and Blinder-Oaxaca Decomposition. *J. Epidemiol. Commun. Health* **2016**, *70*, 367–373. [CrossRef] [PubMed]

86. Paquet, C.; Chaix, B.; Howard, N.; Coffee, N.; Adams, R.; Taylor, A.; Thomas, F.; Daniel, M. Geographic clustering of cardiometabolic risk factors in metropolitan centres in France and Australia. *Int. J. Environ. Res. Public Health* **2016**, *13*, 519. [CrossRef] [PubMed]

87. Alkerwi, A.; Bahi, I.E.; Stranges, S.; Beissel, J.; Delagardelle, C.; Noppe, S.; Kandala, N.B. Geographic variations in cardiometabolic risk factors in Luxembourg. *Int. J. Environ. Res. Public Health* **2017**, *14*, 648. [CrossRef] [PubMed]

88. Smurthwaite, K.; Bagheri, N. Using Geographical Convergence of Obesity, Cardiovascular Disease, and Type 2 Diabetes at the Neighborhood Level to Inform Policy and Practice. *Prev. Chronic Dis.* **2017**, *14*, E91–E91. [CrossRef] [PubMed]

89. Samouda, H.; Ruiz-Castell, M.; Bocquet, V.; Kuemmerle, A.; Chioti, A.; Dadoun, F.; Kandala, N.B.; Stranges, S. Geographical variation of overweight, obesity and related risk factors: Findings from the European Health Examination Survey in Luxembourg, 2013–2015. *PLoS ONE* **2018**, *13*, e0197021. [CrossRef] [PubMed]

90. Australian Bureau of Statistics. *Statistical Geography: Volume 1—Australian Standard Geographical Classification (ASGC), July 2006 (Catalogue No. 1216.0)*; Commonwealth of Australia: Canberra, Autralia, 2006.

91. Australian Bureau of Statistics. TableBuilder Basic. Available online: http://www.abs.gov.au/websitedbs/censushome.nsf/home/tablebuilder (accessed on 31 January 2018).

92. Australian Bureau of Statistics. *Statistical Geography: Volume 2—Census Geographic Areas, 2006 (Catalogue No. 2905.0)*; Commonwealth of Australia: Canberra, Australia, 2006.

93. 45 and Up Study Collaborators. Cohort profile: The 45 and Up Study. *Int. J. Epidemiol.* **2008**, *37*, 941–947. [CrossRef]

94. 45 and Up Study. Researcher Toolkit. Available online: https://www.saxinstitute.org.au/our-work/45-up-study/for-researchers/ (accessed on 31 January 2018).

95. The 45 and Up Study. The 45 and Up Study Data Book—December 2011 Release. Available online: https://www.saxinstitute.org.au/our-work/45-up-study/data-book/ (accessed on 31 January 2018).

96. Australian Bureau of Statistics. *Socio-Economic Indexes for Areas (SEIFA)—Technical Paper, 2006*; Australian Bureau of Statistics: Canberra, Australia, 2008.

97. WHO Expert Committee on Physical Status. *Physical Status: The Use and Interpretation of Anthropometry. Report of a WHO Expert Committee*; WHO Technical Report Series 854; World Health Organisation: Geneva, Switzerland, 1995.

98. Ng, S.P.; Korda, R.; Clements, M.; Latz, I.; Bauman, A.; Bambrick, H.; Liu, B.; Rogers, K.; Herbert, N.; Banks, E. Validity of self-reported height and weight and derived body mass index in middle-aged and elderly individuals in Australia. *Aust. N. Z. J. Public Health* **2011**, *35*, 557–563. [CrossRef] [PubMed]

99. Van Dyck, D.; Cerin, E.; Conway, T.L.; De Bourdeaudhuij, I.; Owen, N.; Kerr, J.; Cardon, G.; Frank, L.D.; Saelens, B.E.; Sallis, J.F. Perceived neighborhood environmental attributes associated with adults' transport-related walking and cycling: Findings from the USA, Australia and Belgium. *Int. J. Behav. Nutr. Phys. Act.* **2012**, *9*, 70. [CrossRef] [PubMed]

100. Van Dyck, D.; Cerin, E.; Conway, T.L.; De Bourdeaudhuij, I.; Owen, N.; Kerr, J.; Cardon, G.; Frank, L.D.; Saelens, B.E.; Sallis, J.F. Perceived neighborhood environmental attributes associated with adults' leisure-time physical activity: Findings from Belgium, Australia and the USA. *Health Place* **2013**, *19*, 59–68. [CrossRef] [PubMed]

101. Sallis, J.F.; Cerin, E.; Conway, T.L.; Adams, M.A.; Frank, L.D.; Pratt, M.; Salvo, D.; Schipperijn, J.; Smith, G.; Cain, K.L. Physical activity in relation to urban environments in 14 cities worldwide: A cross-sectional study. *Lancet* **2016**, *387*, 2207–2217. [CrossRef]

102. Astell-Burt, T.; Feng, X.; Kolt, G.S. Greener neighborhoods, slimmer people? Evidence from 246,920 Australians. *Int. J. Obes.* **2014**, *38*, 156, doi:10.1038/ijo.2013.64. [CrossRef] [PubMed]

103. Buchmueller, T.C.; Johar, M. Obesity and health expenditures: Evidence from Australia. *Econ. Hum. Biol.* **2015**, *17*, 42–58, doi:10.1016/j.ehb.2015.01.001. [CrossRef] [PubMed]

104. Charlton, K.; Kowal, P.; Soriano, M.; Williams, S.; Banks, E.; Vo, K.; Byles, J. Fruit and Vegetable Intake and Body Mass Index in a Large Sample of Middle-Aged Australian Men and Women. *Nutrients* **2014**, *6*, 2305. [CrossRef] [PubMed]

105. Creatore, M.I.; Glazier, R.H.; Moineddin, R.; Fazli, G.S.; Johns, A.; Gozdyra, P.; Matheson, F.I.; Kaufman-Shriqui, V.; Rosella, L.C.; Manuel, D.G. et al. Association of neighborhood walkability with change in overweight, obesity, and diabetes. *JAMA* **2016**, *315*, 2211–2220. [CrossRef] [PubMed]

106. Joshy, G.; Korda, R.J.; Attia, J.; Liu, B.; Bauman, A.E.; Banks, E. Body mass index and incident hospitalisation for cardiovascular disease in 158,546 participants from the 45 and Up Study. *Int. J. Obes.* **2014**, *38*, 848. [CrossRef] [PubMed]

107. Joshy, G.; Korda, R.J.; Bauman, A.; Van Der Ploeg, H.P.; Chey, T.; Banks, E. Investigation of Methodological Factors Potentially Underlying the Apparently Paradoxical Findings on Body Mass Index and All-Cause Mortality. *PLoS ONE* **2014**, *9*, e88641. [CrossRef] [PubMed]

108. Korda, R.J.; Liu, B.; Clements, M.S.; Bauman, A.E.; Jorm, L.R.; Bambrick, H.J.; Banks, E. Prospective cohort study of body mass index and the risk of hospitalisation: Findings from 246,361 participants in the 45 and Up Study. *Int. J. Obes.* **2013**, *37*, 790. [CrossRef] [PubMed]

109. Korda, R.J.; Joshy, G.; Paige, E.; Butler, J.R.G.; Jorm, L.R.; Liu, B.; Bauman, A.E.; Banks, E. The Relationship between Body Mass Index and Hospitalisation Rates, Days in Hospital and Costs: Findings from a Large Prospective Linked Data Study. *PLoS ONE* **2015**, *10*, e0118599. [CrossRef] [PubMed]

110. Magee, C.A.; Caputi, P.; Iverson, D.C. Is Sleep Duration Associated With Obesity in Older Australian Adults? *J. Aging Health* **2010**, *22*, 1235–1255. [CrossRef] [PubMed]

111. Magee, C.A.; Iverson, D.C.; Caputi, P. Sleep Duration and Obesity in Middle-aged Australian Adults. *Obesity* **2010**, *18*, 420–421. [CrossRef] [PubMed]

112. Nguyen, B.; Bauman, A.; Ding, D. Incident Type 2 Diabetes in a Large Australian Cohort Study: Does Physical Activity or Sitting Time Alter the Risk Associated With Body Mass Index? *J. Phys. Act. Health* **2017**, *14*, 13–19. [CrossRef] [PubMed]

113. Pedisic, Z.; Grunseit, A.; Ding, D.; Chau, J.Y.; Banks, E.; Stamatakis, E.; Jalaludin, B.B.; Bauman, A.E. High sitting time or obesity: Which came first? Bidirectional association in a longitudinal study of 32,787 Australian adults. *Obesity* **2014**, *22*, 2126–2130. [CrossRef] [PubMed]

114. Kessler, R.C.; Andrews, G.; Colpe, L.J.; Hiripi, E.; Mroczek, D.K.; Normand, S.L.T.; Walters, E.E.; Zaslavsky, A.M. Short screening scales to monitor population prevalences and trends in non-specific psychological distress. *Psychol. Med.* **2002**, *32*, 959–976. [CrossRef] [PubMed]

115. Australian Bureau of Statistics. Use of the Kessler Psychological Distress Scale in ABS Health Surveys, Australia, 2007-08 (Catalgue No. 4817.0.55.001). Available online: http://www.abs.gov.au/ausstats/abs@.nsf/mf/4817.0.55.001 (accessed on 31 January 2018).

116. Australian Bureau of Statistics. *National Survey of Mental Health and Wellbeing: Summary of Results*; Commonwealth of Australia: Canberra, Australia, 2007.

117. Australian Bureau of Statistics. Australian Health Survey: Users' Guide, 2011-13 (Catalogue No. 4363.0.55.001). Available online: http://www.abs.gov.au/ausstats/abs@.nsf/mf/4363.0.55.001 (accessed on 31 January 2018).

118. Ware, J. E., J.; Sherbourne, C.D. The MOS 36-item short-form health survey (SF-36). I. Conceptual framework and item selection. *Med. Care* **1992**, *30*, 473–483. [CrossRef] [PubMed]

119. Ware, J.E.; Snow, K.K.; Kosinski, M.; Gandek, B. *SF-36 Health Survey: Manual and Interpretation Guide*; The Health Institute, New England Medical Center: Boston, MA, USA, 1993.

120. Banks, E.; Jorm, L.; Rogers, K.; Clements, M.; Bauman, A. Screen-time, obesity, ageing and disability: Findings from 91,266 participants in the 45 and Up Study. *Public Health Nutr.* **2011**, *14*, 34–43. [CrossRef] [PubMed]

121. Waller, L.; Carlin, B. Disease Mapping. In *Handbook of Spatial Statistics*; Gelfand, A.E., Diggle, P.J., Feuentes, M., Guttorp, P., Eds.; Chapman & Hall/CRC Handbooks of Modern Statistical Methods; CRC Press: Boca Raton, FL, USA, 2010; pp. 217–244.

122. Leroux, B.G.; Lei, X.; Breslow, N. Estimation of Disease Rates in Small Areas: A new Mixed Model for Spatial Dependence. In *Statistical Models in Epidemiology, The Environment, and Clinical Trials*; Halloran, M.E., Berry, D., Eds.; Springer: New York, NY, USA, 2000; pp. 179–191.

123. Klassen, A.C.; Kulldorff, M.; Curriero, F. Geographical clustering of prostate cancer grade and stage at diagnosis, before and after adjustment for risk factors. *Int. J. Health Geogr.* **2005**, *4*, 1. [CrossRef] [PubMed]

124. Waldhoer, T.; Wald, M.; Heinzl, H. Analysis of the spatial distribution of infant mortality by cause of death in Austria in 1984 to 2006. *Int. J. Health Geogr.* **2008**, *7*, 21. [CrossRef] [PubMed]

125. Besag, J.; York, J.; Mollié, A. Bayesian image restoration, with two applications in spatial statistics. *Ann. Inst. Stat. Math.* **1991**, *43*, 1–20. [CrossRef]

126. Cowles, M.K.; Carlin, B.P. Markov Chain Monte Carlo Convergence Diagnostics: A Comparative Review. *J. Am. Stat. Assoc.* **1996**, *91*, 883–904. [CrossRef]

127. Spiegelhalter, D.J.; Best, N.G.; Carlin, B.P.; Van Der Linde, A. Bayesian measures of model complexity and fit. *J. R. Stat. Soc. Ser. B Stat. Methodol.* **2002**, *64*, 583–639. [CrossRef]

128. Cramb, S.M.; Mengersen, K.L.; Baade, P.D. Developing the atlas of cancer in Queensland: Methodological issues. *Int. J. Health Geogr.* **2011**, *10*, 9. [CrossRef] [PubMed]

129. Holowaty, E.J.; Norwood, T.A.; Wanigaratne, S.; Abellan, J.J.; Beale, L. Feasibility and utility of mapping disease risk at the neighbourhood level within a Canadian public health unit: An ecological study. *Int. J. Health Geogr.* **2010**, *9*, 21. [CrossRef] [PubMed]

130. Mealing, N.M.; Banks, E.; Jorm, L.R.; Steel, D.G.; Clements, M.S.; Rogers, K.D. Investigation of relative risk estimates from studies of the same population with contrasting response rates and designs. *BMC Med. Res. Methodol.* **2010**, *10*, 1–12. [CrossRef] [PubMed]

131. Mayne, D.J.; Morgan, G.G.; Jalaludin, B.B.; Bauman, A.E. Is it worth the weight? Adjusting physical activity ratio estimates for individual-level non-response is not required in area-level spatial analyses of the 45 and Up Study cohort. In Proceedings of the 45 and Up Study Annual Forum, Sydney, Australia, 24 October 2017.

132. The 45 and Up Study. The 45 and Up Study Data Book—April 2010 Release. Available online: https://www.saxinstitute.org.au/our-work/45-up-study/data-book/ (accessed on 31 January 2018).

133. Wasfi, R.A.; Dasgupta, K.; Orpana, H.; Ross, N.A. Neighborhood Walkability and Body Mass Index Trajectories: Longitudinal Study of Canadians. *Am. J. Public Health* **2016**, *106*, 934–940. [CrossRef] [PubMed]

134. James, P.; Kioumourtzoglou, M.A.; Hart, J.E.; Banay, R.F.; Kloog, I.; Laden, F. Interrelationships Between Walkability, Air Pollution, Greenness, and Body Mass Index. *Epidemiololgy* **2017**, *28*, 780–788. [CrossRef] [PubMed]

135. Kowaleski-Jones, L.; Brown, B.B.; Fan, J.X.; Hanson, H.A.; Smith, K.R.; Zick, C.D. The joint effects of family risk of obesity and neighborhood environment on obesity among women. *Soc. Sci. Med.* **2017**, *195*, 17–24. [CrossRef] [PubMed]

136. Loo, C.K.J.; Greiver, M.; Aliarzadeh, B.; Lewis, D. Association between neighbourhood walkability and metabolic risk factors influenced by physical activity: A cross-sectional study of adults in Toronto, Canada. *BMJ Open* **2017**, *7*. [CrossRef] [PubMed]

137. Méline, J.; Chaix, B.; Pannier, B.; Ogedegbe, G.; Trasande, L.; Athens, J.; Duncan, D.T. Neighborhood walk score and selected Cardiometabolic factors in the French RECORD cohort study. *BMC Public Health* **2017**, *17*, 960. [CrossRef] [PubMed]

138. Australian Urban Research Infrastructure Network (AURIN). Walkability Tools. Available online: https: //docs.aurin.org.au/portal-help/analysing-your-data/walkability-tools/ (accessed on 6 February 2019).

139. Frank, L.D.; Kerr, J.; Sallis, J.F.; Miles, R.; Chapman, J. A hierarchy of sociodemographic and environmental correlates of walking and obesity. *Prev. Med.* **2008**, *47*, 172–178. [CrossRef] [PubMed]

140. Rutt, C.D.; Coleman, K.J. Examining the relationships among built environment, physical activity, and body mass index in El Paso, TX. *Prev. Med.* **2005**, *40*, 831–841. [CrossRef] [PubMed]

141. Lunn, D.; Jackson, C.; Best, N.; Thomas, A.; Spiegelhalter, D. *The BUGS Book: A Practical Introduction to Bayesian Analysis*; Texts in Statistical Science; CRC Press: Boca Raton, FL, USA, 2012.

142. Latouche, A.; Guihenneuc-Jouyaux, C.; Girard, C.; Hémon, D. Robustness of the BYM model in absence of spatial variation in the residuals. *Int. J. Health Geogr.* **2007**, *6*, 1–8. [CrossRef] [PubMed]

143. Fotheringham, A.S.; Brunsdon, C.; Charlton, M. *Quantitative Geography: Perspectives on Apatial Data Analysis*; Sage Publications: London, UK, 2000; p. xii, 270p.

144. Fitzpatrick, J.; Griffiths, C.; Goldblatt, P. Introduction to the Volume. In *Geographic Variations in Health*; Griffiths, C., Fitzpatrick, J., Eds.; Office for National Statistics: London, UK, 2001.

145. Fontaine, K.R.; Cheskin, L.J.; Barofsky, I. Health-related quality of life in obese persons seeking treatment. *J. Fam. Pract.* **1996**, *43*, 265–270. [PubMed]

146. Katz, D.A.; McHorney, C.A.; Atkinson, R.L. Impact of obesity on health-related quality of life in patients with chronic illness. *J. Gen. Intern. Med.* **2000**, *15*, 789–796. [CrossRef] [PubMed]

147. Jia, H.; Lubetkin, E.I. The impact of obesity on health-related quality-of-life in the general adult US population. *J. Public Health* **2005**, *27*, 156–164. [CrossRef] [PubMed]

148. Frühbeck, G.; Toplak, H.; Woodward, E.; Yumuk, V.; Maislos, M.; Oppert, J.M. Obesity: The Gateway to Ill Health—An EASO Position Statement on a Rising Public Health, Clinical and Scientific Challenge in Europe. *Obes. Facts* **2013**, *6*, 117–120. [CrossRef] [PubMed]

149. Booth, H.P.; Prevost, A.T.; Gulliford, M.C. Impact of body mass index on prevalence of multimorbidity in primary care: Cohort study. *Fam. Pract.* **2014**, *31*, 38–43. [CrossRef] [PubMed]

150. Jackson, C.A.; Dobson, A.; Tooth, L.; Mishra, G.D. Body mass index and socioeconomic position are associated with 9-year trajectories of multimorbidity: A population-based study. *Prev. Med.* **2015**, *81*, 92–98. [CrossRef] [PubMed]

151. Kivimäki, M.; Kuosma, E.; Ferrie, J.E.; Luukkonen, R.; Nyberg, S.T.; Alfredsson, L.; Batty, G.D.; Brunner, E.J.; Fransson, E.; Goldberg, M.; et al. Overweight, obesity, and risk of cardiometabolic multimorbidity: Pooled analysis of individual-level data for 120 813 adults from 16 cohort studies from the USA and Europe. *Lancet Public Health* **2017**, *2*, e277–e285. [CrossRef]

152. Katikireddi, S.V.; Skivington, K.; Leyland, A.H.; Hunt, K.; Mercer, S.W. The contribution of risk factors to socioeconomic inequalities in multimorbidity across the lifecourse: A longitudinal analysis of the Twenty-07 cohort. *BMC Med.* **2017**, *15*, 152. [CrossRef] [PubMed]

153. Stafford, M.; Hemingway, H.; Marmot, M. Current obesity, steady weight change and weight fluctuation as predictors of physical functioning in middle aged office workers: The Whitehall II study. *Int. J. Obes.* **1998**, *22*, 23–31. [CrossRef]

154. Dowd, J.B.; Zajacova, A. Long-term obesity and physical functioning in older Americans. *Int. J. Obes.* **2015**, *39*, 502–507. [CrossRef] [PubMed]

155. Academy of Medical Sciences. *Multimorbidity: A Priority for Global Health Research*; Academy of Medical Sciences: London, UK, 2018.

156. Byles, J.E.; Gallienne, L.; Blyth, F.M.; Banks, E. Relationship of age and gender to the prevalence and correlates of psychological distress in later life. *Int. Psychogeriatr.* **2012**, *24*, 1009–1018. [CrossRef] [PubMed]

157. Byles, J.E.; Robinson, I.; Banks, E.; Gibson, R.; Leigh, L.; Rodgers, B.; Curryer, C.; Jorm, L. Psychological distress and comorbid physical conditions: Disease or disability? *Depress Anxiety* **2014**, *31*, 524–532. [CrossRef] [PubMed]

158. Ormel, J.; Rijsdijk, F.V.; Sullivan, M.; van Sonderen, E.; Kempen, G.I.J.M. Temporal and Reciprocal Relationship Between IADL/ADL Disability and Depressive Symptoms in Late Life. *J. Gerontol. B Psychol. Sci. Soc. Sci.* **2002**, *57*, P338–P347. [CrossRef] [PubMed]

159. Gaddey, H.L.; Holder, K. Unintentional weight loss in older adults. *Am. Fam. Physician* **2014**, *89*, 718–22. [PubMed]

160. Andrews, G.; Slade, T. Interpreting scores on the Kessler Psychological Distress Scale (K10). *Aust. N. Z. J. Public Health* **2001**, *25*, 494–497. [CrossRef] [PubMed]

161. Criqui, M.H. Response bias and risk ratios in epidemiologic studies. *Am. J. Epidemiol.* **1979**, *109*, 394–399. [CrossRef] [PubMed]

162. Nohr, E.A.; Frydenberg, M.; Henriksen, T.B.; Olsen, J. Does low participation in cohort studies induce bias? *Epidemiology* **2006**, *17*, 413–418. [CrossRef] [PubMed]

163. Centre for Epidemiology and Evidence. Adult Population Health Survey. Available online: http://www.health.nsw.gov.au/surveys/adult/Pages/default.aspx (accessed on 12 December 2018).

164. Department of Finance, Services and Innovation. NSW Open Data Policy. Available online: https://www.digital.nsw.gov.au/policy/data-information/making-data-open/nsw-open-data-policy (accessed on 4 February 2019).

165. Plantinga, A.J.; Bernell, S. The association between urban sprawl and obesity: Is it a two-way street? *J. Reg. Sci.* **2007**, *47*, 857–879. [CrossRef]

166. Eid, J.; Overman, H.G.; Puga, D.; Turner, M.A. Fat city: Questioning the relationship between urban sprawl and obesity. *J. Urban Econ.* **2008**, *63*, 385–404. [CrossRef]

167. Mokhtarian, P.L.; Cao, X. Examining the impacts of residential self-selection on travel behavior: A focus on methodologies. *Trans. Res. Part B Methodol.* **2008**, *42*, 204–228. [CrossRef]

168. Cao, X.; Mokhtarian, P.L.; Handy, S.L. Examining the Impacts of Residential Self-Selection on Travel Behaviour: A Focus on Empirical Findings. *Transp. Rev.* **2009**, *29*, 359–395. [CrossRef]

169. Kowaleski-Jones, L.; Zick, C.; Smith, K.R.; Brown, B.; Hanson, H.; Fan, J. Walkable neighborhoods and obesity: Evaluating effects with a propensity score approach. *SSM Popul. Health* **2018**, *6*, 9–15. [CrossRef] [PubMed]

170. Smith, K.R.; Zick, C.D.; Kowaleski-Jones, L.; Brown, B.B.; Fan, J.X.; Yamada, I. Effects of neighborhood walkability on healthy weight: Assessing selection and causal influences. *Soc. Sci. Res.* **2011**, *40*, 1445–1455. [CrossRef] [PubMed]

171. Smith, K.R.; Hanson, H.A.; Brown, B.B.; Zick, C.D.; Kowaleski-Jones, L.; Fan, J.X. Movers and stayers: How residential selection contributes to the association between female body mass index and neighborhood characteristics. *Int. J. Obes.* **2016**, *40*, 1384–1391. [CrossRef] [PubMed]

172. Hausman, J.A.; Abrevaya, J.; Scott-Morton, F.M. Misclassification of the dependent variable in a discrete-response setting. *J. Econ.* **1998**, *87*, 239–269. [CrossRef]

173. Tennekoon, V.; Rosenman, R. Systematically misclassified binary dependent variables. *Commun. Stat. Theory Method.* **2016**, *45*, 2538–2555. [CrossRef] [PubMed]

174. Openshaw, S.; Taylor, P.J. A Million or so Correlation Coefficients: Three Experiments on the Mmodifiable Areal Unit Problem. In *Statistical Applications in the Spatial Sciences*; Wrigley, N., Ed.; Pion: London, UK, 1979; pp. 127–144.

175. Openshaw, S. *The Modifiable Areal Unit Problem*; (CATMOG 38); Geo Books: Norwich, UK, 1984.

176. Greenland, S. Avoiding power loss associated with categorization and ordinal scores in dose-response and trend analysis. *Epidemiology* **1995**, *6*, 450–454. [CrossRef] [PubMed]

177. Bennette, C.; Vickers, A. Against quantiles: Categorization of continuous variables in epidemiologic research, and its discontents. *BMC Med. Res. Methodol.* **2012**, *12*, 21. [CrossRef] [PubMed]

178. Goovaerts, P.; Gebreab, S. How does Poisson kriging compare to the popular BYM model for mapping disease risks? *Int. J. Health Geogr.* **2008**, *7*, 1–25. [CrossRef] [PubMed]

179. Huque, M.H.; Anderson, C.; Walton, R.; Ryan, L. Individual level covariate adjusted conditional autoregressive (indiCAR) model for disease mapping. *Int. J. Health Geogr.* **2016**, *15*, 25. [CrossRef] [PubMed]

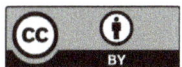

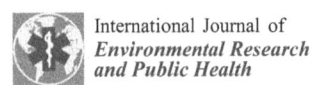
International Journal of
*Environmental Research and Public Health*

*Article*

# Children's Transport Built Environments: A Mixed Methods Study of Associations between Perceived and Objective Measures and Relationships with Parent Licence for Independent Mobility in Auckland, New Zealand

Melody Smith [1,*], Rebecca Amann [1], Alana Cavadino [1], Deborah Raphael [1], Robin Kearns [2], Roger Mackett [3], Lisa Mackay [4], Penelope Carroll [5], Euan Forsyth [2], Suzanne Mavoa [6], Jinfeng Zhao [1], Erika Ikeda [4] and Karen Witten [5]

[1] School of Nursing, The University of Auckland, Auckland 1142, New Zealand; rama919@aucklanduni.ac.nz (R.A.); a.cavadino@auckland.ac.nz (A.C.); d.raphael@auckland.ac.nz (D.R.); jinfeng.zhao@auckland.ac.nz (J.Z.)
[2] School of Environment, The University of Auckland, Auckland 1142, New Zealand; r.kearns@auckland.ac.nz (R.K.); e.forsyth@auckland.ac.nz (E.F.)
[3] Department of Civil, Environmental and Geomatic Engineering, University College London, London WC1E 6BT, UK; roger.mackett@ucl.ac.uk
[4] Human Potential Centre, Auckland University of Technology, Auckland 1142, New Zealand; Lisa.mackay@aut.ac.nz (L.M.); erika.ikeda@aut.ac.nz (E.I.)
[5] Social and Health Outcomes Research and Evaluation (SHORE), Massey University, Auckland 1142, New Zealand; P.A.Carroll@massey.ac.nz (P.C.); k.witten@massey.ac.nz (K.W.)
[6] Melbourne School of Population and Global Health, The University of Melbourne, Melbourne 3010, Australia; suzanne.mavoa@unimelb.edu.au
* Correspondence: melody.smith@auckland.ac.nz

Received: 15 March 2019; Accepted: 13 April 2019; Published: 16 April 2019

**Abstract:** Children's independent mobility is declining internationally. Parents are the gatekeepers of children's independent mobility. This mixed methods study investigates whether parent perceptions of the neighbourhood environment align with objective measures of the neighbourhood built environment, and how perceived and objective measures relate to parental licence for children's independent mobility. Parents participating in the Neighbourhood for Active Kids study ($n = 940$) answered an open-ended question about what would make their neighbourhoods better for their child's independent mobility, and reported household and child demographics. Objective measures of the neighbourhood built environment were generated using geographic information systems. Content analysis was used to classify and group parent-reported changes required to improve their neigbourhood. Parent-reported needs were then compared with objective neighbourhood built environment measures. Linear mixed modelling examined associations between parental licence for independent mobility and (1) parent neighbourhood perceptions; and (2) objectively assessed neighbourhood built environment features. Parents identified the need for safer traffic environments. No significant differences in parent reported needs were found by objectively assessed characteristics. Differences in odds of reporting needs were observed for a range of socio-demographic characteristics. Parental licence for independent mobility was only associated with a need for safer places to cycle (positive) and objectively assessed cycling infrastructure (negative) in adjusted models. Overall, the study findings indicate the importance of safer traffic environments for children's independent mobility.

**Keywords:** traffic safety; walking; cycling; infrastructure; active travel; active transport

---

## 1. Introduction

Physical activity is fundamental to optimal growth, development, and health in children. It is recommended that children and youth aged 5–17 years should participate in at least 60 minutes of moderate-to-vigorous intensity physical activity (MVPA) daily to gain important benefits for their musculoskeletal, cardiovascular, neuromuscular, metabolic, and mental health and development [1]. Yet physical activity levels are low globally [2], including in New Zealand, where a third of children and youth are insufficiently active for health [3].

### 1.1. Children's Independent Mobility

Children's independent mobility can provide important opportunities for children's physical activity accumulation. Independent mobility was first defined in the early 1990s as having the freedom to travel to destinations or engage in outdoor play without adult supervision [4]. Since that time, numerous definitions, associated metrics, and methods (e.g., parent vs. child reports) have been employed [5–7]. For the most part, literature has focused on parental licence for independent mobility, capturing a range of 'licences' to be independent outside the home environment. To a lesser extent, actualized independent mobility has also been explored, with a dominant focus on active travel (e.g., walking, scootering, or cycling) to school or neighbourhood destinations without adult accompaniment. Irrespective of the metric used, a growing evidence base has consistently demonstrated links between independent mobility and active travel to school [8], objectively-assessed physical activity [9–12], and less sedentary behaviour [12].

Independent mobility also plays an unparalleled role in contributing to children's development of social, cognitive, and spatial processing skills and enhanced environmental awareness. Children who travel and play freely in their neighbourhood socialise more frequently with their peers and adults [13–15] and develop a sense of belonging to their community [16] which is important for developing social skills and a sense of identity. Cognitive and psychological development is promoted through spatial awareness and processing [17], learning about risk and its management [13], and engagement with the natural and physical environment [13,14,18,19].

Despite its benefits, independent mobility has been declining globally over the past several decades [4,20,21]. By way of example, in Australia, repeated cross-sectional studies indicate the proportion of children travelling home from school independently halved from 68% in 1991 to 31% in 2012 [20]. Longitudinal data on independent mobility in the New Zealand context are not available. Looking at active travel in general (irrespective of accompaniment) the average time children spent in active travel modes decreased from 130 minutes per week to 72 minutes per week in the two decades prior to 2011. Latest household travel statistics show 70% of travel time for children is spent as a car passenger, and 10% is spent in active travel modes [20]. Less than half of New Zealand youth actively travel to school [3]. Accordingly, there has been increasing interest in understanding factors related to children's active travel in general as well as their independent mobility.

### 1.2. Factors Associated with Children's Independent Mobility

A socio-ecological perspective is helpful to understand the complexity of children's independent mobility [6,22]. In particular, the systems model proposed by Badland and colleagues [23] provides a robust framework for understanding factors related to children's independent mobility. The model encompasses policy and societal norms, as well as factors at the individual and neighbourhood level, which are described briefly below.

#### 1.2.1. Child and Household Characteristics

Parental licence for their child's independent mobility is strongly related to children's actualised independent mobility [24]. Parents are the 'gatekeepers' who determine the travel mode of their children and the degree of freedom they have to independently move in the neighbourhood [6,25].

Although children seek to influence their mobility licence [26], parents' views are invariably stronger than children's in determining independent mobility [27–29].

Individual factors that are associated with children moving independently in their environment include age and sex. Children who are older, especially after 12 years of age, are more likely to have licence from their parents to engage in independent mobility [9,24,30–32]. Many studies indicate that boys have higher rates of independent mobility compared to girls and tend to gain mobility licence earlier than girls [9,32,33]. This difference could be due to the higher parental fear of danger from strangers for girls [34,35].

More broadly, household and family factors such as car ownership, having older siblings [36], competing family schedules and trip chaining [37], and neighbourhood self-selection (i.e., a preference for residing in an environment that is characterized as being more or less walkable) [38–40] may also play important roles in actualizing children's independent mobility.

### 1.2.2. Parental Neighbourhood Perceptions

Parents' perceptions of the neighbourhood environment are associated with whether or not they grant their children independent mobility licence [41]. Parents who view their neighbourhood as safe are more inclined to encourage their children to be physically active outdoors [42]. Perceived safety of the neighbourhood environment may be an especially important indicator for parental licence for independent mobility [30,43], particularly regarding traffic safety and "stranger danger" [35,44]. If parents perceive their neighbourhoods as unsafe they are less likely to allow their children to be independent [45]. Conversely, a positive parental perception of safety from crime in the neighbourhood is associated with greater mobility licence [30,32]. "Stranger danger" has been noted as a concern for parents and has been linked to limited licence for independent mobility [9,34,35,46]. On the other hand, social interactions with neighbours [47] and social cohesion and trust [31,32,48] could contribute to creating a neighbourhood that 'looks out for children' and thus encourages independent mobility.

Safety from traffic is a key priority for parents [24,49]. Numerous studies have shown that parental fear of traffic danger is associated with limiting children's independent mobility licence [21,32,35,36,45,50,51]. Wolfe and McDonald [32] concluded that parents who had a positive view of traffic safety in their neighbourhood were more likely to grant their children licence for independent mobility. Parents who lived on busy roads [51], who had concerns about high traffic volumes [32], or who lived in less urbanised areas [35] had more traffic safety concerns and their children had less independent mobility. On the other hand, safe road crossings were associated with increased independent mobility of boys in a study of Australian children [51].

Moving beyond neighbourhood safety, a number of built environment features, as perceived by parents, have been related to independent active travel and physical activity of children [28]. Specifically, perceived accessibility to destinations, high land use mix, short distance to school, residential density, and well-maintained walking and cycling infrastructure have all been positively associated with children's independent active travel.

### 1.2.3. Objective Measures of the Environment

The objectively-assessed built environment has also been significantly associated with children's independent mobility [51]. Sharmin and Kamruzzaman [52] argue that changes in children's independent mobility are related to the built environment context (e.g., distance to destination and availability of facilities), urban structure (e.g., urban vs. suburban) or urban form alterations (e.g., intersection density, traffic safety infrastructure). However, to date the evidence remains sparse and inconsistent, thus this section also includes some relevant literature on active travel and physical activity.

Street connectivity has been positively associated with active travel [53,54] and independent mobility [55] in some studies. Conversely, there is also evidence that culs-de-sac (dead end streets) are strongly associated with independent mobility [52]. To some extent, this may be a function of the metric of independent mobility used. For example, where independent active travel is the focus, street connectivity would be expected to have a significant role in understanding independent mobility. Conversely, where independent play is of interest, prevalence of neighbourhood culs-de-sac in which to play may be of greater importance. Linked with street connectivity, accessibility to destinations such as schools, parks, and other local settings has been positively associated with active travel and independent mobility [45,54]. Villanueva and colleagues [51] concluded that, in addition to the proximity of destinations, the aesthetics and appeal of destinations are also important features of the built environment that facilitate independent mobility.

Studies in Portugal have shown that when comparing rural and urban areas, increased urbanisation leads to decreased independent mobility of children [24,35]. On the other hand, a meta-analysis by Sharmin and Kamruzzaman [52] concluded that urban–suburban residential location type, and a higher proportion of commercial and residential land use are positively associated with children's independent mobility. To some extent these mismatches may be because these broad environmental measures are not sufficiently fine-grained or population-specific to be relevant to parental decision-making around their child's independent mobility. The field is advancing, however, with examples being the development of new child-specific measures for walkability [56] and destination accessibility [57].

There is also some uncertainty and inconsistency about how objective built environment measures and parent perceptions of the built environment relate, especially in regard to traffic safety. Carver and colleagues [27] identified that there is vagueness as to whether the neighbourhood traffic safety perceptions of parents impact children's physical activity more than objective road safety measures. To date, this has not been clear. Marzi and colleagues [41] concluded in their systematic review that parents' perception of neighbourhood, including that of traffic safety, have a greater impact on children's independent mobility than related built environmental measures. In contrast, Uys and colleagues' study in South Africa concluded that the objective built environment was more strongly associated with out-of-school physical activity of children [58].

### 1.3. Study Aim and Objectives

It is likely that both objective and perceived environmental factors are important in understanding children's independent mobility. Hence, how they relate to each other and with parental licence for independent mobility needs to be better understood to guide and inform future research and practice. The overall aim of this study was to provide new knowledge about factors associated with parental licence for children's independent mobility. Study objectives were: (1) to identify key factors of importance from parent perspectives that would support children's independent neighbourhood active travel, (2) to contextualise parent perceptions in relation to objectively assessed variables around the individual household address, and (3) to determine associations between parental licence for independent mobility and objective neighbourhood built environment measures and parent-reported needs.

## 2. Materials and Methods

### 2.1. Protocol and Study Context

Neighbourhoods for Active Kids was a cross-sectional study of children residing in Auckland, New Zealand. Auckland is New Zealand's largest city with a population of 1.4 million people, a third of New Zealand's total population [59]. The urban landscape of Auckland is comprised largely of suburban neighbourhoods, however there is a move to more compact city housing due to pressures of increasing population and lack of affordable housing [60].

The full study methods are described elsewhere [61]. In brief, addresses of all intermediate schools (junior high school, years 7–8, approximate ages 10–13) in Auckland were geocoded and child-specific measures of walkability [56] and destination accessibility [57] generated for each school. A matrix of walkability, destination accessibility, and school decile (a measure of area-level socioeconomic status [62]) was then used to select schools for invitation, with the aim of ensuring heterogeneity in these factors across the study neighbourhoods. Ensuring heterogeneity in geographic location (north, south, east, west, and central Auckland) was also prioritised. For each intermediate school, a contributing primary school (elementary school, years 1–6, approximate ages 5–11 years) was also invited to participate in the study, resulting in a primary-intermediate school dyad in each neighbourhood.

Either Principal or Board of Trustees (governing body of school) consent for their school to participate was required before initiating participant recruitment. Research team members visited each school to explain the study protocols to teachers and students, and deliver child and parent information sheets, child assent forms, and parent/caregiver consent forms for their child and themselves to participate. Those interested in participating were asked to return the signed forms to the school within two weeks (during which time children and their families were invited to ask the research team any questions they had about the study). A signed assent form and signed parent/caregiver consent form were required for a child to participate in the study.

Researchers visited schools during school time to undertake an online participatory mapping survey to capture children's neighbourhood use and perceptions, measure school routes and perceptions of the school route, and capture measures of food purchasing and consumption of unhealthy foods. Height, weight, and waist circumference were measured by trained researchers at this time and children were provided with an accelerometer on a belt and instructions on how to wear the units for the next seven days. Post collection of the accelerometers, a computer-aided telephone interview (CATI) was conducted with parents/caregivers of participating children. The CATI collected sociodemographic information about the child and household, parent neighbourhood perceptions, licence for their child's independent mobility, and reports of their child's activity and nutrition behaviours. For each school, a face-to-face (or telephone-based) semi-structured interview was conducted with the school Principal or delegate to capture contextual information about supports for active travel to school and related policies and initiatives. Objective measures of the built environment for physical activity and nutrition were generated around the home neighbourhood environment, school neighbourhood environment [63], school route [8,64], and home-school neighbourhood [65]. Measures specific to the current study are described below.

Data were collected between February 2015 and December 2016. Ethical approval to conduct the study was provided by the host institution ethics committees (AUTEC, 14/263, 3 September 2014; MUHECN 3 September 2014; UAHPEC 9 September 2014).

*2.2. Measures*

2.2.1. Socio-Demographic Information

Parents reported on the biological sex (male, female) of their child and main ethnic group in the CATI survey. Ethnicity variables were adapted to combine 'Middle Eastern/Latin America/African' ($n = 17$) 'other' ($n = 4$), and 'not stated' ($n = 158$) due to low frequencies. School level (primary, intermediate) was recorded during the school-based data collection and used as a proxy for age. Parents were asked how many working cars they had available to them in their household. Area-level socio-economic status was determined using the NZDep2013, an index of deprivation comprising Census-derived measures of income, housing tenure, employment, educational qualifications, family structure, household crowding, access to transport, and communications at the meshblock level (smallest Census-area unit) [66]. Deciles were aggregated into categories of low deprivation (decile 1–3), medium deprivation (decile 4–7), and high deprivation (decile 8–10).

2.2.2. Independent Mobility Licence

Licence for independent mobility was assessed using six items from the Policy Studies Institute study of children's independent mobility [21]. Parents were asked whether their child was allowed to travel home from school alone, cross main roads on their own, cycle on main roads alone, go out alone after dark, and go on local public transport on their own. Response options were: always, often, sometimes, and never. Parents were also asked whether their child was usually taken or allowed to go alone to places other than school that were within walking distance. Response options were: usually goes alone, varies, and usually taken. All six items were considered in principal components analysis to generate a measure of independent mobility licence. Bartlett's test of sphericity ($p < 0.001$), and the Kaiser–Meyer–Olkin measure of sampling adequacy (0.697) were deemed acceptable. One component was extracted which explained 32.5% of the variance. A higher score indicated higher licence for independent mobility.

### 2.2.3. Parent-Reported Needs

Parents were asked "What would make your neighbourhood a better place for (Child Name) to walk, bike or scooter by (Himself/Herself)?" Responses were open-ended and parents could mention more than one factor, or choose not to respond.

### 2.2.4. Objectively-Assessed Neighbourhood Built Environment Features

Objective measures were calculated in ArcMap 10.5 (Environmental Systems Research Institute, Redlands, CA, USA) using an 800 m pedestrian street network buffer around each child participant's residential address only. Within the pedestrian network, all motorways and state highway segments were removed to best reflect the pedestrian environment. Unless otherwise specified, spatial data were sourced from the Auckland Council, via the University of Auckland's GeoData Hub database.

#### Ratio of High- to Low-Speed Roads

Traffic speed exposure was measured as the ratio of high speed (>60 km/hour) road length (HSRL) to low speed (<60 km/hour) road lengths (LSRL) within the neighbourhood boundary [56]. The ratio was calculated as HSRL/LSRL, with a higher ratio indicating a greater number of high-speed roads relative to low-speed roads, and thus greater exposure to vehicular traffic.

#### Number of Signalised Crossings

Data on pedestrian crossings at controlled intersections (i.e., with a crossing light) were downloaded from Auckland Transport's Open GIS Data platform (https://data-atgis.opendata.arcgis.com/). A spatial join between each neighbourhood buffer and the pedestrian crossing points was implemented, with the sum count of points intersecting each buffer returned.

#### Ratio of Cycle Path Lengths to Road Lengths

Data for Auckland's cycle lane network were drawn from Auckland Transport's Open GIS Data platform (https://data-atgis.opendata.arcgis.com/). Total cycle lane length (CLL; km) within the neighbourhood buffer was divided by all road lengths (ARL; km), regardless of speed limits to generate a ratio of CLL/ARL, where a higher ratio indicates more cycle lane availability relative to roads.

#### Pedestrian Network Connectivity (PedShed)

PedShed was measured as the ratio of reachable pedestrian network area (network buffer area; NBA) to the maximum possible area (Euclidean buffer area; EBA) within a given distance of each participant's residence [56]. The NBA was derived using the pedestrian street network buffer, and the EBA via a Euclidian buffering of the residence point. The pedestrian network connectivity variable was calculated as NBA/EBA, with a higher ratio indicating that a greater proportion of the maximum possible distance can be reached through the pedestrian network and, therefore, a more connected pedestrian network.

### 2.3. Data Analysis

#### 2.3.1. Objective 1

Content analysis was performed on parent responses to the CATI question "What would make your neighbourhood a better place for (Child Name) to walk, bike or scooter by (Himself/Herself)?" The lead author undertook initial coding with 40% of responses to develop a coding framework for key topics and subtopics (saturation was achieved). Deborah Raphael then independently coded all responses using the framework. Finally, the lead author randomly cross-checked 20% of the full coded dataset. Any disagreements were resolved, and decisions made from this process were used to determine the final coding framework used to code the data. Descriptive statistics for whether or not a subtopic was mentioned by parents were calculated. These were summed to calculate overall frequency of key topics being reported by parents.

IBM SPSS Statistics 24 (IBM Corp, Armonk, NY, USA) was used for all descriptive and inferential analyses. From the content analysis, four topics were identified (based on ranking first and secondly on availability of related objective measures) and recalculated as binary outcomes (i.e., whether parent had reported the topic or not).

#### 2.3.2. Objective 2

Mixed effects logistic regression modelling was employed to examine whether there were any significant differences in parent-reported needs by their corresponding objectively-assessed neighbourhood features (outlined in Table 1). All models were adjusted for school level, sex of child, child ethnicity, and deprivation, with neighbourhood included as a random effect. All ratio measures were reclassified into binary variables using the median value to classify variables as low or high [56]. A $p$-value threshold of 0.05 was used to determine statistical significance.

**Table 1.** Parent reported need and corresponding objective measure of the neighbourhood built environment.

| Parent-Reported Needs | Objectively-Assessed Neighbourhood Features | Key Considerations Regarding Making Direct Comparisons |
|---|---|---|
| Less, slower, and safer traffic | Ratio of high to low speed roads | Objective measure provides an estimate only of traffic safety based on road hierarchy (and does not account for actual driver behavior irrespective of regulatory environment); parent-reported traffic safety needs included a broad range of strategies to reduce speeds and volume of traffic |
| More and safer crossings | Number of signalised crossings | Objective measure only takes signalled crossings into account; parent-reported needs included comments about non-signalled crossings |
| Safer and designated cycle lanes | Ratio of cycle path lengths to road lengths | Objective measure is limited to data available for the cycle network; parent-reported needs included bike paths and also the quality of places to cycle safely |
| More and better walking paths | PedShed | Objective measure provides an indication of the relative prevalence of places to walk only; parent-reported needs noted additional considerations such as wider and better-maintained footpaths |

#### 2.3.3. Objective 3

Differences in parental licence for independent mobility were tested for socio-demographic variables using Mann–Whitney U Tests (for sex and school level) and Kruskal–Wallis H Test (for ethnicity and deprivation). Non-parametric tests were used due to non-normal distribution of independent mobility licence. Mixed-effects linear models were used to examine relationships with parental licence for their child's independent mobility, including the corresponding perceived and objective measures simultaneously in each model. Sex of child, school level, child ethnicity, and deprivation were all included as fixed effects and neighbourhood was included as a random effect. Interactions between objective and perceived measures were also tested. A *p*-value threshold of 0.05 was used to determine statistical significance.

## 3. Results

Overall, 19 schools across 9 neighbourhoods in Auckland participated in the study. In total, 940 parents participated in the study, providing information about their household, child, and neighbourhood perceptions. Nine cases were eliminated from the analysis due to missing data, yielding a final sample of 931 parents.

### 3.1. Objective 1: Parent-Reported Needs

Parents' responses to the question "What would make your neighbourhood a better place for (Child Name) to walk, bike or scooter by (Himself/Herself)?" fell broadly under nine key areas as outlined in Table 2. A majority of parents (88.1%) thought there were physical and social environmental aspects that could make their neighbourhood better for their children to be able to walk, cycle, and scooter around. Three percent of parents made positive comments about their neighbourhoods such as:

"I feel that this area is very community focused and it feels quite safe and feels quite child friendly."

Over half of parents (50.3%) mentioned a need for a safer transport environment (less, slower, and safer traffic; and having safe places to cross, cycle, and walk), with the greatest need being less, slower, and safer traffic (19.9%). Specifically, parents consistently noted a need for the following:

Slower and safer drivers, for example: "If people keep to the speed limit it would make me feel safer"

Less traffic: "The road traffic is busy and too hard for the kids to use."

more traffic-calming infrastructure: "More speed bumps and more signs near the schools so people can see them and slow down."

Lower speed limits: "Lower speed limits or speed bumps around the area as the people tend to speed down the road and there are a lot of kids in the area that play near the roads."

Signage such as "kids around" to slow traffic and encourage safe driver behaviour: "More caution signs on [X] Road where we live as the traffic whizzes through … More caution signs in the hope that people will pay attention to these signs."

Safer places to cross: "More pedestrian crossings on the roads as cars speed around the area"

Safer places to cycle: "I'd like to see a dedicated cycle lanes attached to the footpaths that link up to the school."

Safer places to walk: "Decent footpaths as we have no footpaths on our side of the road and so this is a big deterrent. Also cycle ways would be great as in the bays here we have narrow winding roads."

The social environment of the neighbourhood was also significant for parents. Twelve percent of parents reported that safety from others (in particular reduced sense of "stranger danger", increased community surveillance, reduced drug and gang related crimes, fewer roaming dogs and less bullying from youth) would make their neighbourhood better. A more connected community and having more people 'out and about' in their neighbourhood was considered important by 3.5% of the parents, for example:

"I guess if we all get together as a neighbourhood and get to know each other very well then we could all look out for each other's kids and we would get to trust each other."

**Table 2.** Descriptive statistics for key topics derived from parent responses to the question "What would make your neighbourhood a better place for (Child Name) to walk, bike or scooter by (Himself/Herself)?" (*n* = 931).

| Topic and Subtopics | *n* [a] | % [a] |
|---|---|---|
| **Safety from traffic: Less, slower, and safer traffic** | **185** | **19.9** |
| Less busy traffic | 65 | 7.0 |
| Slower speeds | 56 | 6.0 |
| Traffic calming infrastructure (e.g., humps) | 38 | 4.1 |
| Lowering speed limits | 37 | 4.0 |
| Reducing dangerous driving | 34 | 3.7 |
| Improving traffic safety in general | 19 | 2.0 |
| Signage to slow traffic (e.g., "kids around", "slow down") | 6 | 0.6 |
| **Safety from traffic: More and safer crossings** | **125** | **13.4** |
| More and safer pedestrian crossings | 121 | 13.0 |
| Lights at pedestrian crossings | 4 | 0.4 |
| Supervised crossings | 1 | 0.1 |
| **Safety from traffic: Safer and designated cycle lanes** | **91** | **9.8** |
| Cycle lanes—designated, away from road, on footpaths | 66 | 7.1 |
| Bike tracks and paths | 26 | 2.8 |
| **Safety from traffic: More and better walking paths** | **67** | **7.2** |
| **Safety from others** | **112** | **12.0** |
| Reduced "stranger danger" | 50 | 5.4 |
| Community surveillance | 43 | 4.6 |
| Reduced crime (drugs and gang activity) | 19 | 2.0 |
| Fewer roaming dogs | 12 | 1.3 |
| Reduced perceived danger from others especially youth | 9 | 1.0 |
| Less bullying | 4 | 0.4 |
| **More and better destinations** | **37** | **4.0** |
| More destinations in the neighbourhood | 23 | 2.5 |
| More and better facilities at the destinations | 16 | 1.7 |
| **Better social environment** | **33** | **3.5** |
| More connected community | 25 | 2.7 |
| More children/people out and about | 9 | 1.0 |
| **Others** | **232** | **24.9** |
| Better street lighting | 56 | 6.0 |
| Child too young | 45 | 4.8 |
| Nothing | 38 | 4.1 |
| Positive Comments | 31 | 3.3 |
| Less hilly | 14 | 1.5 |
| Safer neighbourhood | 12 | 1.3 |
| Other | 10 | 1.1 |
| More public transport and school buses | 9 | 1.0 |

**Table 2.** *Cont.*

| Topic and Subtopics | $n$ [a] | % [a] |
|---|---|---|
| Fewer cars parked on street | 8 | 0.9 |
| Better general infrastructure | 8 | 0.9 |
| More walking school buses (adult accompanying group of children to school) | 7 | 0.8 |
| Better upkeep of public spaces | 6 | 0.6 |
| Better visibility of the streets | 4 | 0.4 |
| Improved connectivity | 3 | 0.3 |
| Uncodeable | 3 | 0.3 |

[a] Data are presented for the number and percentage of parents who noted these topics and subtopics. Note: $n$ and % of topics do not equate to the total of all the subtopics due to some parents mentioning more than one subtopic in one topic.

### 3.2. Quantitative Modelling

#### 3.2.1. Descriptive Characteristics

Sociodemographic characteristics of children were relatively evenly distributed with the exception of ethnicity, where a majority were of New Zealand European/Pākehā/Other European ethnicity (42.3%) (Table 3). Parental licence for independent mobility scores were positively skewed, ranging from 3.30 to 10.72 with a mean of 5.28 (*SD* = 1.67). Boys had significantly higher licence for independent mobility than girls ($p < 0.001$). Similarly, older children had significantly higher licence for independent mobility than their younger peers ($p < 0.001$). There was a significant difference in licence for independent mobility between ethnic groups with Pacific children having lower independent mobility than other groups ($p = 0.001$). Almost all parents (98.4%) reported having at least one working car available in their household, with 78% reporting availability of two or more cars. Descriptive information for the objectively assessed neighbourhood environmental features is provided in Table 4.

**Table 3.** Socio-demographic characteristics of children and their licence for independent mobility ($n = 931$).

| Socio-Demographic Variables | $n$ | % | Licence for Independent Mobility Mean (SD) | $p$-Value |
|---|---|---|---|---|
| **Sex** | | | | <0.001 [c] |
| Male | 469 | 50.4 | 5.65 (1.73) | |
| Female | 462 | 49.6 | 5.00 (1.67) | |
| **School level** | | | | <0.001 [c] |
| Primary (years 5–6) | 486 | 52.2 | 4.58 (1.32) | |
| Intermediate (years 7–8) | 445 | 47.8 | 6.04 (1.69) | |
| **Ethnicity** | | | | 0.001 [d] |
| New Zealand European/Pākehā/Other European | 394 | 42.3 | 5.41 (1.61) | |
| Māori | 112 | 12.0 | 5.49 (1.67) | |
| Pacific | 125 | 13.4 | 4.94 (1.73) | |
| Asian | 120 | 12.9 | 5.04 (1.62) | |
| MELAA [a]/Other/Not stated | 180 | 19.3 | 5.25 (1.77) | |
| **Area-level deprivation [b]** | | | | 0.106 [d] |
| Low Deprivation (decile 1–3) | 357 | 38.3 | 5.36 (1.67) | |
| Medium Deprivation (decile 4–7) | 324 | 34.8 | 5.31 (1.65) | |
| High Deprivation (decile 8–10) | 250 | 26.9 | 5.13 (1.71) | |

[a] MELAA = Middle Eastern, Latin American, or African; [b] NZDep13 score calculated for each individual household at the meshblock level; [c] $p$-value from Mann-Whitney U Test; [d] $p$-value from Kruskal-Wallis H Test.

**Table 4.** Descriptive information for objectively-assessed neighbourhood features (*n* = 931).

| Objectively-Assessed Neighbourhood Features [a] | Minimum | Maximum | Mean (SD) |
|---|---|---|---|
| Ratio of high to low speed roads | 0.00 | 1.00 | 0.37 (0.11) |
| Number of signalised crossings | 0.00 | 7.00 | 1.01 (1.40) |
| Ratio of cycle paths to road lengths | 0.00 | 0.74 | 0.12 (0.13) |
| PedShed [b] | 0.01 | 0.63 | 0.32 (0.11) |

[a] Variable corresponding to parent-reported need; derived within the 800 m street network individual neighbourhood buffer using Geographic Information Systems; [b] Ratio of reachable pedestrian network area to the maximum possible area; a higher ratio indicates a more connected pedestrian network.

### 3.2.2. Objective 2: Differences in Objectively-Assessed Neighbourhood Features by Parent-Reported Needs

Given the parental focus on transport-related topics (and the availability of corresponding objective data), the following four variables were considered in further analyses related to objective measures and parental licence for independent mobility: less, slower, and safer traffic; more and safer crossings; safer and designated cycle lanes; and more and better walking paths.

Results from mixed effects logistic regression models testing for differences in odds of reporting a need by objectively-assessed neighbourhood built environment and socio-demographic characteristics are presented in Table 5. Taking socio-demographic factors and neighbourhood into account, no statistically significant differences in parent reported needs were observed between those residing in a more or less supportive neighbourhood (objectively assessed). Differences in odds of reporting needs were observed for a range of socio-demographic characteristics. Parents of primary school-aged children had significantly higher odds of reporting a need for less, slower, and safer traffic (OR 1.54, *p* = 0.014), and significantly lower odds of reporting a need for safer and designated cycle lanes (OR 0.48, *p* = 0.003). Compared with those of New Zealand/other European ethnicity, parents of children of Pacific ethnicity had significantly lower odds of reporting needing less, slower, and safer traffic; more and safer crossings; and safer and designated cycle lanes (ORs 0.06 to 0.36, all *p* < 0.01). All ethnic groups were significantly less likely to report a need for safer and designated cycle lanes compared with the reference group (NZ European/pākehā/other European; ORs 0.06 to 0.51, all *p* < 0.05). Differences in deprivation were only observed for reporting a need for more and better walking paths, with those from medium or high deprivation areas significantly less likely to report this need compared with those residing in areas of lower deprivation.

**Table 5.** Differences in parent-reported needs by objectively-assessed neighbourhood built environment characteristics and socio-demographic factors (n = 931).

| Parent-Reported Need [a] n (% of Parents Reporting Need) | Less, Slower, and Safer Traffic n = 185 (19.9%) | | More and Safer Crossings n = 125 (13.4%) | | Safer and Designated Cycle Lanes n = 91 (9.8%) | | More and Better Walking Paths n = 67 (7.2%) | |
|---|---|---|---|---|---|---|---|---|
| Objective Measure | Ratio of High to Low Speed Roads | | Number of Signalised Crossings | | Ratio of Cycle Path to Road Lengths | | PedShed [b] | |
| | OR (95% CI) [c] | p-Value | OR (95% CI) [c] | p-Value | OR (95% CI) [c] | p-Value | OR (95% CI) [c] | p-Value |
| Objective measure (higher vs. lower) [d] | | | | | | | | |
| Lower | Reference | | Reference | | Reference | | Reference | |
| Higher | 0.79 (0.54, 1.14) | 0.208 | 0.90 (0.72, 1.11) | 0.314 | 1.02 (0.56, 1.87) | 0.944 | 0.77 (0.34, 1.73) | 0.527 |
| Sex | | | | | | | | |
| Male | Reference | | Reference | | Reference | | Reference | |
| Female | 0.93 (0.67, 1.31) | 0.693 | 0.73 (0.49, 1.09) | 0.125 | 0.78 (0.49, 1.24) | 0.296 | 0.87 (0.47, 1.60) | 0.527 |
| School level | | | | | | | | |
| Intermediate (years 7–8) | Reference | | Reference | | Reference | | Reference | |
| Primary (years 5–6) | 1.54 (1.09, 2.19) | 0.014 | 1.01 (0.67, 1.52) | 0.980 | 0.48 (0.29, 0.77) | 0.003 | 1.41 (0.66, 3.00) | 0.372 |
| Ethnicity | | | | | | | | |
| NZ European/Pākehā/Other European | Reference | | Reference | | Reference | | Reference | |
| Māori | 0.78 (0.43, 1.44) | 0.432 | 0.60 (0.27, 1.34) | 0.214 | 0.12 (0.03, 0.52) | 0.004 | 0.30 (0.06, 1.53) | 0.147 |
| Pacific | 0.36 (0.17, 0.76) | 0.008 | 0.13 (0.03, 0.59) | 0.008 | 0.06 (0.01, 0.50) | 0.009 | 0.29 (0.05, 1.55) | 0.148 |
| Asian | 0.61 (0.34, 1.10) | 0.103 | 0.48 (0.22, 1.03) | 0.058 | 0.28 (0.11, 0.75) | 0.012 | 0.37 (0.07, 1.82) | 0.220 |
| MELAA [a]/Other/Not stated | 0.85 (0.51, 1.42) | 0.543 | 0.93 (0.49, 1.75) | 0.816 | 0.51 (0.26, 1.00) | 0.049 | 2.01 (0.73, 5.52) | 0.174 |
| Area-level deprivation [b] | | | | | | | | |
| Low | Reference | | Reference | | Reference | | Reference | |
| Medium | 1.08 (0.72, 1.61) | 0.708 | 0.83 (0.53, 1.28) | 0.396 | 0.84 (0.51, 1.39) | 0.504 | 0.15 (0.07, 0.33) | <0.001 |
| High | 1.08 (0.60, 1.96) | 0.796 | 0.50 (0.22, 1.18) | 0.113 | 0.40 (0.15, 1.08) | 0.071 | 0.22 (0.07, 0.67) | 0.008 |

[a] Variable corresponding to parent-reported need; derived within the 800 m street network individual neighbourhood buffer using Geographic Information Systems; [b] Measure of walking path availability; area of network buffer/area of radial buffer; [c] Estimates from mixed effects logistic regression with random intercept for neighbourhood; [d] Objective measures are included in each model as binary variables to compare those with 'higher' and 'lower' objective measures, defined as being above or below the median value for each.

### 3.2.3. Objective 3: Relationships between Parental Licence for Independent Mobility and Objective Neighbourhood Features and Parent-Reported Needs

Results from linear mixed models of relationships between objectively-assessed neighbourhood features and parent-reported needs and parental licence for independent mobility are presented in Table 6. No significant interactions between objective neighbourhood environment variables and parent reported needs were observed. In the fully adjusted models, both parent-reported need for safe cycling infrastructure (positive) and objectively-assessed cycle infrastructure (negative) were significantly related to parental licence for independent mobility. Children of parents who thought more dedicated and safer cycle lanes in their neighbourhood would make it better for their children to walk, bike, and scooter, had 0.56 higher parental independent mobility licence score on average, compared to parents who did not mention safer places to cycle ($p = 0.001$). Parent licence for their child's independent mobility was an average of 0.46 lower for those residing in areas with a higher ratio of cycle path to road length compared with those who lived in areas with a lower ratio of cycle path to road length.

**Table 6.** Mutually adjusted association of parent reported needs and related objective neighbourhood features with children's licence for independent mobility ($n = 931$).

| Neighbourhood Variables in Model | Comparison | Estimate (95% CI) [a] | *p*-Value |
|---|---|---|---|
| Ratio of high to low speed roads [b] | Higher vs. lower | −0.05 (−0.26, 0.17) | 0.682 |
| Less, slower, and safer traffic [c] | Parent reported vs. didn't report need | −0.03 (−0.2, 0.21) | 0.811 |
| Number of signalised crossings [b] | Per additional crossing | −0.04 (−0.15, 0.06) | 0.421 |
| More and safer crossings [c] | Parent reported vs. didn't report need | 0.01 (−0.27, 0.29) | 0.944 |
| Ratio of cycle path to road lengths [b] | Higher vs. lower | −0.46 (−0.71, −0.20) | 0.001 |
| Safer and designated cycle lanes [c] | Parent reported vs. didn't report need | 0.56 (0.24, 0.88) | 0.001 |
| PedShed [b,d] | Higher vs. lower | 0.20 (−0.01, 0.41) | 0.058 |
| More and better walking paths [c] | Parent reported vs. didn't report need | −0.14 (−0.55, 0.27) | 0.506 |

[a] Linear mixed models with random intercept for neighbourhood to account for neighbourhood clustering, including the objectively-assessed neighbourhood feature and the related parent-reported need, and adjusted for sex of child, school year level, ethnicity, and meshblock-level deprivation; [b] Objectively assessed variable corresponding to parent-reported need; derived within the 800 m street network individual neighbourhood buffer using Geographic Information Systems; [c] Parent-reported need; [d] Measure of walking path availability; area of network buffer/area of radial buffer.

## 4. Discussion

The aim of this study was to understand factors related to parental licence for their child's independent mobility in a large sample of parents of children aged 8–13 years residing in Auckland, New Zealand. A sequential approach was taken using mixed methods. Firstly, data derived from parent interviews were used to determine factors that parents perceived would make their neighbourhood better for their child to be independently mobile. Secondly, objective neighbourhood built environment variables were generated and examined in relation to parent reported needs. Finally, associations between parental licence for their child's independent mobility were determined with key objective and perceived neighbourhood variables. Key findings were that: (1) parents identified a need for safer traffic environments for their child's independent mobility; (2) no significant differences were observed between objective neighbourhood built environment measures and parents' reported neighbourhood needs; and (3) parental licence for their child's independent mobility was positively associated with parent perceptions that dedicated and safer places to bike were needed in their neighbourhood and negatively associated with residing in an area with a higher ratio of cycle path to road lengths. These findings are discussed in detail below and contextualized within independent mobility literature, supplemented by evidence for children's active travel where relevant.

### 4.1. Objective 1: Parents' Perceptions on What Would Make Their Neighbourhood Better for Independent Mobility

Content analysis of parents' answers to the question "what would make their neighbourhoods better for their child to walk, cycle and scooter in?" showed that a majority of the parents believed aspects of their neighbourhood could be improved. A key finding was that parents identified a safer traffic environment as a major need for their children's independent mobility (50.3% of parents overall). Particularly, less, slower, and safer traffic (19.9%); more pedestrian crossings (13.4%); more designated cycle lanes (9.8%); and more and better walking paths (7.2%) were considered important aspects.

Traffic safety is consistently a parental concern and limiting factor for children's independent mobility [35,67,68] and active travel in general. The current study findings aligned closely with the body of work in this field, for example in the early focus group research of Ahlport and colleagues [69], parents identified high traffic volume, dangerous drivers, and busy intersections as specific barriers to their child's active travel.

For the most part, findings related to perceptions of transport infrastructure also aligned with previous research. For example, parental concern for lack of pedestrian crossings was related to less active travel in a study of Australian children [29] and presence of pedestrian crossings was associated with more independent travel in a later study [49]. On the contrary, Evers and colleagues [70] found that traffic lights, marked crossings, and bump-out crossings did not influence parents' concern for their children crossing the road. However, these results were based on whether the parent would let an eight-year-old child cross the road unsupervised, and the age of the child may have been a bigger influence on parental concerns than the crossing infrastructure. In the current study, almost 5% of parents noted that age of their child was the key driver of their child's independent mobility licence, rather than the neighbourhood environment. There is likely an age and stage threshold below which infrastructure and neighbourhood perceptions are irrelevant in determining whether a child is allowed to be independently mobile.

Parents also highlighted the need for safe places to walk and cycle as key environmental considerations. These findings add to a small evidence base about the importance of availability and condition (e.g., uneven surfaces, obstacles, overgrown vegetation) of walking paths for children's independent mobility [70]. As well as providing a safe place to walk, the availability of walking paths may be important as this can reduce the need to cross roads to reach a destination [69]. In an adult sample, half of the respondents believed that lack of sidewalks in their neighbourhood was a problem and was a barrier to them being physically active [71]. Parents also noted the condition of walking paths, specifically that paths should be well maintained and wide enough for children to safely walk and cycle away from the road.

Safe places to cycle were also identified by parents as key infrastructural features that would create a supportive environment for children to be independently mobile. Specifically, parents mentioned the need for cycle lanes that are dedicated and separated from the road. This preference aligns with earlier research reporting on parental views on the importance of cycling infrastructure [28,72]. More specifically, cycle lanes that are separated from road traffic are perceived vital to cycling safety by parents. When considering relative importance of varying traffic infrastructure, one study reported that parents' perceived physical separation of child cyclists and the road was more important than a lower speed limit [73].

Safety from others was also raised by 12% of parents, with a focus on concerns about "stranger danger" (5.4% of parents) and a need for greater community surveillance (4.6%). To a lesser extent, criminal and gang activity, roaming dogs, other "undesirables", and bullying were also identified as factors limiting children's independent mobility. Concern about safety from strangers is an established barrier to parents granting licence for independent mobility to their child [9,34,46] as is the fear of crime [32]. Increased perceived social cohesion is associated with greater independent licence as it may support the perception of a safer neighbourhood for children [31]. However, Foster and colleagues [34] found no association between informal social control and decreased fear of strangers, indicating that the these perceptions are multifaced and may not be alleviated simply by a more supportive neighbourhood community.

### 4.2. Objective 2: Perceived and Objective Aspects of the Neighbourhood Transport Environment

In fully adjusted models, no statistically significant differences were observed in parent reported needs by different levels of the objective measures. In other words, no significant association was found between the objectively-assessed neighbourhood features and reporting a need. This finding was somewhat expected, considering that while the perceived and objective measures were theorized to relate to each other, they were not assessing the same environmental dimensions exactly (as detailed in Table 1). Additionally, a growing body of evidence has shown that adult perceptions do not always align with objective measures of the neighbourhood environment [71,74,75]. Rothman and colleagues [76] concluded that there are some differences between parents' perception and objective measures of traffic safety along school routes. However, some specific measures such as road crossings were related to lower parental perceived traffic danger. McGinn and colleagues [71] also found no agreement between perceived fast and heavy traffic and objectively measured speed and traffic volume. It is likely that both approaches provide valuable insights, and the triangulation of multiple data sources is optimal to gain a comprehensive understanding of environmental features of importance. Indeed, past research examining objective and perceived measures of the neighbourhood environment in relation to independent mobility has shown mixed results. Marzi and colleagues [41] concluded from their systematic review that parental perceptions of traffic have a greater influence in determining children's independent mobility compared with objective measures of the physical environment. Looking across the lifespan, perceptions were stronger indicators than objective measures for physical activity in preschoolers [77], active travel to school in children [78], and adults walking in their neighbourhood [79]. On the contrary, there is evidence that adults' physical activity is supported by urban design features regardless of their perception of the neighbourhood [80]. In adult populations, both McGinn and colleagues [71] and Lee and Dean [81] concluded that it may be necessary that both perceptions and objective measures of the neighbourhood environment are used to understand the complexity of the relationship between the built environment, walkability, and physical activity.

After adjusting for all other factors, differences in parents' perceived needs by socio-demographic characteristics were observed, including child's school level (less, slower, and safer traffic; cycling infrastructure), ethnicity (all variables except walking infrastructure), and area level deprivation (walking infrastructure only). These novel findings highlight the link between socio-demographic factors and neighbourhood perceptions as well as aiding understanding relationships between perceived and objective environments. Parents of younger children had 1.5 times the odds of reporting a need for less, slower, and safer traffic compared with those of older children. This implies the age of a child influences parent traffic safety perceptions, more so than the actual traffic environment. Compared with older children, a higher traffic safety threshold may be required for younger children in order for parents to perceive their environment as being safe. Conversely, parents of younger children were half as likely to report a need for safer and designated cycling infrastructure. It is possible this is due to lower levels of cycling in younger children compared with older children in this study (data not reported here) and thus cycling infrastructure being less relevant for these parents. In a similar manner, all ethnic groups were significantly less likely to report a need for safer and designated cycle lanes compared with parents of children who identified as being of New Zealand European/Pākehā/Other European ethnicity. National travel survey data suggest significantly higher rates in those of New Zealand European ethnicity compared with other ethnic groups (and low rates of cycling overall) [82]. Parents of children of Pacific ethnicity also had significantly lower odds of reporting needing less, slower, and safer traffic; more and safer crossings. It is unclear why these differences existed—further work examining ethnic differences in neighbourhood perceptions would be worthwhile.

Differences in deprivation were only observed for reporting a need for more and better walking paths, with those from higher deprivation areas significantly less likely to report this need compared with those residing in higher deprivation. It is possible this is a reflection of the New Zealand context, where positive relationships have been found consistently between walkability elements (e.g., destination accessibility) and deprivation [83].

### 4.3. Objective 3: Factors Associated with Parent Licence for Independent Mobility

Independent mobility licence was significantly related to both parent-reported need for safer cycling infrastructure and objectively-assessed cycle infrastructure. Children had a higher independent mobility licence when their parents mentioned that their neighbourhood needed more dedicated and safer cycle lanes, compared with children of parents who did not mention cycling infrastructure. This finding aligns with earlier work by Timperio and colleagues [29] indicating it is possible that parents are more aware of their traffic environment when they grant their children more independent mobility licence. Specifically, if children cycle in their neighbourhood, parents may notice the lack of cycle lanes available for their children, while in comparison parents who grant low mobility licence may not identify the need for more cycling lanes. Neighbourhood self-selection [39] may play a role in understanding parent perceptions. It is possible that parents who prefer neighbourhoods with safer transport infrastructure have chosen to live in neighbourhoods that align with this preference, yet their own personal preferences are still not being met sufficiently.

In terms of objectively measured cycling infrastructure, children with higher parental licence for independent mobility lived in areas with lower cycle lane availability. This finding could be due to parents allowing their children to be independently mobile, but more so for walking rather than cycling. Indeed, Moran and colleagues [53] concluded that walking is a more common form of independent mobility than cycling, and that different built environmental features are associated with each type of active travel mode.

No other significant associations with independent mobility were found. Inconsistent findings have been observed in earlier literature with regard to links between parental perceptions and children's independent mobility. Traffic safety perceptions of parents was positively associated with adolescent active travel [84] and independent mobility in girls [72]. Conversely, Santos and colleagues [43] found no association with traffic safety and independent mobility. Perceived poor availability of road crossings has been associated with decreased independent mobility for boys [51] and decreased active travel in children, generally [85,86]. In other studies, parent perceptions of available walking paths was a predictor for independent mobility [43] and active travel [28].

A recent meta-analysis identified a number of built environment features related to children's independent mobility (operationalized as independent mobility time, independent mobility to destinations, territorial range, or licence for independent mobility) [52]. Positive associations were found for proportion of residential land, proportion of commercial land, residential location type, and dead-end streets. Negative associations were observed for vehicular street width, road density, street connectivity, proportion of major roads, land use mix, availability of recreational facilities, residential density, and distance to destinations. Situating the current study findings with the extant literature, it is clear that understanding determinants of children's independent mobility is a complex challenge. Factors exist across the socio-ecological spectrum [23], and the role of parenting practices, beliefs, and perceptions in this context cannot be underestimated [87]. Nuances may also exist, whereby differences in relationships might be expected by neighbourhood social and built environment contexts and spatio-temporal factors may also play a role. For example, earlier work with Auckland children showed that active travel was associated with destination accessibility on weekdays only, and differential relationships between activity and built environment characteristics were also observed between weekend days and weekdays [54].

### 5. Strengths and Limitations

This study was cross-sectional and conducted in one city in New Zealand only. Findings cannot be generalized to other environments, and causality cannot be inferred. Parental licence for their child's independent mobility was employed in the current study to align with the majority of literature in this field. However, it is important to recognise this measure does not necessarily encompass all facets of children's independent mobility (e.g., time, range, destinations) and that children may also report their independence differently from their parents. Had different measures of independent mobility been used in the current study, it is possible alternative findings might have been identified. It is also worth noting that broader family and household characteristics may play an important role in children's independent mobility, including having older siblings, household car ownership, competing family schedules, and neighbourhood self-selection. The latter three variables were not measured in this examination. The almost universal access to a working car in this study hindered any ability to detect the effect of not having access to a car on children's independent mobility. The pervasiveness of the car is consistent with national data. New Zealand has one of the highest rates of car ownership internationally and rates have continued to rise in recent years [88]. It is possible these broader factors are more likely to be linked to children's actualized independent mobility, rather than parental licence for independent mobility, and further work in this area is needed. It is also possible that other parent psychological factors and experiences may have contributed to understanding children's independent mobility and parent neighbourhood perceptions, however these were not examined in the current investigation. For example, factors such as anxiety, values around child independence, incidences or 'near misses', and local narratives about past incidents related to child independent mobility could all play a role in how a parent perceives their environment and thus impact the independence granted to their child.

No agreed upon approach for determining neighbourhood buffers for children's independent mobility exists. Previous examinations in Neighbourhoods for Active Kids have used a range of study-specific buffers to determine environments of importance including 800 m around schools only for outdoor advertising [63], 800 m around home plus school (less any overlap) for children's body size [65], and school route only using 80 m on each side of the street centre line for active school travel [64]. The "home only" buffer was determined for the current study to align with the study's focus on parent perceptions about their neighbourhood and their child's independence in the neighbourhood. Not all children lived within close proximity to school, so including a school buffer to characterize the objective built environment and examine this in relation to parent perceptions would have reduced sensitivity and specificity. Previous research with Auckland children supported a 1000 m buffer to capture levels of MVPA [54]. Conversely, a Canadian study showed 500 m was optimal to measure associations with girls' MVPA, and 800 m was best for boys' MVPA [89]. An 800 m buffer was chosen in the current study as a pragmatic approach to capture sufficient environmental features that might be 'front of mind' for parents when considering their neighbourhood and their child's independent mobility, and to allow comparability with previous research [51,54,89]. Future research would benefit from the use of more individually-centred measures such as activity spaces [90].

## 6. Conclusions

Through the use of mixed methods with a large sample of parents, this study provides a comprehensive examination of children's independent mobility licence, parent neighbourhood perceptions, and objectively assessed neighbourhood built environments. For the first time, objective pedestrian crossing and cycle lane availability has been examined in relation to children's independent mobility, contributing to improving sensitivity and specificity in neighbourhood built environment measures. Novel findings on relationships between socio-demographic characteristics and parent neighbourhood perceptions can help interpret research exploring differences between perceived and objectively-assessed neighbourhood features. Further research is needed to explore the complex relationships between parent psychological characteristics, family and household context, perceived and objective neighbourhood environments and children's actualized independent mobility and licence for independent mobility across a range of settings. Novel findings demonstrate the importance of measuring both perceived and objective characteristics, and exploring why these do not always align. Overall, this novel study demonstrates the importance of providing safer traffic environments, particularly safer places to cycle, for children's independent mobility.

**Author Contributions:** M.S., K.W., S.M., R.K., R.M. and P.C. conceptualised and developed the Neighbourhoods for Active Kids study, and secured funding for the study. M.S., K.W., P.C., L.M. and E.I. were involved in participant recruitment and data collection. M.S. and D.R. led the qualitative data coding and framework development. R.A. and A.C. led the quantitative data modelling and interpretation. S.M., J.Z. and E.F. led the development of objective neighbourhood built environment factors. M.S. and R.A. prepared the full draft manuscript. All authors contributed to interpretation of research findings. All authors read, contributed edits to, and approved the final manuscript.

**Funding:** Neighbourhoods for Active Kids was supported by the Health Research Council of New Zealand (grant number 14/436). R.A. was supported by a University of Auckland Faculty of Medical and Health Sciences summer research scholarship. M.S. is supported by a Health Research Council of New Zealand Sir Charles Hercus Research Fellowship (grant number 17/013). S.M. is supported by an Australian National Health and Medical Research Council Early Career Fellowship (grant number 1121035).

**Acknowledgments:** The authors would like to acknowledge the support and time of children who participated in the Neighbourhoods for Active Kids Study, their parents and caregivers, and schools.

**Conflicts of Interest:** The authors declare no conflict of interest.

## References

1. Strong, W.B.; Malina, R.M.; Blimkie, C.J.; Daniels, S.R.; Dishman, R.K.; Gutin, B.; Hergenroeder, A.C.; Must, A.; Nixon, P.A.; Pivarnik, J.M.; et al. Evidence based physical activity for school-age youth. *J. Pediatr.* **2005**, *146*, 732–737. [CrossRef]

2. Aubert, S.; Barnes, J.D.; Abdeta, C.; Abi Nader, P.; Adeniyi, A.F.; Aguilar-Farias, N.; Andrade Tenesaca, D.S.; Bhawra, J.; Brazo-Sayavera, J.; Cardon, G.; et al. Global Matrix 3.0 Physical Activity Report Card Grades for Children and Youth: Results and Analysis from 49 Countries. *J. Phys. Act. Health* **2018**, *15*, S251–S273. [CrossRef]

3. Smith, M.; Ikeda, E.; Hinckson, E.; Duncan, S.; Maddison, R.; Meredith-Jones, K.; Walker, C.; Mandic, S. Results from New Zealand's 2018 Report card on Physical Activity for Children and Youth. *J. Phys. Act. Health* **2018**, *15*, S390–S392. [CrossRef]

4. Hillman, M.; Adams, J.; Whitelegg, J. *One False Move ... A Study of Children's Independent Mobility*; Policy Studies Institute: London, UK, 1990; ISBN 0853744947.

5. Chaudhury, M.; Oliver, M.; Badland, H.M.; Mavoa, S. Public Open Spaces, Children's Independent Mobility. In *Play, Recreation, Health and Well Being, Geographies of Children and Young People*; Evans, B., Horton, J., Eds.; Springer Science: Singapore, 2015; Volume 9, pp. 315–335.

6. Marzi, I.; Reimers, A.K. Children's Independent Mobility: Current Knowledge, Future Directions, and Public Health Implications. *Int. J. Environ. Res. Public Health* **2018**, *15*, 2441. [CrossRef]

7. Riazi, N.A.; Faulkner, G. Children's Independent Mobility. In *Children's Active Transportation*, 1st ed.; Larouche, R., Ed.; Elsevier: Amsterdam, The Netherlands, 2018; pp. 77–87.

8. Ikeda, E.; Hinckson, E.; Witten, K.; Smith, M. Assessment of direct and indirect associations between children active school travel and environmental, household and child factors using structural equation modelling. *Int. J. Behav. Nutr. Phys. Act.* **2019**, *16*, 32. [CrossRef]

9. Mitra, R.; Faulkner, G.E.; Buliung, R.N.; Stone, M.R. Do parental perceptions of the neighbourhood environment influence children's independent mobility? Evidence from Toronto, Canada. *Urban Stud.* **2014**, *51*, 3401–3419. [CrossRef]

10. Oliver, M.; Parker, K.; Witten, K.; Mavoa, S.; Badland, H.M.; Donovan, P.; Chaudhury, M.; Kearns, R. Children's Out-of-School Independently Mobile Trips, Active Travel, and Physical Activity: A Cross-Sectional Examination from the Kids in the City Study. *J. Phys. Act. Health* **2016**, *13*, 318–324. [CrossRef]

11. Schoeppe, S.; Duncan, M.J.; Badland, H.; Oliver, M.; Curtis, C. Associations of children's independent mobility and active travel with physical activity, sedentary behaviour and weight status: A systematic review. *J. Sci. Med. Sport* **2013**, *16*, 312–319. [CrossRef]

12. Stone, M.R.; Faulkner, G.E.; Mitra, R.; Buliung, R.N. The freedom to explore: Examining the influence of independent mobility on weekday, weekend and after-school physical activity behaviour in children living in urban and inner-suburban neighbourhoods of varying socioeconomic status. *Int. J. Behav. Nutr. Phys. Act.* **2014**, *11*, 5. [CrossRef]

13. Bento, G.; Dias, G. The importance of outdoor play for young children's healthy development. *Porto Biomed. J.* **2017**, *2*, 157–160. [CrossRef]

14. Pooley, C.; Whyatt, D.; Walker, M.; Davies, G.; Coulton, P.; Bamford, W. Understanding the school journey: Integrating data on travel and environment. *Environ. Plan. A* **2010**, *42*, 948–965. [CrossRef]

15. Prezza, M.; Pilloni, S.; Morabito, C.; Sersante, C.; Alparone, F.R.; Giuliani, M.V. The influence of psychosocial and environmental factors on children's independent mobility and relationship to peer frequentation. *J. Community Appl. Soc. Psychol.* **2001**, *11*, 435–450. [CrossRef]

16. Prezza, M.; Pacilli, M.G. Current fear of crime, sense of community, and loneliness in italian adolescents: The role of autonomous mobility and play during childhood. *J. Community Psychol.* **2007**, *35*, 151–170. [CrossRef]

17. Rissotto, A.; Tonucci, F. Freedom of Movement and Environmental Knowledge in Elementary School Children. *J. Environ. Psychol.* **2002**, *22*, 65–77. [CrossRef]

18. Mitchell, H.; Kearns, R.; Collins, D.C.A. Nuances of neighbourhood: Children's perceptions of the space between home and school in Auckland, New Zealand. *Geoforum* **2007**, *38*, 614–627. [CrossRef]

19. Mackett, R.; Brown, B.; Gong, Y.; Kitazawa, K.; Paskins, J. Children's Independent Movement in the Local Environment. *Built Environ.* **2007**, *33*, 454–468. [CrossRef]

20. Schoeppe, S.; Tranter, P.; Duncan, M.J.; Curtis, C.; Carver, A.; Malone, K. Australian children's independent mobility levels: Secondary analyses of cross-sectional data between 1991 and 2012. *Child.'s Geogr.* **2016**, *14*, 408–421. [CrossRef]

21. Shaw, B.; Bicket, M.; Elliott, B.; Fagan-Watson, B.; Mocca, E.; Hillman, M. *Children's Independent Mobility: An International Comparison and Recommendations for Action*; Policy Studies Institute: London, UK, 2015; ISBN 9780853740148.

22. Sallis, J.F.; Cervero, R.B.; Ascher, W.; Henderson, K.A.; Kraft, M.K.; Kerr, J. An ecological approach to creating active living communities. *Annu. Rev. Public Health* **2006**, *27*, 297–322. [CrossRef]

23. Badland, H.; Kearns, R.; Carroll, P.; Oliver, M.; Mavoa, S.; Donovan, P.; Parker, K.; Chaudhury, M.; Lin, E.Y.; Witten, K. Development of a systems model to visualise the complexity of children's independent mobility. *Child.'s Geogr.* **2016**, *14*, 91–100. [CrossRef]

24. Cordovil, R.; Lopes, F.; Neto, C. Children's (in)dependent mobility in Portugal. *J. Sci. Med. Sport* **2015**, *18*, 299–303. [CrossRef]

25. Egli, V.; Ikeda, E.; Stewart, T.; Smith, M. Interpersonal Correlates of Active Transportation. In *Children's Active Transportation*, 1st ed.; Larouche, R., Ed.; Elsevier: Amsterdam, The Netherlands, 2018; pp. 115–125.

26. Crawford, S.B.; Bennetts, S.K.; Hackworth, N.J.; Green, J.; Graesser, H.; Cooklin, A.R.; Matthews, J.; Strazdins, L.; Zubrick, S.R.; D'Esposito, F.; et al. Worries, 'weirdos', neighborhoods and knowing people: A qualitative study with children and parents regarding children's independent mobility. *Health Place* **2017**, *45*, 131–139. [CrossRef]

27. Carver, A.; Timperio, A.; Crawford, D. Playing it safe: The influence of neighbourhood safety on children's physical activity—A review. *Health Place* **2008**, *14*, 217–227. [CrossRef]

28. De Meester, F.; Van Dyck, D.; De Bourdeaudhuij, I.; Cardon, G. Parental perceived neighborhood attributes: Associations with active transport and physical activity among 10–12 year old children and the mediating role of independent mobility. *BMC Public Health* **2014**, *14*, 631. [CrossRef]

29. Timperio, A.; Crawford, D.; Telford, A.; Salmon, J. Perceptions about the local neighborhood and walking and cycling among children. *Prev. Med.* **2004**, *38*, 39–47. [CrossRef]

30. Janssen, I.; Ferrao, T.; King, N. Individual, family, and neighborhood correlates of independent mobility among 7 to 11-year-olds. *Prev. Med. Rep.* **2016**, *3*, 98–102. [CrossRef]

31. Schoeppe, S.; Duncan, M.J.; Badland, H.M.; Alley, S.; Williams, S.; Rebar, A.L.; Vandelanotte, C. Socio-demographic factors and neighbourhood social cohesion influence adults' willingness to grant children greater independent mobility: A cross-sectional study. *BMC Public Health* **2015**, *15*, 690. [CrossRef]

32. Wolfe, M.K.; McDonald, N.C. Association between neighborhood social environment and children's independent mobility. *J. Phys. Act. Health* **2016**, *13*, 970–979. [CrossRef]

33. Carver, A.; Panter, J.R.; Jones, A.P.; van Sluijs, E.M.F. Independent mobility on the journey to school: A joint cross-sectional and prospective exploration of social and physical environmental influences. *J. Transp. Health* **2014**, *1*, 25–32. [CrossRef]

34. Foster, S.; Villanueva, K.; Wood, L.; Christian, H.; Giles-Corti, B. The impact of parents' fear of strangers and perceptions of informal social control on children's independent mobility. *Health Place* **2014**, *26*, 60–68. [CrossRef]

35. Lopes, F.; Cordovil, R.; Neto, C. Children's independent mobility in Portugal: Effects of urbanization degree and motorized modes of travel. *J. Transp. Geogr.* **2014**, *41*, 210–219. [CrossRef]

36. Lin, E.Y.; Witten, K.; Smith, M.; Carroll, P.; Asiasiga, L.; Badland, H.; Parker, K. Social and built-environment factors related to children's independent mobility: The importance of neighbourhood cohesion and connectedness. *Health Place* **2017**, *46*, 107–113. [CrossRef]

37. Carver, A.; Barr, A.; Singh, A.; Badland, H.; Mavoa, S.; Bentley, B. How are the built environment and household travel characteristics associated with children's active transport in Melbourne, Australia? *J. Transp. Health* **2019**, *12*, 115–129. [CrossRef]

38. Heinen, E.; van Wee, B.; Panter, J.; Mackett, R.; Ogilvie, D. Residential self-selection in quasi-experimental and natural experimental studies: An extended conceptualization of the relationship between the built environment and travel behavior. *J. Transp. Land Use* **2018**, *11*, 939–959. [CrossRef]

39. Levine, J.; Inam, A.; Torng, G.-W. A Choice-Based Rationale for Land Use and Transportation Alternatives. *J. Plan. Educ. Res.* **2005**, *24*, 317–330. [CrossRef]

40. Oliver, M.; Badland, H.; Mavoa, S.; Witten, K.; Kearns, R.; Ellaway, A.; Hinckson, E.; Mackay, L.; Schluter, P.J. Environmental and socio-demographic associates of children's active transport to school: A cross-sectional investigation from the URBAN Study. *Int. J. Behav. Nutr. Phys. Act.* **2014**, *11*, 70. [CrossRef]

41. Marzi, I.; Demetriou, Y.; Reimers, A.K. Social and physical environmental correlates of independent mobility in children: A systematic review taking sex/gender differences into account. *Int. J. Health Geogr.* **2018**, *17*, 24. [CrossRef]

42. Nicksic, N.E.; Salahuddin, M.; Butte, N.F.; Hoelscher, D.M. Associations Between Parent-Perceived Neighborhood Safety and Encouragement and Child Outdoor Physical Activity Among Low-Income Children. *J. Phys. Act. Health* **2018**, *15*, 317–324. [CrossRef]

43. Santos, M.P.; Pizarro, A.N.; Mota, J.; Marques, E.A. Parental physical activity, safety perceptions and children's independent mobility. *BMC Public Health* **2013**, *12*, 584. [CrossRef]

44. Giles-Corti, B.; Kelty, S.F.; Zubrick, S.R.; Villanueva, K.P. Encouraging walking for transport and physical activity in children and adolescents: How important is the built environment? *Sports Med.* **2009**, *39*, 995–1009. [CrossRef]

45. Christian, H.E.; Klinker, C.D.; Villanueva, K.; Knuiman, M.W.; Foster, S.A.; Zubrick, S.R.; Divitini, M.; Wood, L.; Giles-Corti, B. The effect of the social and physical environment on children's independent mobility to neighborhood destinations. *J. Phys. Act. Health* **2015**, *12*, S84–S93. [CrossRef]

46. Francis, J.; Martin, K.; Wood, L.; Foster, S. 'I'll be driving you to school for the rest of your life': A qualitative study of parents' fear of stranger danger. *J. Environ. Psychol.* **2017**, *53*, 112–120. [CrossRef]

47. Ikeda, E.; Hinckson, E.; Witten, K.; Smith, M. Associations of children's active school travel with perceptions of the physical environment and characteristics of the social environment: A systematic review. *Health Place* **2018**, *54*, 118–131. [CrossRef]

48. Carroll, P.; Witten, K.; Kearns, R.; Donovan, P. Kids in the City: Children's use and experiences of urban neighbourhoods in Auckland, New Zealand. *J. Urban Des.* **2015**, *20*, 417–436. [CrossRef]

49. Johansson, M. Environment and parental factors as determinants of mode for children's leisure travel. *J. Environ. Psychol.* **2006**, *26*, 156–169. [CrossRef]

50. Kyttä, M. The extent of children's independent mobility and the number of actualized affordances as criteria for child-friendly environments. *J. Environ. Psychol.* **2004**, *24*, 179–198. [CrossRef]

51. Villanueva, K.; Giles-Corti, B.; Bulsara, M.; Timperio, A.; McCormack, G.; Beesley, B.; Trapp, G.; Middleton, N. Where Do Children Travel to and What Local Opportunities Are Available? The Relationship Between Neighborhood Destinations and Children's Independent Mobility. *Environ. Behav.* **2012**, *45*, 679–705. [CrossRef]

52. Sharmin, S.; Kamruzzaman, M. Association between the built environment and children's independent mobility: A meta-analytic review. *J. Transp. Geogr.* **2017**, *61*, 104–117. [CrossRef]

53. Moran, M.R.; Plaut, P.; Baron-Epel, O. Do children walk where they bike? Exploring built environment correlates of children's walking and bicycling. *J. Transp. Land Use* **2015**, *9*, 43–65. [CrossRef]

54. Oliver, M.; Mavoa, S.; Badland, H.; Parker, K.; Donovan, P.; Kearns, R.A.; Lin, E.Y.; Witten, K. Associations between the neighbourhood built environment and out of school physical activity and active travel: An examination from the Kids in the City study. *Health Place* **2015**, *36*, 57–64. [CrossRef]

55. Villanueva, K.; Giles-Corti, B.; Bulsara, M.; Trapp, G.; Timperio, A.; McCormack, G.; Van Niel, K. Does the walkability of neighbourhoods affect children's independent mobility, independent of parental, socio-cultural and individual factors? *Child.'s Geogr.* **2014**, *12*, 393–411. [CrossRef]

56. Giles-Corti, B.; Wood, G.; Pikora, T.; Learnihan, V.; Bulsara, M.; Van Niel, K.; Timperio, A.; McCormack, G.; Villanueva, K. School site and the potential to walk to school: The impact of street connectivity and traffic exposure in school neighborhoods. *Health Place* **2011**, *17*, 545–550. [CrossRef]

57. Badland, H.; Donovan, P.; Mavoa, S.; Oliver, M.; Chaudhury, M.; Witten, K. Assessing neighbourhood destination access for children: Development of the NDAI-C audit tool. *Environ. Plan. B Plan. Des.* **2015**, *42*, 1148–1160. [CrossRef]

58. Uys, M.; Broyles, S.T.; Draper, C.E.; Hendricks, S.; Rae, D.; Naidoo, N.; Katzmarzyk, P.T.; Lambert, E.V. Perceived and objective neighborhood support for outside of school physical activity in South African children. *BMC Public Health* **2016**, *16*, 462. [CrossRef]

59. Statistics New Zealand. 2013 Census QuickStats About a Place: Auckland Region. Available online: http://archive.stats.govt.nz/Census/2013-census/profile-and-summary-reports/quickstats-about-a-place.aspx?request_value=13170&tabname= (accessed on 10 April 2019).

60. Witten, K.; Kearns, R.; Carroll, P.; Asiasiga, L. Children's everyday encounters and affective relations with place: Experiences of hyperdiversity in Auckland neighbourhoods. *Soc. Cult. Geogr.* **2017**, *9365*, 1–18. [CrossRef]

61. Oliver, M.; McPhee, J.; Carroll, P.; Ikeda, E.; Mavoa, S.; Mackay, L.; Kearns, R.A.; Kyttä, M.; Asiasiga, L.; Garrett, N.; et al. Neighbourhoods for Active Kids: Study protocol for a cross-sectional examination of neighbourhood features and children's physical activity, active travel, independent mobility and body size. *BMJ Open* **2016**, *6*, e013377. [CrossRef]

62. Ministry of Education. School Deciles. Available online: https://www.education.govt.nz/school/running-a-school/resourcing/operational-funding/school-decile-ratings/ (accessed on 10 April 2019).

63. Egli, V.; Zinn, C.; Mackay, L.; Donnellan, N.; Villanueva, K.; Mavoa, S.; Exeter, D.J.; Vandevijvere, S.; Smith, M. Viewing obesogenic advertising in children's neighbourhoods using Google Street View. *Geogr. Res.* **2018**, *57*, 84–97. [CrossRef]

64. Ikeda, E.; Mavoa, S.; Hinckson, E.; Witten, K.; Donnellan, N.; Smith, M. Differences in child-drawn and GIS-modelled routes to school: Impact on space and exposure to the built environment in Auckland, New Zealand. *J. Transp. Geogr.* **2018**, *71*, 103–115. [CrossRef]

65. Egli, V. *Neighbourhoods for Healthy Kids: A Child-Centred Investigation into the Role of the Built Environment on Child Body Size*; Auckland University of Technology: Auckland, New Zealand, 2019.

66. Atkinson, J.; Salmond, C.; Crampton, P. *NZDep2013 Index of Deprivation*; Department of Public Health, University of Otago: Wellington, New Zealand, 2014.

67. Fyhri, A.; Hjorthol, R.; Mackett, R.; Fotel, T.N.; Kyttä, M. Children's active travel and independent mobility in four countries: Development, social contributing trends and measures. *Transp. Policy* **2011**, *8*, 703–710. [CrossRef]

68. Jago, R.; Thompson, J.L.; Page, A.S.; Brockman, R.; Cartwright, K.; Fox, K.R. Licence to be active: Parental concerns and 10–11-year-old children's ability to be independently physically active. *J. Public Health* **2009**, *31*, 472–477. [CrossRef] [PubMed]

69. Ahlport, K.N.; Linnan, L.; Vaughn, A.; Evenson, K.R.; Ward, D.S.; Carmen Head, B.J. Barriers to and Facilitators of Walking and Bicycling to School: Formative Results From the Non-Motorized Travel Study. *Health Educ. Behav.* **2008**, *35*, 221–244. [CrossRef]

70. Evers, C.; Boles, S.; Johnson-Shelton, D.; Schlossberg, M.; Richey, D. Parent Safety Perceptions of Child Walking Routes. *J. Transp. Health* **2014**, *1*, 108–115. [CrossRef] [PubMed]

71. McGinn, A.P.; Evenson, K.R.; Herring, A.H.; Huston, S.L.; Rodriguez, D.A. Exploring Associations between Physical Activity and Perceived and Objective Measures of the Built Environment. *J. Urban Health* **2007**, *84*, 162–184. [CrossRef]

72. Ghekiere, A.; Deforche, B.; Carver, A.; Mertens, L.; de Geus, B.; Clarys, P.; Cardon, G.; De Bourdeaudhuij, I.; Van Cauwenberg, J. Insights into children's independent mobility for transportation cycling—Which socio-ecological factors matter? *J. Sci. Med. Sport* **2017**, *20*, 267–272. [CrossRef]

73. Nevelsteen, K.; Steenberghen, T.; Van Rompaey, A.; Uyttersprot, L. Controlling factors of the parental safety perception on children's travel mode choice. *Accid. Anal. Prev.* **2012**, *45*, 39–49. [CrossRef] [PubMed]
74. Lee, S.M.; Conway, T.L.; Frank, L.D.; Saelens, B.E.; Cain, K.L.; Sallis, J.F. The Relation of Perceived and Objective Environment Attributes to Neighborhood Satisfaction. *Environ. Behav.* **2017**, *49*, 136–160. [CrossRef]
75. Schüle, S.; Nanninga, S.; Dreger, S.; Bolte, G.; Schüle, S.A.; Nanninga, S.; Dreger, S.; Bolte, G. Relations between Objective and Perceived Built Environments and the Modifying Role of Individual Socioeconomic Position. A Cross-Sectional Study on Traffic Noise and Urban Green Space in a Large German City. *Int. J. Environ. Res. Public Health* **2018**, *15*, 1562. [CrossRef] [PubMed]
76. Rothman, L.; Buliung, R.; To, T.; Macarthur, C.; Macpherson, A.; Howard, A. Associations between parents perception of traffic danger, the built environment and walking to school. *J. Transp. Health* **2015**, *2*, 327–335. [CrossRef]
77. Eichinger, M.; Schneider, S.; De Bock, F. Subjectively and objectively assessed social and physical environmental correlates of preschoolers' accelerometer-based physical activity. *Int. J. Behav. Nutr. Phys. Act.* **2017**, *14*, 1–13. [CrossRef]
78. Kerr, J.; Rosenberg, D.; Sallis, J.F.; Saelens, B.E.; Frank, L.D.; Conway, T.L.; Rosenberg, D.; Sallis, J.F.; Saelens, B.E.; Frank, L.D.; et al. Active Commuting to School: Associations with Environment and Parental Concerns. *Am. Coll. Sports Med.* **2006**, *38*, 787–794. [CrossRef]
79. Koohsari, M.J.; Badland, H.; Sugiyama, T.; Mavoa, S.; Christian, H.; Giles-Corti, B. Mismatch between Perceived and Objectively Measured Land Use Mix and Street Connectivity: Associations with Neighborhood Walking. *J. Urban Health* **2015**, *92*, 242–252. [CrossRef]
80. Cerin, E.; Conway, T.L.; Adams, M.A.; Barnett, A.; Cain, K.L.; Owen, N.; Christiansen, L.B.; van Dyck, D.; Mitáš, J.; Sarmiento, O.L.; et al. Objectively-assessed neighbourhood destination accessibility and physical activity in adults from 10 countries: An analysis of moderators and perceptions as mediators. *Soc. Sci. Med.* **2018**, *211*, 282–293. [CrossRef]
81. Lee, E.; Dean, J. Perceptions of walkability and determinants of walking behaviour among urban seniors in Toronto, Canada. *J. Transp. Health* **2018**, *9*, 309–320. [CrossRef]
82. Shaw, C.; Russell, M. *Benchmarking Cycling and Walking in Six New Zealand Cities*; New Zealand Centre for Sustainable Cities, University of Otago: Wellington, New Zealand, 2016.
83. Witten, K.; Pearce, J.; Day, P. Neighbourhood Destination Accessibility Index: A GIS tool for measuring infrastructure support for neighbourhood physical activity. *Environ. Plan. A* **2011**, *43*, 205–223. [CrossRef]
84. Esteban-Cornejo, I.; Carlson, J.A.; Conway, T.L.; Cain, K.L.; Saelens, B.E.; Frank, L.D.; Glanz, K.; Roman, C.G.; Sallis, J.F. Parental and adolescent perceptions of neighbourhood safety related to adolescents' physical activity in their neighborhood. *Res. Q. Exerc. Sport* **2016**, *87*, 191–199. [CrossRef]
85. Hume, C.; Timperio, A.; Salmon, J.; Carver, A.; Giles-Corti, B.; Crawford, D. Walking and Cycling to School Predictors of Increases Among Children and Adolescents. *Am. J. Prev. Med.* **2009**, *36*, 195–200. [CrossRef]
86. Timperio, A.; Ball, K.; Salmon, J.; Roberts, R.; Giles-Corti, B.; Simmons, D.; Baur, L.A.; Crawford, D. Personal, Family, Social, and Environmental Correlates of Active Commuting to School. *Am. J. Prev. Med.* **2006**, *30*, 45–51. [CrossRef]
87. Witten, K.; Kearns, R.; Carroll, P.; Asiasiga, L.; Tava'e, N. New Zealand parents' understandings of the intergenerational decline in children's independent outdoor play and active travel. *Child.'s Geogr.* **2013**, *11*, 215–229. [CrossRef]
88. Environmental Health Indicators New Zealand. Number of Motor Vehicles in New Zealand. Available online: http://www.ehinz.ac.nz/assets/Factsheets/Released-2017/NumberOfVehiclesInNZ2000-2016-release201710.pdf (accessed on 15 March 2019).
89. Mitchell, C.A.; Clark, A.F.; Gilliland, J.A. Built environment influences of children's physical activity: Examining differences by neighbourhood size and sex. *Int. J. Environ. Res. Public Health* **2016**, *13*, 130. [CrossRef]
90. Hasanzadeh, K.; Laatikainen, T.; Kyttä, M. A place-based model of local activity spaces: Individual place exposure and characteristics. *J. Geogr. Syst.* **2018**, *20*, 227–252. [CrossRef]

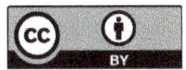

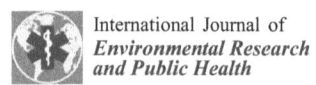

International Journal of
*Environmental Research and Public Health*

*Article*

# How Do Neighbourhood Definitions Influence the Associations between Built Environment and Physical Activity?

Suzanne Mavoa [1,2,*], Nasser Bagheri [3], Mohammad Javad Koohsari [4,5], Andrew T. Kaczynski [6], Karen E. Lamb [7], Koichiro Oka [4], David O'Sullivan [8] and Karen Witten [1]

[1]  SHORE and Whariki Research Centre, School of Public Health, Massey University, P.O. Box 6137, Auckland 1141, New Zealand; K.Witten@massey.ac.nz

[2]  Melbourne School of Population and Global Health, The University of Melbourne, Melbourne, VIC 3010, Australia

[3]  The Visualisation and Decision Analytics (VIDEA) lab, Centre for Mental Health Research, Research School of Population Health, College of Health and Medicine, The Australian National University, Canberra, ACT 2601, Australia; nasser.bagheri@anu.edu.au

[4]  Faculty of Sport Sciences, Waseda University, Saitama 359-1192, Japan; Javad.Koohsari@baker.edu.au (M.J.K.); koka@waseda.jp (K.O.)

[5]  Behavioural Epidemiology Laboratory, Baker IDI Heart and Diabetes Institute, Melbourne, VIC 3004, Australia

[6]  Prevention Research Center, Arnold School of Public Health, University of South Carolina, Columbia, SC 29208, USA; ATKACZYN@mailbox.sc.edu

[7]  Murdoch Children's Research Institute, Melbourne, VIC 3052, Australia; karen.lamb@mcri.edu.au

[8]  School of Geography, Environment and Earth Sciences, Victoria University, Wellington 6012, New Zealand; david.osullivan@vuw.ac.nz

*  Correspondence: suzanne.mavoa@unimelb.edu.au

Received: 8 April 2019; Accepted: 19 April 2019; Published: 28 April 2019

**Abstract:** Researchers investigating relationships between the neighbourhood environment and health first need to decide on the spatial extent of the neighbourhood they are interested in. This decision is an important and ongoing methodological challenge since different methods of defining and delineating neighbourhood boundaries can produce different results. This paper explores this issue in the context of a New Zealand-based study of the relationship between the built environment and multiple measures of physical activity. Geographic information systems were used to measure three built environment attributes—dwelling density, street connectivity, and neighbourhood destination accessibility—using seven different neighbourhood definitions (three administrative unit boundaries, and 500, 800, 1000- and 1500-m road network buffers). The associations between the three built environment measures and five measures of physical activity (mean accelerometer counts per hour, percentage time in moderate–vigorous physical activity, self-reported walking for transport, self-reported walking for recreation and self-reported walking for all purposes) were modelled for each neighbourhood definition. The combination of the choice of neighbourhood definition, built environment measure, and physical activity measure determined whether evidence of an association was detected or not. Results demonstrated that, while there was no single ideal neighbourhood definition, the built environment was most consistently associated with a range of physical activity measures when the 800-m and 1000-m road network buffers were used. For the street connectivity and destination accessibility measures, associations with physical activity were less likely to be detected at smaller scales (less than 800 m). In line with some previous research, this study demonstrated that the choice of neighbourhood definition can influence whether or not an association between the built environment and adults' physical activity is detected or not. This study additionally highlighted the importance of the choice of built environment attribute and physical activity measures. While we identified the 800-m and 1000-m road network buffers as the neighbourhood definitions most consistently associated with a range of physical activity measures, it is important that researchers carefully consider the most appropriate type of neighbourhood definition and scale for the particular aim and participants, especially at smaller scales.

**Keywords:** neighbourhood; scale; built environment; physical activity; walking

---

## 1. Introduction

Many studies have investigated associations between the neighbourhood-built environment attributes and the physical activity of residents, with evidence accumulating on the health benefits of living in higher density neighbourhoods with well-connected street networks and pedestrian access to a range of amenities [1–3]. Within this area of research, an important methodological challenge is how to define a "neighbourhood" [4–6]. A neighbourhood refers to the geographical area within which environmental attributes are investigated in relation to physical activity. It is hypothesised that residents are only able to walk within such geographical areas of their homes. The challenge of defining a neighbourhood is also shared by the wider neighbourhood research field and has been regularly highlighted over the past decade [4,5,7–9]. Currently, researchers have been using a variety of neighbourhood definitions and there is little consensus as to the most appropriate geographic scales [10,11]. This is a problem because using different neighbourhood definitions can change the results [5,10–15] and the lack of standardisation makes it difficult to compare and combine evidence across studies [10]. Furthermore, identifying the most appropriate geographical scales at which built environments may influence health behaviours is an important step in translating the evidence into urban design and public health practice [16]. For example, evidence that the proximity of public open spaces is associated with better health behaviours and outcomes is useful but not sufficient for those that (re)design the built environment or write environmental policy. Urban design policy makers and practitioners also need to know how far away the public open spaces need to be located from people's homes to maximise their amenity value and health outcomes. In other words, a better understanding of the distances and geographical scales at which the built environment influences health could inform more effective urban design and policy interventions [10,16,17].

Neighbourhood is commonly conceptualised as the home neighbourhood and operationalised using geographic information systems (GIS). The dimensions of a neighbourhood are determined by the type of boundary applied and its size or geographical scale. There are three main types of neighbourhood definitions used in built environments and public health research: administrative units, circular buffers, and road network buffers. Administrative units (e.g., census tracts, postal codes) allow researchers to link their data with secondary data sources. However, they are subject to the modifiable areal unit problem (MAUP) where results can vary depending on the division of the study area, a zonation or aggregation effect [18], and the size of the units used, a scale effect [19]. Circular (or Euclidean) buffers are circles of a defined radius centred on an address, whereas road network buffers are calculated by drawing an area around an address that is accessible by travelling a defined distance along roads. Circular buffers are simpler to calculate, but road network buffers are conceptually more appealing because they better represent where people may travel, particularly in areas with features such as rivers, lakes, or a poorly connected road network [20]. Both circular and road network buffers address the zonation effect of the MAUP but are still subject to scale effects. A further issue is that appropriate geographical scales are likely to vary for different population groups, different built environment measures, and different outcomes [4,5]. In practice, built environment and physical activity researchers use a variety of geographical scales ranging from 100–8050 m [4].

The impact of neighbourhood definition on research results has been frequently demonstrated in the wider literature, and more recently in several studies focused on the built environment and physical activity [10,12,15,21]. While researchers have struggled to identify optimal neighbourhood definitions, some of the existing built environment and physical activity research suggests that larger buffers might best explain objectively measured moderate-to-vigorous physical activity in children [21], and self-reported walking for transport in adults [10]. Existing research has tended to focus on single measures of physical activity, yet it is possible that the choice of neighbourhood definition may differ for different aspects of physical activity. Furthermore, appropriate neighbourhood definitions are likely to vary for different aspects of the built environment and in different contexts. Therefore, it is important to investigate this issue across a range of exposure measures, outcome measures (e.g., walking for transport, walking for recreation moderate–vigorous physical activity, overall physical activity), population groups, and locations.

Given these considerations, the main purpose of this paper is to test the hypothesis that neighbourhood definitions of different types and geographical scales will determine whether or not evidence of an association between the built environment and physical activity is identified in statistical models. While this question has been explored in existing studies, to our knowledge no study has examined this issue in the context of associations between the built environment and objectively measured physical activity in adults, nor has any research yet examined how the choice of neighbourhood definition differentially impacts associations between different physical activity measures (e.g., self-report versus objective, recreational versus transport walking). Therefore, we also test the hypothesis that detection of an association will vary with different neighbourhood definitions, built environment measures, and physical activity measures.

## 2. Materials and Methods

### 2.1. Study Background

This study is based on data collected within the Understanding the Relationship Between Physical Activity and Neighbourhood (URBAN) study [22]. The URBAN is part of the International Physical Activity and Environment Network (IPEN) Adult study, an observational, cross-sectional study in 12 countries [23]. The present study uses data from New Zealand and uses IPEN protocols for exposure and outcome measures [24,25]. Ethical approval was granted by the Auckland University of Technology and Massey University ethics committees (AUTEC: 07/126, MUHECN: 07/045). All participants provided written informed consent.

The URBAN study recruited 2033 adults aged 20–65 years from 24 high- and 24 low-walkability neighbourhoods in four New Zealand cities: Waitakere, North Shore, Wellington and Christchurch (12 neighbourhoods in each city). Compared to the other eleven IPEN countries, the neighbourhoods in these four New Zealand cities tended to be less walkable with lower street connectivity (i.e., more cul-de-sacs), lower residential density, and lower land-use mix [25]. Walkability scores were calculated for each census meshblock using GIS and included measures of residential dwelling density, street connectivity, land-use mix, and retail floor area ratio [22]. The meshblock is the smallest spatial statistical unit in New Zealand, containing on average 110 people in urban areas and varying in size. Meshblocks with walkability scores in the highest tertile were defined as highly walkable, while meshblocks with walkability scores in the lowest tertile were defined as having low walkability. Meshblocks with average walkability scores were deliberately excluded to maximise variability as prescribed by IPEN protocols. The URBAN study neighbourhoods comprised five-plus contiguous meshblocks with consistently high- or low-walkability scores. All eligible neighbourhoods within each city were identified. Where there were more neighbourhoods than required, the URBAN study research team purposefully selected neighbourhoods based on local knowledge.

The 48 neighbourhoods were mainly suburban (*n* = 36) and dominated by residential land use with large areas of open space. Ten neighbourhoods were located within or adjacent to an activity centre with a mix of land uses—including retail, open space, institutional, and light industrial—but still dominated by residential land use. Two neighbourhoods were located on the outskirts of the Wellington central business district (CBD). These neighbourhoods were dominated by a mix of retail, commercial, institutional, and light industrial, with residual areas of residential and open space land use. Table 1 presents summary statistics describing the neighbourhood demographics. The NZ deprivation score is a value between 1 and 10, with 10 indicating that an area is more deprived [26]. The CBD neighbourhoods were more deprived and had a larger number of people and dwellings than suburban and activity centre-based neighbourhoods.

**Table 1.** Summary of neighbourhood demographics.

| Neighbourhood Type | Average Usual Resident Population 2006 (Range) | Average Number of Occupied Dwellings 2006 (Range) | Average NZ Deprivation Score (Range) |
|---|---|---|---|
| Suburban neighbourhoods (*n* = 36) | 773.4 (435–1218) | 282.1 (153–414) | 3.8 (1–10) |
| Neighbourhoods near activity centres (*n* = 10) | 811.5 (495–1251) | 306.9 (192–561) | 4.8 (1–10) |
| central business district (CBD) neighbourhoods (*n* = 2) | 898.5 (771–1026) | 405 (357–453) | 7.9 (6–10) |

For this study, 44 participants were excluded due to accelerometer exclusion criteria (see below) and the inability to locate residential addresses, leaving a total of 1989 participants. The methodology relevant to the present paper is described below. Detailed methods and participant demographics for the broader study are described elsewhere [22,27].

### 2.2. Physical Activity Measures

Objective physical activity was measured using Actical accelerometers (Mini-Mitter, Sunriver, OR, USA), which participants wore on their hips for seven consecutive days during waking hours. Accelerometers sense frequency and intensity of movement [28] and can distinguish between less intense physical activity such as walking and more intense physical activity such as riding a bicycle or running.

The accelerometers were set to record every 30 seconds. The raw output from the accelerometer is a unitless measure called a count [29], with higher counts indicating more intense physical activity. Periods of greater than 59 minutes of consecutive zero counts (indicating likely non-wear time) or where the accelerometer was worn for less than 60 minutes were excluded from analysis. Days with less than 10-hours-per-day wear time were also excluded.

Self-report physical activity data were collected using the International Physical Activity Questionnaire—Long Form (IPAQ-LF; [30]). Three self-reported measures of physical activity measures were created based on this questionnaire: self-reported walking for transport, self-reported walking for recreation, and total self-reported minutes walking for all purposes.

### 2.3. Neighbourhood Definitions

Overall, seven different neighbourhood definitions were created for each participant at a range of geographical scales. Three of the seven areas were based on the administrative units: the meshblock, the census area unit, which is comprised of meshblocks in urban areas and contains between 3000—5000 people [31], and the URBAN study neighbourhoods (see Table 1 for relative neighbourhood sizes). The four remaining neighbourhood definitions were road network buffers centred on participants' geocoded residential addresses and calculated at four geographical scales commonly used in built environment and health research [4]: 500 m, 800 m, 1000 m and 1500 m. The road network buffers were created using the Service Area function in ArcGIS version 9.3 (ESRI, Redmond, WA, USA) [32]. The road network was supplied by territorial authorities and excluded pedestrian-only paths due to a lack of data. Roads that are inaccessible to pedestrians (i.e., motorways and motorway on and off ramps) were removed prior to analysis. The relative sizes of the neighbourhoods are illustrated in Figure 1, which shows the different neighbourhood definitions for an exampleparticipant.

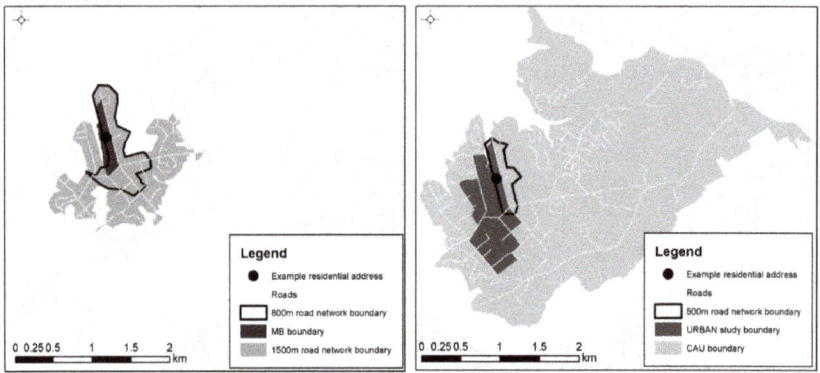

**Figure 1.** An example of neighbourhood boundaries for a participant. Road data shown in this figure were sourced from Land Information New Zealand (Creative Commons Attribution 3.0 New Zealand) and the neighbourhood boundary data were created as part of this study.

*2.4. Built Environment Attributes*

Three built environment attributes—dwelling density, street connectivity, and destination accessibility—were calculated for each participant within each of the seven neighbourhood definitions. These three attributes were chosen because they have been frequently found to be associated with physical activity within many studies across different contexts [33–35], and they were also shown to be associated with physical activity within the same dataset [27].

Dwelling density was calculated by dividing the number of occupied private dwellings by the residential land area, which was obtained from zoning datasets provided by territorial authorities. Dwelling numbers were sourced from the 2006 New Zealand census at the meshblock level. Since meshblock boundaries align with all administrative neighbourhoods, the number of private occupied dwellings is easily calculated for this type of neighbourhood definition. However, meshblock boundaries do not align with road network buffer boundaries. Therefore, the number of private occupied dwellings within each road network buffer was estimated by calculating a weighted average based on the land area of contributing meshblocks. Street connectivity was calculated by dividing the number of intersections (three or more ways) within the neighbourhood by the area in square kilometres. The calculation of dwelling density and street connectivity measures followed IPEN GIS protocols [24].

Destination accessibility was assessed using the neighbourhood destination accessibility index (NDAI; [27,36]). The NDAI is a measure of access to 31 neighbourhood destinations in eight domains (education, transport, recreation, social and cultural, food retail, financial, health, and other retail). The destination data used to calculate the NDAI were obtained from a range of sources including government (New Zealand Ministry of Education, New Zealand Ministry of the Environment and Land, New Zealand Ministry of Health, Territorial authorities, Liquor Licensing Authority), private spatial data suppliers (Terra Link International, GeoSmart) and an online business directory (www.zenbu.co.nz).

Most NDAI domains were calculated by assigning a score based on the presence of destinations within a neighbourhood. However, the transport and recreation domain scores were based on the density of destinations. The final NDAI score was calculated by summing the weighted domain scores, producing a value between 0 and 31, with a higher score representing better walking access to services and amenities. Since the NDAI was based on the presence/absence of destinations, it will necessarily increase with increased neighbourhood size.

*2.5. Demographics, Neighbourhood Preference and Neighbourhood Socioeconomic Deprivation*

Information on participants' age, gender, ethnicity, marital status, household income, educational qualifications, occupation, household car access, and preferences for living in a more or less walkable neighbourhood were collected in face-to-face computer-assisted personal interviews (CAPI).

Individuals may choose to live in neighbourhoods that support physical activity, introducing the possibility that individual neighbourhood preference may confound associations between neighbourhood environments and physical activity [27]. Therefore, neighbourhood preference was measured using items developed by Levine et al. [37]. Participants were provided with illustrations and verbal descriptions of two types of neighbourhoods—a lower-density suburban neighbourhood with common destinations accessible by car and a higher-density urban neighbourhood with most destinations accessible by walking or public transport. Participants indicated which of the two neighbourhood types they would prefer to live in—assuming similar housing costs, school quality and a mix of people in both neighbourhoods—using a five-point scale (strongly prefer walkable, moderately prefer walkable, neutral, moderately prefer less walkable, strongly prefer less walkable) [37].

Neighbourhood socio-economic deprivation was measured using the New Zealand Deprivation Index 2006 provided at the meshblock level [26].

*2.6. Statistical Analysis*

The associations between the built environment and physical activity measures were modelled using linear multi-level mixed-effect models to take into account the clustering of individuals within neighbourhoods (defined as the URBAN study neighbourhood) and cities. The multi-level mixed-effect model was chosen to assess the effect of neighbourhood characteristics on individual physical activity level. The appropriateness of the multilevel structure was tested by applying the likelihood ratio (LR) test to compare an empty model with and without adjustment for clustering (URBAN study neighbourhood nested in cities). The model's fit was significantly improved ($p < 0.001$) with the inclusion of the neighbourhood level variables, so the multilevel structure was maintained. The association between built environment exposures and physical activity were assessed through three models and progressively adjusted for confounders. All outcome variables were log transformed to have a normal distribution and aid comparison across models. The regression coefficients when exponentiated are the ratio or relative change in the outcome measure for each unit change in the exposure variable. Therefore, regression coefficients were exponentiated and reported as a relative change in the results.

The association between each of the three built environment measures and each of the five physical activity measures was modelled separately for each of the seven neighbourhood definitions. Each association was assessed by adjusting for individual-level factors (sex, age, ethnicity, income, marital status, education, employment and car access), neighbourhood socioeconomic deprivation and neighbourhood preference. All models reported in this paper were fully adjusted for these covariates. Adjusted intraclass correlation coefficients (ICCs) were calculated for null models (constant term in the fixed part) for each outcome. The goodness-of-fit of each model was estimated by calculating the marginal $R^2$ (proportion of variance explained by fixed factors alone) and conditional $R^2$ (proportion of variance explained by both fixed and random effects) [38]. Statistical analyses were conducted in R [39] using the "lme4" package to fit the linear mixed models and the "MuMIn" package to calculate goodness-of-fit [40,41].

## 3. Results

Descriptive statistics for the outcome measures are presented in Table 2. To put the mean accelerometer counts per hour measure into context: a participant who is washing dishes for an hour might record counts in the order of 600 (~10 counts per minute), while a participant who is continuously playing basketball for an hour might record counts in the order of 282,000 (~4700 per minute) [42].

**Table 2.** Descriptive statistics for the physical activity outcome measures assessed over a 7-day period.

| Physical Activity Outcome | Low Walkability | | | High Walkability | | | Adjusted Intraclass Correlation Coefficient (ICC) for Null Model |
|---|---|---|---|---|---|---|---|
| | Mean | Median | SD | Mean | Median | SD | |
| Self-reported walking for transport (total minutes) | 80.0 | 40 | 125.2 | 109.4 | 50 | 154.7 | 0.136 |
| Self-reported walking for recreation (total minutes) | 82.5 | 30 | 125.0 | 83.8 | 30 | 128.6 | 0.011 |
| Self-reported overall walking (total minutes) | 161.8 | 100 | 191.6 | 192.4 | 120 | 220.5 | 0.120 |
| Mean accelerometer counts per hour | 8701.1 | 8040.0 | 4215.0 | 9426.6 | 8586.7 | 4692.6 | 0.048 |
| % time spend in moderate-vigorous physical activity (MVPA) | 12.3 | 11 | 6.6 | 12.5 | 11 | 6.9 | 0.080 |

Descriptive statistics for the size of the seven neighbourhood definitions are shown in Table 3. The meshblock is the smallest neighbourhood, with a median area almost one quarter the size of that of the next smallest area (500-m road network buffer). The URBAN study neighbourhood is closest in size to the 500-m road network buffer, and the census area unit falls between the 1000-m and 1500-m road network buffers.

**Table 3.** Neighbourhood boundary size descriptive statistics.

| Boundary TYPE | Neighbourhood Boundary | N | Median (km$^2$) | Range (km$^2$) | IQR [a] (km$^2$) |
|---|---|---|---|---|---|
| Administrative unit | Meshblock | 272 | 0.05 | 1.43 | 0.05 |
| Contiguous administrative units | URBAN neighbourhood | 48 | 0.30 | 1.03 | 0.20 |
| Administrative unit | Census area unit | 67 | 1.83 | 8.96 | 1.37 |
| Road network buffer | 500-m road network buffer | 1989 | 0.28 | 1.03 | 0.13 |
| Road network buffer | 800-m road network buffer | 1989 | 0.64 | 0.98 | 0.31 |
| Road network buffer | 1000-m road network buffer | 1989 | 1.00 | 1.63 | 0.51 |
| Road network buffer | 1500-m road network buffer | 1989 | 2.26 | 3.41 | 0.95 |

[a] Interquartile range (IQR), [b] Understanding the Relationship between physical Activity and Neighbourhood (URBAN) study.

Table 4 displays the descriptive statistics for the built environment measures for each neighbourhood definition. The median street connectivity and dwelling density measures decreased consistently with increasing neighbourhood size. In contrast, NDAI measures consistently increased with increasing neighbourhood size. This is expected because the NDAI measure is calculated solely on the presence and number of destinations, meaning that an increase in neighbourhood size will always result in either no change or an increase in the NDAI score.

The results of the fully adjusted models presented in Table 5 indicate that whether or not an association between the built environment and physical activity was detected depends on the choice of neighbourhood definition, built environment measure and physical activity measure. Coefficients for all models are provided in Supplementary Tables S1–S5. For all models, the URBAN study neighbourhood and city were modelled as random effects and all other explanatory variables were modelled as fixed effects. The results are reported as the percentage change in the physical activity measure unit per unit increase in the built environment measure (Table 5). Bold text indicates results where there was some evidence (confidence intervals did not cross zero) to support an association between the built environment and physical activity. As expected in built environment research, the effect sizes were small as individual outcomes are more strongly associated with individual predictors.

Table 4. Built environment descriptive statistics for neighbourhood boundaries (n = 1989 adults).

| Neighbourhood Boundary | Dwelling Density (dwellings/Ha) | | | Street Connectivity (Intersections/km$^2$) | | | Neighbourhood Destination Accessibility Index (NDAI) (Score 0–31) | | |
|---|---|---|---|---|---|---|---|---|---|
| | Median | Range | IQR | Median | Range | IQR | Median | Range | IQR |
| Meshblock | 11.9 | 0.6–80.8 | 8.8–15.4 | 25.4 | 0–311.4 | 3.2–48.0 | 2.0 | 0–10.8 | 0.6–5.0 |
| URBAN neighbourhood | 11.8 | 2.1–58.3 | 8.0–15.1 | 33.2 | 3.7–111.7 | 14.9–40.2 | 5.9 | 2.5–18.9 | 4.2–8.1 |
| Census area unit | 8.8 | 1.3–32.1 | 5.8–11.0 | 25.6 | 3.6–92.3 | 15.3–33.8 | 9.3 | 2.2–24.1 | 6.1–13.4 |
| 500-m road network buffer | 10.2 | 1.1–42.0 | 8.4–12.5 | 34.1 | 0–101.1 | 24.8–42.5 | 6.4 | 0–24.6 | 4.1–9.4 |
| 800-m road network buffer | 9.8 | 1.9–37.3 | 8.4–11.8 | 32.5 | 0–91.2 | 25.6–39.8 | 10.2 | 0–29.5 | 6.2–14.9 |
| 1000-m road network buffer | 9.6 | 2.4–36.6 | 8.4–11.4 | 31.1 | 0–90.6 | 25.6–38.7 | 13.9 | 0–34.5 | 7.9–19.4 |
| 1500-m road network buffer | 9.3 | 2.5–33.0 | 8.3–11.0 | 29.6 | 0–76.5 | 25.3–38.2 | 20.7 | 0–40.2 | 14.6–7.4 |

Table 5. Percentage change (95% CI) in fully adjusted models of physical activity, for a one unit change in the built environment measures for the seven neighbourhood boundaries. All models were fully adjusted for sex, age, ethnicity, income, marital status, education, employment, car access, neighbourhood socioeconomic deprivation and neighbourhood preference. Bold text indicates results where there was some evidence (confidence intervals did not cross zero) to support an association between the built environment and physical activity.

| Built Environment Measure | Neighbourhood Definition | Mean Accelerometer Counts/Hour % Change (95% CI) Marginal R$^2$/Conditional R$^2$ | Percentage Time in MVPA % Change (95% CI) Marginal R$^2$/Conditional R$^2$ | Self-Reported Walking for Transport (Total Minutes) % Change (95% CI) Marginal R$^2$/Conditional R$^2$ | Self-Reported Walking for Recreation (Total Minutes) % Change (95% CI) Marginal R$^2$/Conditional R$^2$ | Self-Reported Overall Walking (Total Minutes) % Change (95% CI) Marginal R$^2$/Conditional R$^2$ |
|---|---|---|---|---|---|---|
| Dwelling density (dwellings/Ha) | MB [a] | **0.63 (0.37–0.89)** 0.08/0.09 | **0.47 (0.07–0.86)** 0.08/0.16 | **2.25 (0.76–3.73)** 0.09/0.16 | **3.10 (1.61–4.59)** 0.07/0.10 | **1.93 (0.60–3.25)** 0.07/0.12 |
| | UN [b] | **0.82 (0.43–1.08)** 0.08/0.09 | 0.65 (−0.05–1.36) 0.08/0.16 | **4.58 (2.21–6.95)** 0.11/0.16 | **4.39 (2.13–6.64)** 0.07/0.10 | **4.07 (2.0–6.1)** 0.10/0.13 |
| | CA [c] | **0.87 (0.24–1.49)** 0.07/0.09 | **1.20 (0.20–2.19)** 0.08/0.16 | **4.85 (1.53–8.16)** 0.09/0.17 | 3.11 (−0.36–6.57) 0.06/0.09 | 1.81 (−1.31–4.92) 0.07/0.13 |
| | B0500 [d] | **1.05 (0.55–1.56)** 0.08/0.10 | **0.98 (0.15–1.80)** 0.08/0.16 | **4.88 (1.92–7.83)** 0.10/0.16 | **4.25 (1.31–7.19)** 0.06/0.09 | **3.93 (1.27–6.59)** 0.08/0.12 |
| | B0800 [e] | **1.16 (0.53–1.78)** 0.08/0.10 | **1.06 (0.02–2.09)** 0.08/0.16 | **5.12 (1.38–8.86)** 0.10/0.16 | **5.59 (1.98–9.20)** 0.07/0.09 | **4.65 (1.31–7.99)** 0.08/0.12 |
| | B1000 [f] | **1.17 (0.46–1.88)** 0.07/0.09 | 0.83 (−0.33–1.97) 0.08/0.16 | **5.20 (0.94–9.45)** 0.09/0.16 | **6.69 (2.61–10.76)** 0.07/0.09 | **4.80 (1.01–8.59)** 0.08/0.12 |
| | B1500 [g] | **1.18 (0.40–1.97)** 0.07/0.09 | −0.01 (−0.76–1.82) 0.07/0.16 | **6.53 (1.71–11.36)** 0.10/0.16 | **7.48 (2.86–12.10)** 0.07/0.10 | **5.75 (1.43–10.06)** 0.08/0.12 |

Table 5. *Cont.*

| Built Environment Measure | Neighbourhood Definition | Mean Accelerometer Counts/Hour % Change (95% CI) Marginal R²/Conditional R² | Percentage Time in MVPA % Change (95% CI) Marginal R²/Conditional R² | Self-Reported Walking for Transport (Total Minutes) % Change (95% CI) Marginal R²/Conditional R² | Self-Reported Walking for Recreation (Total Minutes) % Change (95% CI) Marginal R²/Conditional R² | Self-Reported Overall Walking (Total Minutes) % Change (95% CI) Marginal R²/Conditional R² |
|---|---|---|---|---|---|---|
| Street connectivity (intersections/km²) | MB | 0.02 (−0.01–0.01) 0.06/0.09 | 0.57 (−0.1–0.07) 0.07/0.16 | 0.18 (−0.14–0.51) 0.08/0.17 | 0.05 (−0.30–0.40) 0.05/0.10 | 0.10 (−0.19–0.39) 0.06/0.13 |
| | UN | **0.27 (0.15–0.40) 0.08/0.09** | **0.28 (0.05–0.53) 0.09/0.16** | **1.34 (0.59–2.09) 0.10/0.17** | **1.16 (0.39–1.93) 0.06/0.10** | **1.04 (0.37–1.71) 0.08/0.13** |
| | CA | **0.37 (0.12–0.63) 0.07/0.09** | **0.29 (0.18–0.96) 0.09/0.16** | **2.13 (0.75–3.52) 0.09/0.17** | **1.50 (0.03–1.93) 0.06/0.09** | **1.49 (0.20–2.77) 0.07/0.13** |
| | B0500 | **0.28 (0.09–0.47) 0.07/0.09** | **0.27 (0.00–0.55) 0.08/0.16** | 0.94 (−0.10–1.95) 0.08/0.16 | 0.90 (−0.17–1.96) 0.06/0.09 | **0.99 (0.07–2.37) 0.07/0.12** |
| | B0800 | **0.37 (0.14–0.61) 0.07/0.09** | **0.41 (0.08–0.75) 0.08/0.16** | 0.56 (−0.73–1.85) 0.08/0.16 | **2.08 (0.77–3.38) 0.06/0.10** | **1.22 (0.07–2.37) 0.07/0.12** |
| | B1000 | **0.45 (0.25–0.70) 0.07/0.09** | **0.43 (0.05–0.81) 0.08/0.16** | **1.50 (0.05–2.94) 0.09/0.16** | **2.07 (0.62–3.53) 0.06/0.09** | **1.40 (0.10–2.70) 0.07/0.12** |
| | B1500 | **0.42 (0.19–0.65) 0.07/0.09** | 0.23 (−0.18–0.63) 0.08/0.16 | **2.75 (1.25–4.24) 0.11/0.16** | **2.79 (1.35–4.22) 0.07/0.10** | **1.53 (0.14–2.93) 0.08/0.12** |
| NDAI (Score 0–31) | MB | −1.00 (−2.05–0.05) 0.06/0.09 | −0.88 (−2.91–0.43) 0.07/0.16 | −1.57 (−6.78–3.63) 0.08/0.17 | 1.18 (−4.43–6.80) 0.05/0.10 | 0.05 (−4.69–4.79) 0.06/0.13 |
| | UN | −0.17 (−1.32–0.97) 0.06/0.09 | 1.17 (−0.81–3.14) 0.08/0.16 | −3.61 (−10.06–2.83) 0.08/0.17 | 1.07 (−5.38–7.52) 0.05/0.10 | 1.15 (−4.56–6.97) 0.06/0.13 |
| | CA | **0.88 (0.21–1.55) 0.06/0.09** | 0.41 (−0.67–1.49) 0.07/0.16 | **4.64 (0.91–8.37) 0.08/0.17** | **3.89 (0.09–7.70) 0.06/0.10** | **4.90 (1.68–8.13) 0.07/0.13** |
| | B0500 | 0.52 (−0.01–1.14) 0.06/0.09 | 0.17 (−0.64–0.97) 0.07/0.16 | 1.13 (−2.03–4.29) 0.08/0.17 | 0.92 (−2.47–4.30) 0.05/0.10 | **3.36 (0.53–6.19) 0.06/0.13** |
| | B0800 | **0.81 (0.33–1.28) 0.07/0.09** | **0.82 (0.15–1.49) 0.08/0.15** | **3.51 (1.04–5.98) 0.09/0.16** | 1.39 (−1.29–4.07) 0.05/0.10 | **4.01(1.82–6.20) 0.07/0.13** |
| | B1000 | **0.63 (0.21–1.05) 0.06/0.09** | **0.64 (0.04–1.23) 0.08/0.16** | **3.90 (1.76–6.05) 0.09/0.17** | 1.75 (−0.61–4.11) 0.06/0.10 | **4.08 (2.18–5.97) 0.07/0.13** |
| | B1500 | **0.60 (0.21–0.98) 0.07/0.09** | 0.51 (−0.06–1.07) 0.08/0.16 | **2.80 (0.77–4.82) 0.09/0.17** | 0.96 (−1.24–3.16) 0.05/0.10 | **2.78 (0.98–4.58) 0.06/0.13** |

[a] MB: meshblock, [b] UN: URBAN study neighbourhood, [c] CA: census area unit, [d] B0500: 500-m street network buffer, [e] B0800: 800-m street network buffer, [f] B1000: 1000-m street network buffer, [g] B1500: 1500-m street network buffer. The bold text indicates the results of models where there was evidence supporting an association between the built environment and physical activity.

There was no single neighbourhood definition that resulted in statistical evidence of an association between all built environments and physical activity measures. The meshblock, 500-m and 800-m road network buffers consistently resulted in evidence of an association between dwelling density and all five physical activity measures. For street connectivity, the URBAN neighbourhood, census area unit, and 1000-m road network buffer produced consistent evidence of an association with physical activity. In contrast, there was no single neighbourhood definition that resulted in consistent evidence of an association between NDAI and all five physical activity measures. The neighbourhood definitions where NDAI was most consistently associated with physical activity were the census area unit, 800-m road network buffer and 1000-m road network buffer. Overall, associations between the built environment and physical activity measures were most consistently detected when the 800-m and 1000-m road network buffers/were used.

When comparing models with the same built environment and physical activity measure, the marginal and conditional $R^2$ values were similar. This indicates that the choice of neighbourhood delineation did not meaningfully change the amount of variance explained by the models.

## 4. Discussion

The main aim of this paper was to test the hypothesis that neighbourhood definitions of different types and geographical scales will determine whether or not evidence of an association between the built environment and physical activity is captured in statistical models. Extending existing research, this paper also makes a new contribution by examining whether or not the choice of the physical activity outcome measure also determines whether or not an association is detected. Looking first at the individual models, in general, the magnitude of the effects appears meaningful. For a one dwelling per hectare (dph) increase in dwelling density, the estimates ranged from a 0.63% to 1.18% increase in overall physical activity. As a whole, the size of these effects are meaningful when you consider that the median dwelling density of the neighbourhoods in this study (~10 dph) falls within the "low-density suburban" category (8–12 dph) and to reach the next highest density category would require an increase in the order of 5 dph [43]. An increase of this magnitude would be associated with an increase in overall physical activity in the order of 5%. Although the effect sizes for street connectivity were smaller (0.27% to 0.48%), they also represent a meaningful increase in physical activity given that this is associated with increasing street connectivity by one intersection per square kilometre. For NDAI, the effect sizes (0.60% to 0.88%) relate to a one unit increase in NDAI score, which means adding one more different type of destination within the neighbourhood. For example, adding a convenience store to a neighbourhood where there are currently no convenience stores.

Results from this study supported the main hypothesis: that the choice of neighbourhood definition can determine whether evidence can be found or not. For all three built environment attributes there was evidence of an association for at least one of the seven neighbourhood definitions, yet for both street connectivity and NDAI some neighbourhood definitions had no evidence of an association between the built environment and physical activity. Our results also demonstrated that the choice of built environment and physical activity measures also determined whether or not evidence of an association was found. A neighbourhood delineation that is appropriate for one built environment measure may not be appropriate for all built environment measures. Similarly, different delineations may be more appropriate for different physical activity outcome measures. Therefore, it is important to carefully choose neighbourhood definitions and to report results at a range of geographical scales [4]. Similar to previous research, we were unable to clearly identify a single optimal neighbourhood definition for use in the built environment and physical activity research. However, our study showed that associations between the built environment and physical activity were most consistently detected when the 800-m and 1000-m road network buffers were used.

The lack of evidence of association at the smaller geographical scales makes sense when we consider the different types of measure. Given the neighbourhoods included in the study, we would expect dwellings to be the most common feature and for dwellings to be present at all scales. Therefore, it is not surprising that associations between dwelling density and physical activity were found at the smallest scales. In contrast, the NDAI measure is based on the presence of destinations, which are far less common than dwellings, especially in the study neighbourhoods which were largely suburban.

There may be other explanations for the lack of identified associations at the smallest geographical scales. There is a greater effect of positional accuracy (geocoding and spatial data precision and error) at smaller scales [44]. Furthermore, it is possible that smaller scale neighbourhoods are more relevant to population groups not considered in this study (e.g., non-drivers compared to drivers or children compared to adults). For example, in a study of geographic area and scale on the relationship between food environment and behaviour, Thornton and colleagues [11] found no evidence of an association between the food environment at the smallest geographic area (400-m road network buffer) for the full sample, although it reached significance when only households without cars were assessed; a finding that is consistent with travel survey data that shows that people in non-car households are more likely to use active transport modes than households with access to a car [45–47].

In general, our findings are consistent with those of similar studies investigating the impact of different neighbourhood boundaries on the built environment and physical activity. Clark and Scott [44] who, in a study of the MAUP on the relationship between the built environment and active travel, concluded that while the choice of neighbourhood definition influences coefficient magnitudes and significance, the patterns were inconsistent for different built environment measures. Our findings that the smaller scales were less likely to detect evidence of an association are similar to studies that suggest that larger buffer sizes might be more appropriate when investigating adults walking for transport [10] and children's moderate-to-vigorous physical activity [21].

As mentioned earlier, it has been recommended that researchers report GIS-based built environment measures at a range of scales [4], and our results support this. Not only would this assist with greater consistency and comparison across studies, but it would also help identify optimal built environment thresholds to support health behaviour for a range of built environment measures, population groups and health behaviours and outcomes [16]. However, reporting results at a range of scales may be difficult from a practical perspective. Calculating GIS-based measures of the built environment requires technical staff, specialist software, and sufficient computing power. This can make the calculation of built environment measures at a range of geographical scales prohibitively difficult and expensive. Possible solutions to this problem include sharing GIS resources and knowledge (e.g., sharing scripts and GIS-based models that automatically calculate built environment measures, developing manuals) [48], and the provision of open source tools to calculate built environment measures [49].

Reporting results at a range of geographical scales does not preclude first determining what scales and ranges are appropriate. An important first step is to consider available theoretical and conceptual models that could assist with decisions about what scales are likely to be most relevant [50]. Other data—such as time-use data [51], travel survey data [52,53], GPS data [54,55], public participation GIS [56] and studies on perceived neighbourhood sizes [57,58]—can also be used to inform the choice of scale by providing information on distances people travel and places they spend time.

*Limitations*

One of the strengths of this study was the use of an objective measure of physical activity, thus avoiding some of the issues with self-report measures such as poor respondent memory, recall bias and under-estimation of incidental activities [59]. However, this study had several limitations. First, a limitation of this outcome measure is that the built environment was assessed for the residential neighbourhood, yet the physical activity data were collected everywhere participants went, not only in their residential neighbourhood (non-context specific). Focusing only on the residential neighbourhood is a common issue in the built environment and health research as neighbourhoods are typically defined around the home address. A related issue is that the geographic context in which the built environment influences physical activity behaviours is unknown. This is the uncertain geographic context problem [60], and it means that neighbourhood definitions such as administrative units and road network buffers may not align with the true context whereby the built environment influences physical activity. In response, there have been calls to include the built environments of non-residential neighbourhoods, such as work and school neighbourhoods [61,62], to move from place-based research to person-based research [11,63], and to move to individualised measures of the built environment [11,60].

A limitation that is more important to the conclusions of the study is that the maximum scale did not go beyond 1500 m. It is possible that there is an even larger scale at which the effect of the built environment on physical activity changes. In other words, while our results suggest that buffers ranging from 800–1500 m are likely to be appropriate, it is possible that scales beyond 1500 m are also appropriate. However, as the scale increases, the reduced heterogeneity may lead to difficulty detecting effects [4,11].

There were methodological limitations related to the incomplete representation of where people can travel and imprecise representation of destinations. When creating road network buffers, a lack of pedestrian network data meant that our study used road network data to represent where people can travel. However, this is an incomplete representation of potential travel paths because it excludes non-road networks that people commonly travel along (e.g., pedestrian-only paths, cycle trails). Therefore, the neighbourhood definitions based on road network buffers are likely only subsets of the experienced neighbourhoods. Research has demonstrated that including pedestrian networks can increase the size of the neighbourhood [64,65] and so we would expect that our road network buffers are underestimations of the size of the neighbourhood accessible within a certain distance. Although the importance of including pedestrian paths when defining neighbourhoods has been identified [64,65], the lack of pedestrian network data makes this challenging in practice. While we were not able to include non-road networks in our study, it is likely that pedestrian network data will become increasingly available with the continual development of freely available OpenStreetMap (OSM) data, and also the development of new methods to approximate footpath locations [66] or extract footpaths from remotely sensed imagery [67,68].

Finally, our study was limited by the imprecise representation of destination data. The location of each destination was represented by a single point, whereas in reality, destinations cover areas of varying sizes and in the case of a large park, several access points are likely. This means that compared to administrative units, road network buffers are less likely to accurately capture destinations when they are represented as points.

Future research could address some of these limitations by consider individual factors (e.g., non-car households, bicycle ownership) that might be important in determining the scale at which the built environment influences health outcomes and behaviours. Other methods of measuring the built environment should also be considered. For example, kernel density measures are an underutilized technique in built environment and health research that account for the proximity of built environment features to one another [69]. Yet, in a recent food environment study they showed stronger associations with food behaviours than measures calculated using circular or road network buffers [11].

## 5. Conclusions

In summary, this study demonstrated that the choice of neighbourhood definition can influence whether or not an association between built environment attributes and adults' physical activity is detected. Furthermore, the association with physical activity was robust enough to be detected at a range of scales for all built environment measures. Although like previous researchers, this study was unable to identify a single optimal neighbourhood definition, we did note that associations were less likely to be found when measured using smaller neighbourhoods. The 800-m and 1000-m road network buffers were the neighbourhood definitions where associations between the built environment and physical activity were most consistently detected.

It is important that researchers carefully consider the most appropriate type of neighbourhood boundary and geographical scale. To assist in this decision, more evidence on appropriate neighbourhood types and scales is needed not only in different environments, but also with different population groups, built environment measures, outcome measures, scales and neighbourhood definitions. Given the difficulties in trying to identify a single optimal neighbourhood definition and the policy need for evidence to be provided with an associated scale, we suggest that future work of this nature might aim to identify a range of appropriate neighbourhood definitions. Furthermore, future work should compare a greater range of scales than studied here, especially larger scales.

**Supplementary Materials:** The following are available online at http://www.mdpi.com/1660-4601/16/9/1501/s1, Table S1: Results from the fully adjusted models where the outcome is accelerometer counts. All models are fully adjusted for sex, age, ethnicity, income, marital status, education, employment, car access, neighbourhood socioeconomic deprivation, and neighbourhood preference; Table S2: Results from the fully adjusted models where the outcome is percentage time in MVPA. All models are fully adjusted for sex, age, ethnicity, income, marital status, education, employment, car access, neighbourhood socioeconomic deprivation, and neighbourhood preference; Table S3: Results from the fully adjusted models where the outcome is self reported walking for transport (time in minutes). All models are fully adjusted for sex, age, ethnicity, income, marital status, education, employment, car access, neighbourhood socioeconomic deprivation, and neighbourhood preference; Table S4: Results from the fully adjusted models where the outcome is self reported walking for recreation (time in minutes). All models are fully adjusted for sex, age, ethnicity, income, marital status, education, employment, car access, neighbourhood socioeconomic deprivation, and neighbourhood preference; Table S5: Results from the fully adjusted models where the outcome is self reported overall walking (time in minutes). All models are fully adjusted for sex, age, ethnicity, income, marital status, education, employment, car access, neighbourhood socioeconomic deprivation, and neighbourhood preference.

**Author Contributions:** Conceptualization, S.M., D.O. and K.W.; Data curation, S.M.; Formal analysis, S.M. and N.B.; Funding acquisition, S.M. and K.W.; Investigation, S.M. and M.J.K.; Methodology, S.M., N.B., M.J.K., A.T.K., K.E.L., D.O. and K.W.; Project administration, S.M.; Resources, K.W.; Supervision, D.O. and K.W.; Visualization, S.M.; Writing—original draft, S.M.; Writing—review and editing, S.M., N.B., M.J.K., A.T.K., K.E.L., K.O., D.O. and K.W.

**Funding:** This research received no external funding.

**Acknowledgments:** The Understanding Relationships Between Neighbourhoods and Physical Activity (URBAN) study was funded by the Health Research Council of New Zealand (grant: 07/356). The authors thank the URBAN study team, the participants who completed the study, the research assistants who collected the data and the territorial authorities for providing the GIS datasets. S.M. is supported by an Australian National Health and Medical Research Council Early Career Fellowship (#1121035). M.J.K. was supported by a JSPS Postdoctoral Fellowship for Research in Japan (#17716) from the Japan Society for the Promotion of Science. K.O. is supported by the MEXT-Supported Program for the Strategic Research Foundation at Private Universities, 2015–2019 the Japan Ministry of Education, Culture, Sports, Science and Technology (S1511017).

**Conflicts of Interest:** The authors declare no conflict of interest.

## References

1. Humpel, N.; Owen, N.; Leslie, E. Environmental factors associated with adults' participation in physical activity: A review. *Am. J. Prev. Med.* **2002**, *22*, 188–199. [PubMed]
2. Ding, D.; Sallis, J.F.; Kerr, J.; Lee, S.; Rosenberg, D.E. Neighborhood environment and physical activity among youth: A review. *Am. J. Prev. Med.* **2011**, *41*, 442–455. [CrossRef]
3. McCormack, G.; Giles-Corti, B.; Lange, A.; Smith, T.; Martin, K.; Pikora, T.J. An update of recent evidence of the relationship between objective and self-report measures of the physical environment and physical activity behaviours. *J. Sci. Med. Sport* **2004**, *7*, 81–92. [CrossRef]
4. Brownson, R.C.; Hoehner, C.M.; Day, K.; Forsyth, A.; Sallis, J.F. Measuring the built environment for physical activity: State of the science. *Am. J. Prevent. Med.* **2009**, *36*, S99–S123.e12. [CrossRef]
5. Moudon, A.V.; Lee, C.; Cheadle, A.D.; Garvin, C.; Johnson, D.; Schmid, T.L.; Weathers, R.D.; Lin, L. Operational definitions of walkable neighborhood: Theoretical and empirical insights. *J. Phys. Activity Health* **2006**, *3*, S99–S117. [CrossRef]
6. Villanueva, K.; Knuiman, M.; Nathan, A.; Giles-Corti, B.; Christian, H.; Foster, S.; Bull, F. The impact of neighborhood walkability on walking: Does it differ across adult life stage and does neighborhood buffer size matter? *Health Place* **2014**, *25*, 43–46. [CrossRef] [PubMed]

7.   Diez Roux, A.V. Investigating neighborhood and area effects on health. *Am. J. Public Health* **2001**, *91*, 1783–1789.

8.   Gauvin, L.; Robitaille, É.; Riva, M.; McLaren, L.; Dassa, C.; Potvin, L. Conceptualizing and operationalizing neighbourhoods. *Can. J. Public Health* **2007**, *98*, S18–S26. [PubMed]

9.   Chaix, B.; Merlo, J.; Evans, D.; Leal, C.; Havard, S. Neighbourhoods in eco-epidemiologic research: Delimiting personal exposure areas. A response to Riva, Gauvin, Apparicio and Brodeur. *Soc. Sci. Med.* **2009**, *69*, 1306–1310. [CrossRef]

10.  Learnihan, V.; Van Niel, K.P.; Giles-Corti, B.; Knuiman, M. Effect of scale on the links between walking and urban design. *Geogr. Res.* **2011**, *49*, 183–191. [CrossRef]

11.  Thornton, L.E.; Pearce, J.R.; Macdonald, L.; Lamb, K.E.; Ellaway, A. Does the choice of neighbourhood supermarket access measure influence associations with individual-level fruit and vegetable consumption? A case study from Glasgow. *Int. J. Health Geograph.* **2012**, *11*, 29. [CrossRef]

12.  Mitra, R.; Buliung, R.N. Built environment correlates of active school transportation: Neighborhood and the modifiable areal unit problem. *J. Transport Geogr.* **2012**, *20*, 51–61. [CrossRef]

13.  Messer, L.C.; Vinikoor-Imler, L.C.; Laraia, B.A. Conceptualizing neighborhood space: Consistency and variation of associations for neighborhood factors and pregnancy health across multiple neighborhood units. *Health Place* **2012**, *18*, 805–813. [CrossRef]

14.  Coffee, N.T.; Howard, N.; Paquet, C.; Hugo, G.; Daniel, M. Is walkability associated with a lower cardiometabolic risk? *Health Place* **2013**, *21*, 163–169. [CrossRef]

15.  Boone-Heinonen, J.; Popkin, B.M.; Song, Y.; Gordon-Larsen, P. What neighborhood area captures built environment features related to adolescent physical activity? *Health Place* **2010**, *16*, 1280–1286. [CrossRef]

16.  Koohsari, M.J.; Badland, H.; Giles-Corti, B. (Re) Designing the built environment to support physical activity: Bringing public health back into urban design and planning. *Cities* **2013**, *35*, 294–298. [CrossRef]

17.  Sallis, J.F. Angels in the details: Comment on the relationship between destination proximity, destination mix and physical activity behaviors. *Prev. Med.* **2008**, *46*, 6–7. [CrossRef]

18.  Openshaw, S. Ecological fallacies and the analysis of areal census data. *Environ. Plan. A* **1984**, *16*, 17–31. [CrossRef]

19.  Flowerdew, R.; Manley, D.J.; Sabel, C.E. Neighbourhood effects on health: Does it matter where you draw the boundaries? *Soc. Sci. Med.* **2008**, *66*, 1241–1255. [CrossRef]

20.  Oliver, L.N.; Schuurman, N.; Hall, A.W. Comparing circular and network buffers to examine the influence of land use on walking for leisure and errands. *Int. J. Health Geogr.* **2007**, *6*, 41. [CrossRef]

21.  Van Loon, J.; Frank, L.D.; Nettlefold, L.; Naylor, P.J. Youth physical activity and the neighbourhood environment: Examining correlates and the role of neighbourhood definition. *Soc. Sci. Med.* **2014**, *104*, 107–115. [CrossRef]

22.  Badland, H.M.; Schofield, G.M.; Witten, K.; Schluter, P.J.; Mavoa, S.; Kearns, R.A.; Hinckson, E.A.; Oliver, M.; Kaiwai, H.; Jensen, V.G.; Ergler, C. Understanding the Relationship between Activity and Neighbourhoods (URBAN) Study: Research design and methodology. *BMC Public Health* **2009**, *9*, 224. [CrossRef]

23.  Kerr, J.; Sallis, J.F.; Owen, N.; De Bourdeaudhuij, I.; Cerin, E.; Sugiyama, T.; Reis, R.; Sarmiento, O.; Frömel, K.; Mitáš, J.; Troelsen, J. Advancing science and policy through a coordinated international study of physical activity and built environments: IPEN adult methods. *J. Phys. Activity Health* **2013**, *10*, 581–601. [CrossRef]

24.  Adams, M.A.; Chapman, J.; Sallis, J.F.; Frank, L.D. *Built Environment and Physical Activity: GIS Templates and Variable Naming*; International Physical Activity and Environment Network (IPEN) Study Coordinating Centre: University of California, San Diego, CA, USA, 2012.

25.  Adams, M.A.; Frank, L.D.; Schipperijn, J.; Smith, G.; Chapman, J.; Christiansen, L.B.; Coffee, N.; Salvo, D.; du Toit, L.; Dygrýn, J.; et al. International variation in neighborhood walkability, transit, and recreation environments using geographic information systems: The IPEN adult study. *Int. J. Health. Geogr* **2014**, *13*, 43. [CrossRef] [PubMed]

26.  Salmond, C.; Crampton, P.; Atkinson, J. *NZDep2006 Index of Deprivation*; Department of Public Health, University of Otago Wellington: Wellington, New Zealand, 2007; Volume 5541.

27.  Witten, K.; Blakely, T.; Bagheri, N.; Badland, H.; Ivory, V.; Pearce, J.; Mavoa, S.; Hinckson, E.; Schofield, G. Neighborhood built environment and transport and leisure physical activity: Findings using objective exposure and outcome measures in New Zealand. *Environ. Health Perspect.* **2012**, *120*, 971–977. [CrossRef] [PubMed]

28. Bouten, C.V.; Koekkoek, K.T.; Verduin, M.; Kodde, R.; Janssen, J.D. A triaxial accelerometer and portable data processing unit for the assessment of daily physical activity. *IEEE Trans. Biomed. Eng.* **1997**, *44*, 136–147. [CrossRef] [PubMed]

29. Chen, K.Y.; Bassett, J.D.R. The technology of accelerometry-based activity monitors: Current and future. *Med. Sci. Sport Exerc.* **2005**, *37*, S490–S500. [CrossRef]

30. Craig, C.L.; Marshall, A.L.; Sjöström, M.; Bauman, A.E.; Booth, M.L.; Ainsworth, B.E.; Pratt, M.; Ekelund, U.L.F.; Yngve, A.; Sallis, J.F.; et al. International physical activity questionnaire: 12-country reliability and validity. *Med. Sci. Sport Exerc* **2003**, *35*, 1381–1395. [CrossRef]

31. Statistics New Zealand. Geographic Hierarchy. 2013. Available online: www.stats.govt.nz (accessed on 28 April 2019).

32. ESRI. *ArcGIS 9.3*; ESRI: Redlands, CA, USA, 2009.

33. Sundquist, K.; Eriksson, U.; Kawakami, N.; Skog, L.; Ohlsson, H.; Arvidsson, D. Neighborhood walkability, physical activity, and walking behavior: The Swedish Neighborhood and Physical Activity (SNAP) study. *Soc. Sci. Med.* **2011**, *72*, 1266–1273. [CrossRef]

34. Kligerman, M.; Sallis, J.F.; Ryan, S.; Frank, L.D.; Nader, P.R. Association of neighborhood design and recreation environment variables with physical activity and body mass index in adolescents. *Am. J. Health Promot.* **2007**, *21*, 274–277. [CrossRef]

35. Van Dyck, D.; Cardon, G.; Deforche, B.; Sallis, J.F.; Owen, N.; De Bourdeaudhuij, I. Neighborhood SES and walkability are related to physical activity behavior in Belgian adults. *Prev. Med.* **2010**, *50* (Suppl. 1), S74–S79. [CrossRef] [PubMed]

36. Witten, K.; Pearce, J.; Day, P. Neighbourhood Destination Accessibility Index: A GIS tool for measuring infrastructure support for neighbourhood physical activity. *Environ. Plan. A* **2011**, *43*, 205–223. [CrossRef]

37. Levine, J.; Inam, A.; Torng, G.-W. A choice-based rationale for land use and transportation alternatives: Evidence from Boston and Atlanta. *J. Plan. Educ. Res.* **2005**, *24*, 317–330. [CrossRef]

38. Nakagawa, S.; Schielzeth, H. A general and simple method for obtaining R2 from generalized linear mixed-effects models. *Methods Ecol. Evolut.* **2013**, *4*, 133–142. [CrossRef]

39. R Development Core Team. *R: A Language and Environment for Statistical Computing*; R Foundation for Statistical Computing: Vienna, Austria, 2008.

40. Bates, D.; Maechler, M.; Bolker, B. Lme4: Linear Mixed-Effects Models Using S4 Classes. 2012. Available online: https://CRAN.R-project.org/package=lme4 (accessed on 28 April 2019).

41. Barton, K. MuMIn: Multi-Model Inference. 2015. Available online: https://CRAN.R-project.org/package=MuMIn (accessed on 28 April 2019).

42. Kozey, S.L.; Lyden, K.; Howe, C.A.; Staudenmayer, J.W.; Freedson, P.S. Accelerometer output and MET values of common physical activities. *Med. Sci. Sports Exerc.* **2010**, *42*, 1776–1784.

43. Ghosh, S.; Vale, R. Typologies and basic descriptors of New Zealand residential urban forms. *J. Urban Des.* **2009**, *14*, 507–536. [CrossRef]

44. Clark, A.; Scott, D. Understanding the impact of the modifiable areal unit problem on the relationship between active travel and the built environment. *Urban Stud.* **2014**, *51*, 284–299. [CrossRef]

45. Healy, M.A.; Gilliland, J.A. Quantifying the magnitude of environmental exposure misclassification when using imprecise address proxies in public health research. *Spat. Spatio Temp. Epidemiol.* **2012**, *3*, 55–67. [CrossRef]

46. Barton, H.; Horswell, M.; Millar, P. Neighbourhood accessibility and active travel. *Plan. Pract. Res.* **2012**, *27*, 177–201. [CrossRef]

47. Dieleman, F.M.; Dijst, M.; Burghouwt, G. Urban form and travel behaviour: Micro-level household attributes and residential context. *Urban Stud.* **2002**, *39*, 507–527. [CrossRef]

48. Forsyth, A. NEAT-GIS (Neighborhood Environment for Active Transport) Protocols; An updated version of Environment and Physical Activity: GIS Protocols; Version 5.0. 2010. Available online: http://designforhealth.net/wp-content/uploads/2012/12/NEAT_GIS_V5_0_26Nov2010FIN.pdf (accessed on 28 April 2019).

49. Giles-Corti, B.; Macaulay, G.; Middleton, N.; Boruff, B.; Bull, F.; Butterworth, I.; Badland, H.; Mavoa, S.; Roberts, R.; Christian, H. Developing a research and practice tool to measure walkability: A demonstration project. *Health Promot. J. Austr.* **2014**, *25*, 160–166. [CrossRef]

50. Roux, A.-V.D. Neighborhoods and health: Where are we and were do we go from here? *Revue d'epidemiol. Sante Publique* **2007**, *55*, 13–21. [CrossRef]

51. Millward, H.; Spinney, J.; Scott, D. Active-transport walking behaviour: Destinations, durations, distances. *J. Transport Geogr.* **2013**, *28*, 101–110. [CrossRef]

52. Yang, Y.; Diez-Roux, A.V. Walking distance by trip purpose and population subgroups. *Am. J. Prev. Med.* **2012**, *43*, 11–19. [CrossRef] [PubMed]

53. Burke, M.; Brown, A. Distances people walk for transport. *Road Transport Res. A J. Aust. N. Z. Res. Pract.* **2007**, *16*, 16.

54. Boruff, B.J.; Nathan, A.; Nijënstein, S. Using GPS technology to (re)-examine operational definitions of 'neighbourhood'in place-based health research. *Int. J. Health Geogr.* **2012**, *11*, 22. [CrossRef]

55. Zenk, S.N.; Schulz, A.J.; Matthews, S.A.; Odoms-Young, A.; Wilbur, J.; Wegrzyn, L.; Gibbs, K.; Braunschweig, C.; Stokes, C. Activity space environment and dietary and physical activity behaviors: A pilot study. *Health Place* **2011**, *17*, 1150–1161. [CrossRef] [PubMed]

56. Hasanzadeh, K.; Broberg, A.; Kyttä, M. Where is my neighborhood? A dynamic individual-based definition of home ranges and implementation of multiple evaluation criteria. *Appl. Geogr.* **2017**, *84*, 1–10. [CrossRef]

57. Smith, G.; Gidlow, C.; Davey, R.; Foster, C. What is my walking neighbourhood? A pilot study of English adults' definitions of their local walking neighbourhoods. *Int. J. Behav. Nutr. Phys. Act.* **2010**, *7*, 34. [CrossRef]

58. Coulton, C.J.; Jennings, M.Z.; Chan, T. How big is my neighborhood? Individual and contextual effects on perceptions of neighborhood scale. *Am. J. Community Psychol.* **2013**, *51*, 140–150. [CrossRef] [PubMed]

59. Dollman, J.; Okely, A.D.; Hardy, L.; Timperio, A.; Salmon, J.; Hills, A.P. A hitchhiker's guide to assessing young people's physical activity: Deciding what method to use. *J. Sci. Med. Sport* **2009**, *12*, 518–525. [CrossRef] [PubMed]

60. Kwan, M.-P. The uncertain geographic context problem. *Ann. Associat. Am. Geogr.* **2012**, *102*, 958–968. [CrossRef]

61. Hurvitz, P.M.; Moudon, A.V. Home versus nonhome neighborhood: Quantifying differences in exposure to the built environment. *Am. J. Prev. Med.* **2012**, *42*, 411–417. [CrossRef] [PubMed]

62. Kestens, Y.; Lebel, A.; Daniel, M.; Thériault, M.; Pampalon, R. Using experienced activity spaces to measure foodscape exposure. *Health Place* **2010**, *16*, 1094–1103. [CrossRef] [PubMed]

63. Kwan, M.P. From place-based to people-based exposure measures. *Soc. Sci. Med.* **2009**, *69*, 1311–1313. [CrossRef]

64. Chin, G.K.; Van Niel, K.P.; Giles-Corti, B.; Knuiman, M. Accessibility and connectivity in physical activity studies: The impact of missing pedestrian data. *Prev. Med.* **2008**, *46*, 41–45. [CrossRef] [PubMed]

65. Tal, G.; Handy, S. Measuring nonmotorized accessibility and connectivity in a robust pedestrian network. *Transp. Res. Rec.* **2012**, *2299*, 48–56. [CrossRef]

66. Janssen, I.; Rosu, A. Measuring sidewalk distances using Google Earth. *BMC Med. Res. Methodol.* **2012**, *12*, 39. [CrossRef]

67. Senlet, T.; Elgammal, A. Segmentation of occluded sidewalks in satellite images. In Proceedings of the 21st International Conference on Pattern Recognition (ICPR2012), Tsukuba Science City, Japan, 11–15 November 2012.

68. Smith, V.; Malik, J.; Culler, D. Classification of sidewalks in street view images. In Proceedings of the 2013 International Green Computing Conference Proceedings, Arlington, VA, USA, 27–29 June 2013.

69. King, T.L.; Thornton, L.E.; Bentley, R.J.; Kavanagh, A.M. The use of kernel density estimation to examine associations between neighborhood destination intensity and walking and physical activity. *PLoS ONE* **2015**, *10*, e0137402. [CrossRef]

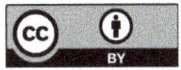

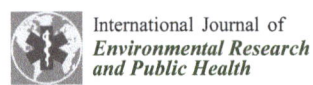

International Journal of
*Environmental Research
and Public Health*

*Article*

# Winter City Urbanism: Enabling All Year Connectivity for Soft Mobility

**David Chapman [1,*], Kristina L. Nilsson [1], Agatino Rizzo [1] and Agneta Larsson [2]**

[1]   Architecture Group, Luleå University of Technology, 971 87 Luleå, Sweden; kristina.l.nilsson@ltu.se (K.L.N.); agatino.rizzo@ltu.se (A.R.)
[2]   Health Sciences, Luleå University of Technology, 971 87 Luleå, Sweden; agneta.larsson@ltu.se
*    Correspondence: david.chapman@ltu.se

Received: 12 March 2019; Accepted: 20 May 2019; Published: 22 May 2019

**Abstract:** This study explores connectivity for soft mobility in the winter season. Working with residents from the sub-arctic city of Luleå, Sweden, the research examines how the interaction between the built environment and winter season affects people's use of the outdoor environment. The research questions for this study are (1) How do residents perceive the effects of winter on an areas spatial structure and pattern of streets and pathways? and (2) What enablers and barriers impact resident soft mobility choices and use of the public realm in winter? Methods used were mental mapping and photo elicitation exercises. These were used to gain a better understanding of people's perception of soft mobility in winter. The results were analysed to identify how soft mobility is influenced by the winter season. The discussion highlights that at the neighbourhood scale, residents perceive that the winter alters an areas spatial structure and pattern of streets and pathways. It was also seen to reduce ease of understanding of the public realm and townscape. In conclusion, it is argued that new and re-tooled town planning strategies, such as extending blue/ green infrastructure planning to include white space could help better enable all year outdoor activity in winter cities.

**Keywords:** soft mobility; walkable environment; physical activity; health outcomes; active living

---

## 1. Introduction

All over the world, the form of the built environment plays a key role in enabling urban outdoor activities such as soft mobility. The public realm can make it more attractive for people to be mobile outdoors and to participate in public life or it can put people off venturing outside.

For the purpose of this study, soft mobility is defined as human-powered, non-motorized ways of getting around, that have a relatively little impact on the environment, while connectivity in the built environment is defined as the degree to which a place and its parts are connected to each other [1]. Together connectivity for soft mobility, which collectively can be defined as how the built environment influences soft mobility choices in the form of walking and cycling, has been linked to a range of town planning agendas. It was been linked to reducing building and transport pollution [2,3] and more efficient use of land [4]. It has been associated with discussions around energy efficient modes of transport and reduced car usage [5]. It has been linked to the human wellbeing agenda by helping facilitate physical activity [6,7]. Today, creating active built environments that enable regular, all year outdoor soft mobility responds to the United Nation's Sustainable Development Goals and the World Health Organization's Global action plan on physical activity 2018–2030 (2018).

While there are many arguments for why connectivity for soft mobility is an essential part of the urban design of settlements, there is currently little knowledge of how it is affected by seasonal climate variation. As such, the aim of this study is to explore how the interaction between the built environment and winter season create barriers and enablers to connectivity for soft mobility.

The main research questions were (1) how do residents perceive the effects of winter on an areas spatial structure and pattern of streets and pathways? and (2) what enablers and barriers impact resident soft mobility choices and use of the public realm in winter?

### 1.1. Climate-Sensitive Urban Design

Settlements are usually discussed as being in a state of constant evolution or change rather than being static or, finished [8]. Equally, for those involved in the design and planning of the built environment, such changes are most commonly associated with physical, social, cultural or economic conditions, rarely are the changes created by seasonal climate investigated.

For urban design connectivity for soft mobility is a common focus, whether it is described as walking and cycling, connectivity, permeability, integration or just merely, ease of movement [9–13]. For most designers and planners, soft mobility is a critical dimension of urban design that has been subject to numerous publications [14]. For a detailed review, see Stephen Marshall's book, *Streets & Patterns* [15]. However, within these studies the implications of seasonal climate on connectivity for soft mobility is less well understood. This is important today because settlements that experience significant seasonal climate variation are challenged with enabling all year outdoor soft mobility as part of a range of town planning and health policy agendas.

For such settlements, seasonal climate variation can significantly complicate the design of urban form and public realm. Here it is often seen that the interaction between the built environment and seasonal climate variation can physically affect the public realm and the levels of connectivity for soft mobility an area can afford.

### 1.2. Winter City Urban Design

Winter settlements are usually places that experience high degrees of seasonal climate variation, temperatures commonly below zero, precipitation that is mainly snow, and limited hours of sunshine and daylight [16]. In such settlements, winter conditions and covers of snow and ice are a regular part of the built environment and can be in place for between 4–6 months of the year.

Research into the design of winter cities has been ongoing since around the middle of the twentieth century and reached a peak in the 1980s and 1990s [17]. Notable advocates of climate-sensitive urban design for winter settlements were the Swedish-English architect Ralph Erskine and the Canadian planner Norman Pressman. Erskine's 1959 'A Grammar for High Latitudes' [18] provides an early example of climate-sensitive design guidelines for winter communities. Here, Erskine highlights the importance of considering the cold, heat, snow, frost, light, wind, vegetation and the microclimate in the design process [18].

Pressman published numerous books and articles on winter cities between 1986 and 2004. While his works looked at a range of different ways of making winter cities more liveable, his work settled and focused on three climate-sensitive design principles for winter cities. Here his microclimatic design ideas focused on maximising solar access, minimising the negative effects of wind and managing snowfall and gathering [19–22].

The work of Erskine, Pressman and others including the Winter Cities institute (wintercities.com) is influential in improving our understanding of winter city urban design and a detailed state of the art of this work can be found in *Updating Winter: The Importance of Climate-Sensitive Urban Design for Winter Settlements*, Arctic Yearbook, 2018 [17]. However, while these works cover many dimensions of winter urbanism, they do not address how people perceive connectivity for soft mobility in winter.

## 2. Materials and Methods

The study focused on a single case study neighborhood where it investigates resident's perceptions of the urban structure and barriers and enablers to soft mobility in streets and spaces in the winter season. A sequential mixed methods design was used [23] combining two qualitative participatory methods; mental mapping and photo-elicitation method. This design was chosen as the combination of the two methods provides a deeper understanding of the topic.

As both methods enables residents to record and reflect their neighborhood, the results from each method can be brought together for a more detailed analysis about how the interaction between the built environment and winter season creates barriers and enablers to connectivity for soft mobility. The results from the mental mapping focuses on the urban scale. Here, the findings will provide an insight into how residents perceive the urban structure of their neighbourhood environment and surroundings in winter conditions, in comparison to summer conditions. The results from the photo-elicitation exercise will deepen these results and explore how the public realm (the streets and spaces) of the neighbourhood are altered by the winter season.

### 2.1. Case Study

The city of Luleå, Sweden is located at 66.5622° N (latitude) just below the Arctic Circle (Figure 1). It is identified in the Köppen–Geiger Climate Classification system as sub-arctic. In the summer temperatures can reach +30 degrees and the sun does not set for significant periods. During the winter, temperatures can reach −30 with minimal daylight hours. The sea freezes annually for 6–7 months. The selected neighbourhood for the research was Mjölkudden, Luleå. Mjölkudden is a mixed-use neighbourhood and has a residential population of 3491. The average age is 46 years and there is an almost equal male to female ratio [24]. The area contains a variety of functions including a healthcare centre, pharmacy, dentist, church, supermarket and leisure facilities. Housing accommodation is both single and multi-family houses.

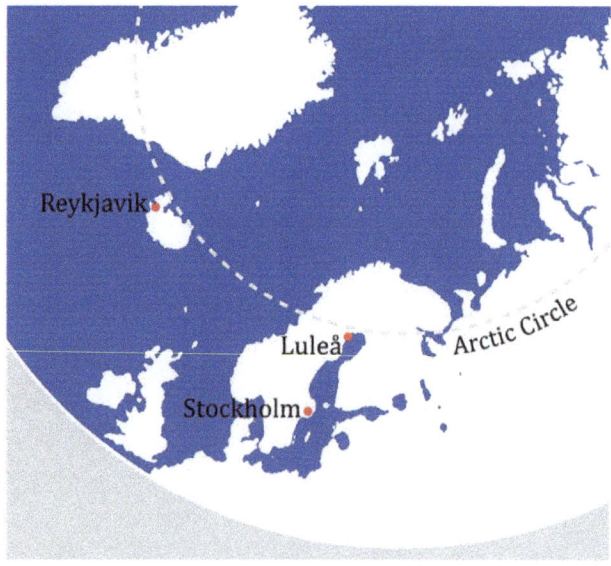

**Figure 1.** Location map for Luleå, Sweden.

### 2.2. Data Collection

The study focused on gathering in-depth data from a group of residents from the case study neighbourhood. Study participants were recruited from staff at the university and the residential home care services unit. An invitation letter containing information about the content and date of workshops and inclusion criteria for the study was provided by email. Criteria for inclusion was being a resident in Mjölkudden and regularly moving by foot or bicycle in the area in wintertime. The ambition was to include a variety of persons with different capacities and ages, to reflect the demographics of residents in the location. In total, 15 residents of the case study neighborhood signed up to take part in the study and of these nine were male and six were female. The range of participants was in active adult age from early twenties to late fifties.

Two sequential workshop sessions led by the first author were conducted in a meeting room at the university. The first meeting focused on introducing the research purpose and the methodology to the participants and the preparation of mental maps. The second meeting focused on the photo elicitation method and semi-structured group discussions. This sequence was repeated twice to offer suitable dates and form groups of 5–9 residents to support creative reflection and dialogue.

The study was performed in accordance with the ethical principles of the Helsinki Declaration, and informed consent was obtained from each participant.

### 2.2.1. Mental Mapping

In the first workshop, each participant was asked to prepare a number of mental maps of the neighbourhood. To ensure that all participants had a clear understanding of what mental maps were and their use in understanding urban form, Kevin Lynch's methods for urban analysis and example mental maps were discussed at the start of the meeting [25,26]. Each participant was asked to draw one winter and one summer mental map for each of the following questions:

- Draw a quick sketch map of Mjölkudden showing the most interesting and important features, and giving a stranger enough knowledge to move about without too much difficulty and avoid major barriers.
- Make a similar sketch of the route and events along a typical trip (using soft mobility) from Mjölkudden to the City Centre.

After this meeting, the main author analysed all of the maps to identify recurring features and patterns. Once, these features and patterns were identified, this information was synthesised into two plan based images of the neighbourhood and surroundings. One map was drawn for the winter neighbourhood and one for summer. All maps were drawn to the same scale and use Lynch's standard notation of Path, Edge, Node, District, and Landmarks [25,26].

### 2.2.2. Photo-Elicitation

At the end of the first meeting, the photo-elicitation method was introduced. For this second workshop, participants were asked to photograph physical aspects of the neighbourhood that they perceived as facilitators or barriers to connectivity for soft mobility in winter. Participants were given two weeks to take these pictures and at the end of this period, they were asked to email their ten most relevant pictures to the principal author. Here participants were left to self-select their preferred images.

At the start of the second meeting, each participant received a full set of A4 prints of his or her photographs. Participants were then asked to write a brief description of the image on the back of each photograph and then rank them in order from most significant barrier to greatest enabler.

This prioritisation was used to encourage participants to identify issues of the most significant importance. Once everyone had ordered their pictures, he or she were asked to lay them out of tables in sequence. The facilitator then led an open discussion around each participant's ordered set of photographs. The dialogue intended to allow for a free exchange of opinions and facilitate critical reflection. Each participant explained their reasoning behind taking each photograph and the message each image was trying to convey. The dialogue was audiotaped and later analysed by the main author in order to identify principal content in terms of emerging issues, recurring themes, and representative quotations.

## 3. Results

### 3.1. Mental Mapping—Urban Scale

The two plan-based images for winter and summer respectively, both highlighted the local center, which houses retail and community facilities, as a node and the church as a landmark. Equally, winter and summer maps illustrated a number of distinct residential areas or districts. Maps also showed the main strategic connections to the city centre and the university area but often lacked the smaller routes that can be found in the neighbourhood. Where the winter and summer maps differed was in the description of the outdoor environment and the landscape. Summer illustration show the green and blue spaces of the neighborhood as separate identified areas, while the winter map shows these areas to merge into one and form one overall white space of snow and ice. Winter illustration also highlighted a range of soft mobility options on the frozen sea. While, the 'ice-road', which is a formal winter route connecting the city's northern and southern harbours via a route along the peninsula, featured prominently, individual participant maps also showed that areas outside the formal route were also used for soft mobility. Here the maps highlighted that in general, the ice parts of this 'white space' enabled soft mobility, whether set out as a formal route or not (Figure 2).

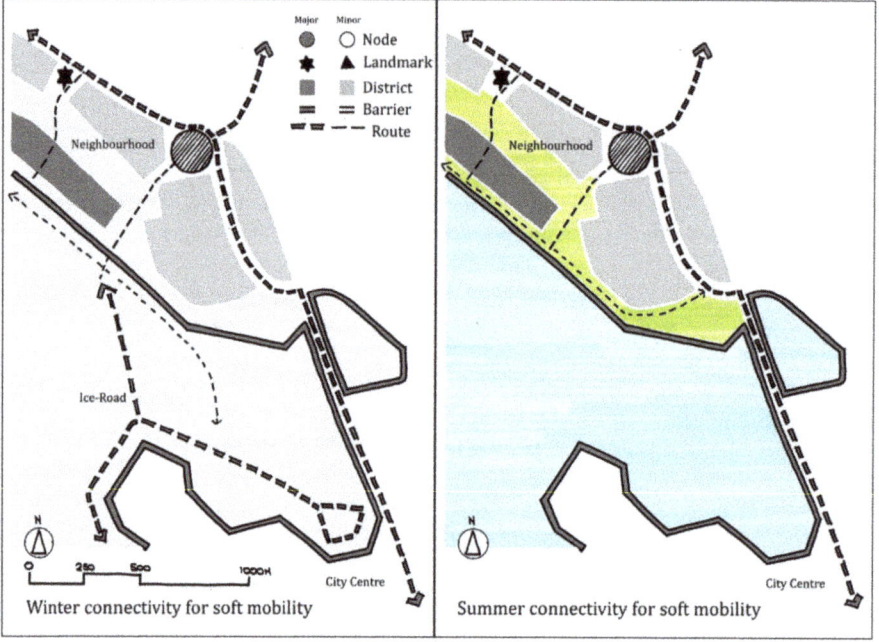

**Figure 2.** Plan based images compiled from participant mental maps show how the neighbourhood's connectivity options for soft mobility change in the winter (left) and summer (right).

### 3.2. Photo-Elicitation—Public Realm

Participant photographs of the neighbourhood deepened the results from the mental mapping and showed how the winter season changed the local network of streets and pathways. Here discussions focused on terrain conditions and how the public realm and townscape changed in the winter season. Participants highlighted that build-ups of snow and ice reduced the usable area of the public realm, altered the local network of pathways in the winter season and changed the townscape of the neighbourhood. At a structural level, participants stated that build-ups changed the neighbourhood's network of pathways and townscape. They highlighted that in the winter, 'walkways disappear and then you need to cycle on the roads'. They also stated that 'summer traffic management solutions coupled with snow piling blocked many pathways' in winter. This was seen to have two impacts for connectivity for soft mobility in the winter season. The first being that the number of routes available for soft mobility was less in winter than summer. The second being that in winter, remaining routes were more likely to be on bigger vehicular routes. Both were seen as detractors for walking and cycling (Figure 3).

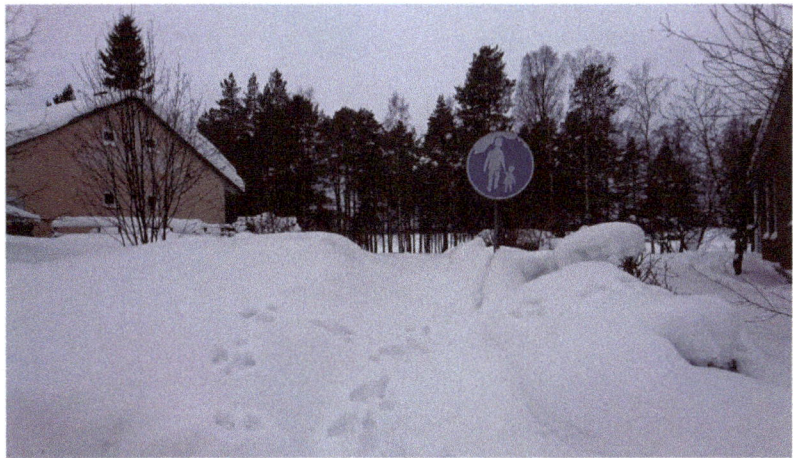

**Figure 3.** A participant's photograph shows how walkways can 'disappear' in the winter season.

Similarly, the winter season were seen to change the townscape of the neighbourhood and the neighbourhoods visual appearance. Here it was suggested that the look of the neighbourhood 'changes every week and it always looks different depending on the snow'. While this was not discussed as a barrier to soft mobility, it was seen to create safety issues for pedestrians and cyclists as it often reduced route visibility and masked vehicle noise (Figure 4).

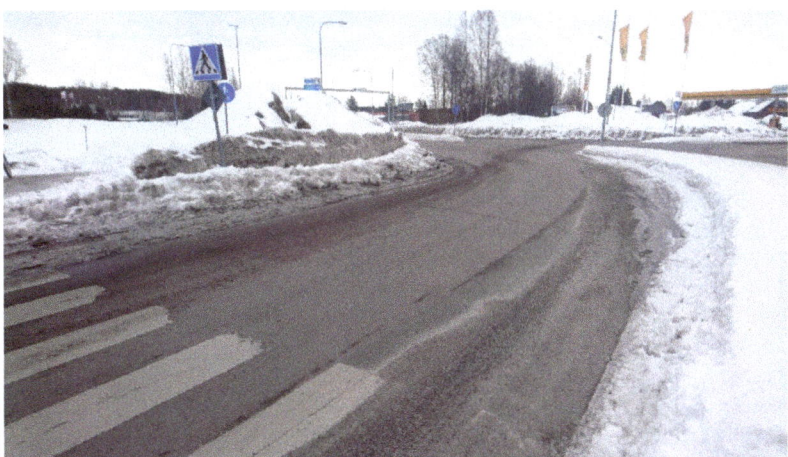

**Figure 4.** A participant's photograph shows how walkways can 'disappear' in the winter season.

The photo elicitation exercise also highlighted that the winter season made it more difficult for people to identify the different elements that make up the public realm. Here the winter season was described as having a 'whiteout effect that made it difficult to understand the area'. For example, participants stated that it was hard to understand where the pedestrian and cycleway were or the extents of the roadway. Participants saw this whiteout effect as a detractor for soft mobility as it made it unclear which modes of transport had priority. On top of this participants highlighted, that for soft mobility, relatively wide pavements in summer became narrower in the winter season. Together the whiteout effect and the reduction in the usable area of the public realm were seen as a significant barriers to soft mobility and potential sources of conflict between different modes of transport (Figure 5).

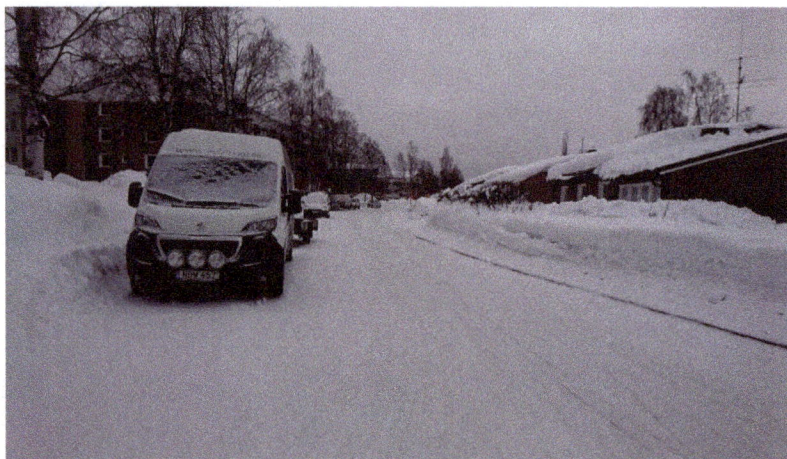

**Figure 5.** A participant's photograph illustrates how the snow can 'white-out' the street and its features.

It was also discussed that, 'if it was very cold, the conditions are OK to go with the bike, the problem is around zero temperatures'. Within reason, coldness was not seen as a barrier to soft mobility. However, many saw that main barriers to soft mobility occurred when temperatures were around zero degrees Celsius. Around this temperature, mixed conditions of snow, ice, slush and water were likely to build on the ground. Participants described this 'as the worst' and this was seen by all to be unpleasant and a significant barrier to soft mobility. Comparatively, participants highlighted few enablers to soft mobility in winter. The removal of snow and the grading of streets and pavements were seen as the major enabler to soft mobility. For cycling, the provision of high-quality cycle storage areas was also highlighted as a significant enabler.

## 4. Discussion

The study aimed to explore how the interaction between the built environment and winter season creates barriers and enablers to connectivity for soft mobility.

The mental mapping exercise showed that broadly speaking people's image of the 'neighbourhood', regards nodes, landmarks and districts was similar in the winter and summer season. However, they also showed that peoples image of the outdoor environment was very different depending on the season. Here the neighbourhood maps showed that the summer and autumn blue and green areas of the neighbourhood became white with the winter season. In winter maps, the frozen sea was seen to support a range of soft mobility choices including walking, cycling, skiing and skating. Mapping also showed that both prepared and unprepared ice can both connect communities and facilitate soft mobility. These outcomes suggest to enable all year outdoor activity, and the health benefits this can bring, such communities need to plan for soft mobility when the outdoor environment is both in its blue and green form and when it becomes white due to the winter season [17,27].

The manner in which participants illustrated the ice-road was significant (Figure 6). In drawings, the route was shown in more detail than other routes and was often annotated. This suggested that the route established a strong image in people's mind and gave a good indication that the route was perceived as an important part of the winter image of the city. However, participant maps clearly showed that the 'ice-road' starting some distance away from the shore. This suggested that participants did not perceive the 'ice-road' as being connected into the neighourhood's land-based networks of streets and pathways. Here, to enable outdoor soft mobility in winter, planners should consider how ephemeral winter routes connect in to the settlements permanent networks of streets and routes.

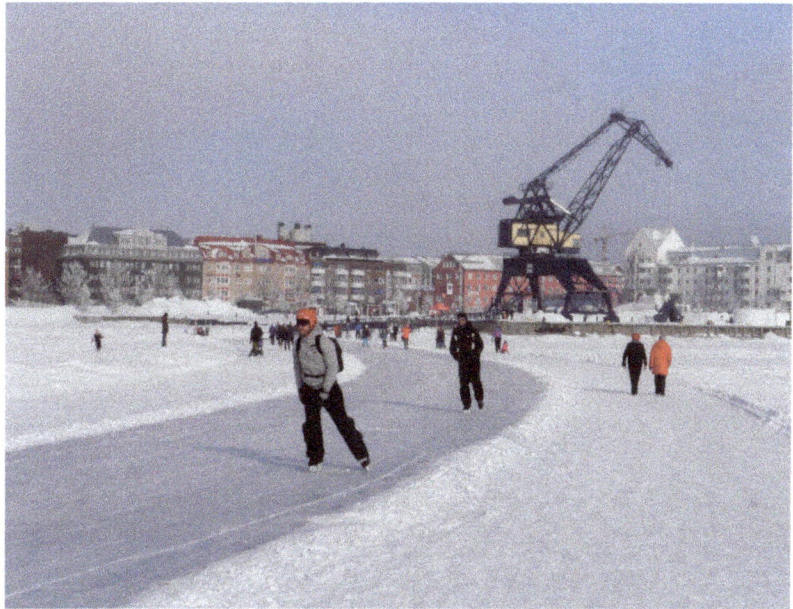

**Figure 6.** Photograph of Luleå's ice road looking back toward the City's southern harbour.

Results from the photo-elicitation highlighted that the interaction between the built environment and winter season created a range of affects to soft mobility. The photographs highlighted that different terrain conditions, such as ice and slush were seen as barriers to soft mobility [28,29]. Importantly, the discussions also established that the winter season was seen to be significant enough to alter the urban structure of the neighbourhood, its public realm and the townscape, and create safety issues [30,31] (Figure 7). Interesting, however, the negative impact by ice and snow on outdoor activity that is commonly reported [32], is challenged by the participants' positive view of the ice road. Which implies that icy and snowy terrain conditions can have different qualities (depending on design and maintenance) [27]. The results also showed that physical barriers to soft mobility were compounded by the 'white-out' effect created by the interaction between the built environment and winter season. Here the terrain covers of ice, snow, or slush and the grading of the public realm was seen to reduce the public realm surface to one large undefined area.

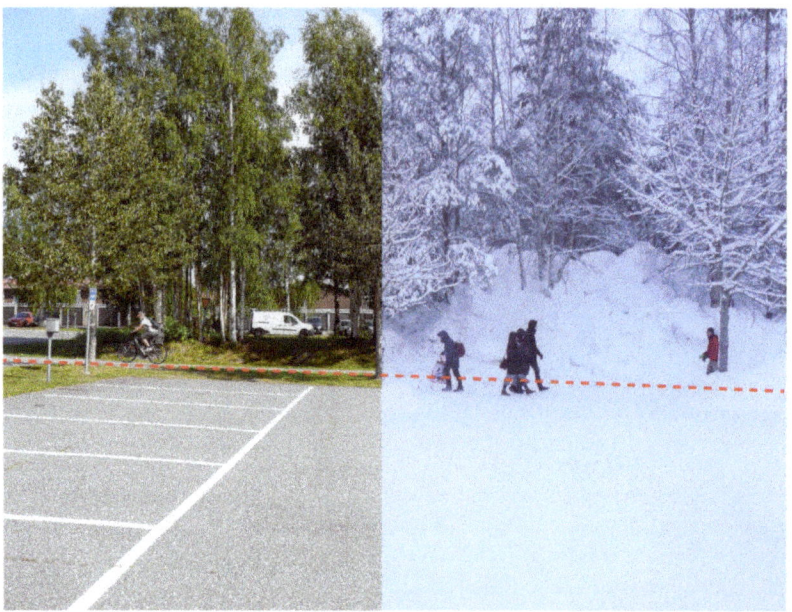

**Figure 7.** An illustration of how the image of the same area in summer (left) and winter (right) can change due to weather conditions (copyright: David Chapman).

### 4.1. Limitations of the Study

To obtain the required results of the study we used a mixed method design with qualitative participatory methods. An advantage with this approach is that it provided a deeper understanding about how residents in the case study location perceive barriers and enablers to soft mobility in winter. The inclusion of a variety of participants suggests that they represent the voices of residents in this location. Also the case study location can be seen as representing a common neighborhood area in a northern Nordic location. However, there are number of factors that may have influenced residents' willingness to participate in this study, which imply that they may differ in some regard from other residents. For example, those perceiving a higher commitment and outdoor activity might have been more inclined to participate. However, increased knowledge of the residents' mental models as basis for individuals' decision making for soft mobility in winter is important, as it reflects the daily use of the network of streets and walkways for mobility. Hereby the results also sheds lights on what is successful or lacking in the planning and maintenance in a common neighborhood area in northern cities in this point of time. The knowledge based on residents perceptions and synthesised by the main author, can form the basis for following workshops with city planner and policy makers. It can also guide the design of an implementation study where the neighborhood is a testbed for experiments.

### 4.2. Practical Implications and Suggestions for Further Research

As the results highlight that people perceive the neighbourhood's structure and appearance to be changed by the winter season, those involved in enabling connectivity for soft mobility should seek to understand these changes and design and plan for winter urban movement strategies. For soft mobility, such places, like their summer equivalents, should focus on creating a desired winter urban structure of connected streets and spaces, with an understandable townscape coupled with a high quality and useable winter public realm. Planners and designers should also focus on reducing ambiguity in the public realm that is created by the winter 'white-out' effect and seek design solutions that reduce confusion about the user priorities in an area. This could be achieved by strategies of elevating movement information above ground level, using snow and ice to define different circulation pathways or using projection and light to define space (Figure 8).

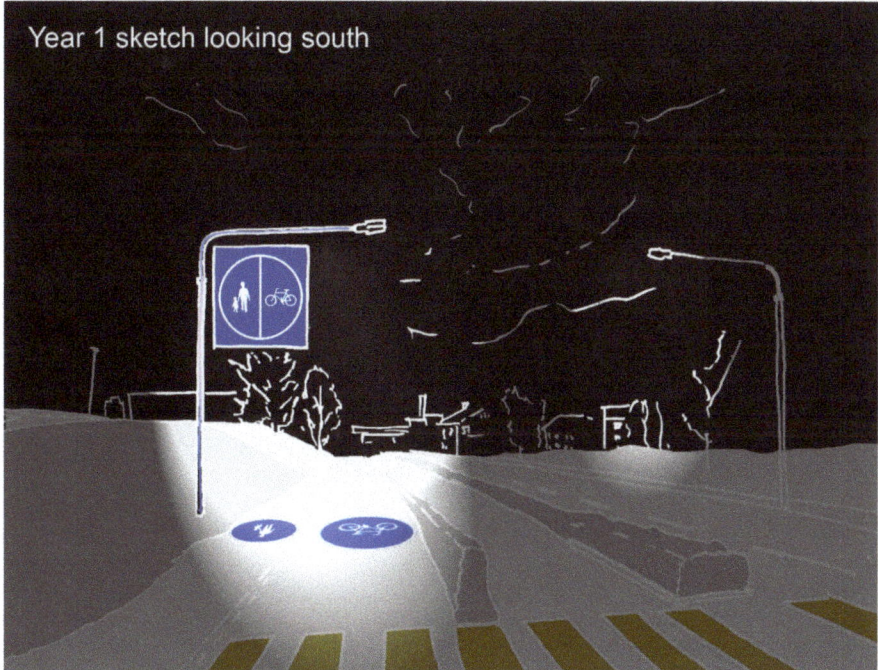

**Figure 8.** An illustration of seasonal winter cycle lanes that are being tested by Lulea University of Technology in Kiruna, Sweden. Here winter cycle lanes are marked out using projected information on to the snow and ice and separated from vehicular traffic by low snow walls (copyright: David Chapman).

For policy-makers and practitioners, the results show three main outcomes regarding the interaction between the built environment and the winter season and the effect on connectivity for soft mobility. These interactions are seen to reduce the spatial structure of an area and the network of streets and pathways that are for soft mobility. It has also been seen to create ambiguity in the public realm and alter a places townscape. All of which have been identified by participants as barriers to soft mobility.

## 5. Conclusions

This study has shown that the winter season creates barriers to outdoor soft mobility in the built environment, which in turn limits the opportunities for the health benefits regular all year outdoor soft mobility can bring. It can be concluded that in winter settlements, focusing solely on the weather and climatic dimensions of the winter season is too limited an approach when designing and planning for these places. Instead, it is important to focus on how the interaction between the winter season and built environment alters the urban structure and public realm of the settlement. That is when blue and green spaces of the outdoor environment are free of snow and ice and, when they have the white cover of the winter season.

This could be done by bringing forward new types of planning strategies for winter settlements and/or re-tooling existing planning methods. For example, blue-green planning strategies can be extended to blue-green-white planning strategies. In winter cities, these strategies would address the structure, function and design of green and blue public areas, spaces, streets and paths when they become white due to snow and ice. These plans would seek to achieve an attractive built environment where transport by walking and biking is prioritised and inviting as an everyday activity throughout the year. These plans would focus equally on winter and summer connections and pathways for soft-mobility, formal vehicular infrastructure and public space maintenance and management. As the winter season is dark they would address the structure, function and design of lighting. At a technical level, these plans would address snow removal and storage [27]. The re-tooling of such strategies for both summer and winter would enable designers and planner to better envisage and design for how the public realm operates in both situations. Both, in turn, would help public policy enable higher levels of outdoor soft mobility in the winter season and help bring the individual health benefits that come from outdoor activity.

**Author Contributions:** Conceptualization, D.C., K.N., A.R., and A.L.; methodology, D.C., K.N., A.R., and A.L.; investigation, D.C.; writing—original draft preparation, D.C.; writing—review and editing, D.C., K.N., A.R., and A.L.; project administration, D.C.

**Funding:** This research received no external funding.

**Conflicts of Interest:** The authors declare no conflicts of interest.

## References

1. Cowan, R. *The Dictionary of Urbanism*; Streetwise Press: Wiltshire, UK, 2005.
2. Gordon, I. Densities, Urban form and travel behavior. *Town Ctry. Plan.* **1997**, *66*, 239–241.
3. Urban Task Force. *Towards an Urban Renaissance*; DETR: London, UK, 1999.
4. DETR. *PPG3: Housing*; HMSO: London, UK, 2000.
5. Jenks, M.; Burton, E.; Williams., K. (Eds.) *The Compact City: A Sustainable Urban Form?* E & FN Spon: London, UK, 1996.
6. U.S. Department of Health and Human Services. *Step It Up! The Surgeon General's Call to Action to Promote Walking and Walkable Communities*; U.S. Department of Health and Human Services: Washington, DC, USA, 2015.
7. World Health Organization. *Global Action Plan on Physical Activity 2018–2030: More Active People for a Healthier World*; WHO: Geneva, Switzerland, 2018.
8. Kostof, S. *The City Assembled*; Thames and Hudson Ltd.: London, UK, 1992.
9. Tibbalds, F. *Making People-Friendly Towns*; Spon Press: London, UK, 1992.
10. CABE. *By Design, Urban Design in the Planning System: Towards Better Practice*; Thomas Telford Publishing: London, UK, 2000.
11. Swedish Transport Administration. *Transport for an Attractive City*; Trafikverket: Borlange, Switzerland, 2015.
12. The Academy of Urbanism. Manifesto. Available online: https://www.academyofurbanism.org.uk/manifesto/ (accessed on 3 July 2018).
13. Congress for the New Urbanism, the Charter of the New Urbanism. Available online: https://www.cnu.org/who-we-are/charter-new-urbanism (accessed on 3 July 2018).
14. Brown, L.; Dixon, D.; Gillham, O. *Urban Design for an Urban Century*; John Wiley & Sons: Hoboken, NJ, USA, 2014.
15. Marshall, S. *Streets & Patterns*; Spon Press: London, UK, 2005.
16. Pressman, N. Final Report, UN/ECE Research Colloquium on Human Settlements in Harsh Living Conditions. *Habitat Int.* **1989**, *13*, 127–137. [CrossRef]
17. Chapman, D.; Nilsson, K.; Rizzo, A.; Larsson, A. Updating winter: The importance of climate-sensitive urban design for winter settlements. *Arct. Yearb.* **2018**, *1*, 86–105.
18. Collymore, P. *The Architecture of Ralph Erskine*; Academy Editions: London, UK, 1994.
19. Pressman, N. *Northern Cityscape*; Winter Cities Association: Michigan, USA, 1995.
20. Urbansystems. *Winter City Design Guidelines*; Urbansystems: Fort St. John, Canada, 2000.
21. Ebrahimabadi, S. Outdoor Comfort in Cold Climates: Integrating Microclimate Factors in Urban Design. Ph.D. Thesis, Lulea University of Technology, Lulea, Sweden, 2015.
22. Edmonton Winter Design Guidelines. Transforming Edmonton into a Great Winter City. Available online: https://www.edmonton.ca/city_government/documents/PDF/WinterCityDesignGuidelines_draft.pdf (accessed on 12 March 2019).

23. Creswell, J.W.; Clark, V.L.P. *Designing and Conducting Mixed Methods Research*, 2nd ed.; Sage Publications: Los Angeles, CA, USA, 2011.
24. Luleå Kommun. Mjölkudden 2017. Available online: http://www.lulea.se/download/18.5933b14813eeba8f7961b8d/1432882995235/Mj%C3%B6lkudden.pdf (accessed on 12 March 2019).
25. Banerjee, T.; Southworth, M. (Eds.) *City Sense and City Design, Writings and Projects of Kevin Lynch*; MIT Press: Cambridge, MA, USA, 1990.
26. Lynch, K. *The Image of the City*; MIT Press: Cambridge, MA, USA, 1992.
27. Chapman, D.; Nilsson, K.; Larsson, A.; Rizzo, A. Climatic barriers to soft-mobility in winter: Lulea, Sweden as case study. *Sustain. Cities Soc.* **2017**, *35*, 574–580. [CrossRef]
28. Clarke, P.; Hirsch, J.A.; Melendez, R.; Winters, M.; Gould, J.S.; Ashe, M.; Furst, S.; McKay, H. Snow and Rain Modify Neighbourhood Walkability for Older Adults. *Can. J. Aging* **2017**, *36*, 159–169. [CrossRef] [PubMed]
29. Clarke, P.; Yan, T.; Keusch, F.; Gallagher, N.A. The Impact of Weather on Mobility and Participation in Older US Adults. *Am. J. Public Health* **2015**, *105*, 1489–1494. [CrossRef] [PubMed]
30. Chaudhury, H.; Mahmood, A.; Michael, Y.; Campo, M.; Hay, K. The influence of neighborhood residential density, physical and social environments on older adults' physical activity: An exploratory study in two metropolitan areas. *J. Aging Stud.* **2012**, *26*, 35–43. [CrossRef]
31. Garvin, T.; Nykiforuk, C.; Johnson, S. Can we get old here? Seniors' perceptions of seasonal constraints of neighbourhood built environments in a northern, winter city. *Geogr. Ann. Ser. B* **2012**, *94*, 369–389. [CrossRef]
32. Wagner, A.L.; Keusch, F.; Yan, T.; Clarke, P.J. The impact of weather on summer and winter exercise behaviors. *J. Sport Health Sci.* **2019**, *8*, 39–45. [CrossRef] [PubMed]

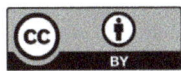

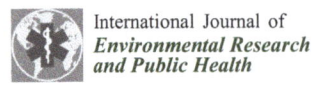

International Journal of
*Environmental Research*
*and Public Health*

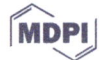

*Article*

# Comparative Associations of Street Network Design, Streetscape Attributes and Land-Use Characteristics on Pedestrian Flows in Peripheral Neighbourhoods

**Ayse Ozbil [1,\*], Tugce Gurleyen [2], Demet Yesiltepe [1] and Ezgi Zunbuloglu [3]**

[1]  Department of Architecture and Built Environment, Northumbria University, Newcastle NE1 8ST, UK; demet.yesiltepe@northumbria.ac.uk
[2]  Department of City and Regional Planning, Istanbul Technical University, Istanbul 34367, Turkey; tugcegurleyen@gmail.com
[3]  Department of Urban Design, Istanbul Technical University, Istanbul 34367, Turkey; ezgi.zunbuloglu@gmail.com
\*  Correspondence: ayse.torun@northumbria.ac.uk; Tel.: +44-191-227-3004

Received: 15 April 2019; Accepted: 21 May 2019; Published: 24 May 2019

**Abstract:** Research has sufficiently documented the built environment correlates of walking. However, evidence is limited in investigating the comparative associations of micro- (streetscape features) and macro-level (street network design and land-use) environmental measures with pedestrian movement. This study explores the relative association of street-level design-local qualities of street environment-, street network configuration –spatial structure of the urban grid- and land-use patterns with the distribution of pedestrian flows in peripheral neighbourhoods. Street design attributes and ground-floor land-uses are obtained through field surveys while street network configuration is evaluated through space syntax measures. The statistical models indicate that the overall spatial configuration of street network proves to be a stronger correlate of walking than local street-level attributes while only average sidewalk width appears to be a significant correlate of walking among the streetscape measures. However, the most significant and consistent correlate of the distribution of flows is the number of recreational uses at the segment-level. This study contributes to the literature by offering insights into the comparative roles of urban design qualities of the street environment and street network layout on pedestrian movement. The findings also offer evidence-based strategies to inform specific urban design and urban master planning decisions (i.e., the provision of more generous sidewalks on streets with relatively higher directional accessibility) in creating lively, walkable environments.

**Keywords:** street network configuration; peripheral neighbourhoods; pedestrian flow; streetscape features; Istanbul

## 1. Introduction

Physical activity is an important lifestyle component of improving long-term health [1]. Walking is the most common form of adult physical activity [1,2]. Earlier studies point to the positive effects of walking on various government priorities including but not limited to, air quality and pollution [3], physical activity, obesity [4], mental health [5] and congestion [6]. Research indicates that walking reduces anxiety, depression, anger and time pressure [7] tension and confusion [8] and increases creativity [9]. Moreover, studies also argue that walking and cycling reduces health and parking costs [10]. Hence, developing walkable environments is key in promoting sustainable urban neighbourhoods [11,12].

Researchers and practitioners alike agree on the importance of the built environment in facilitating or restraining walking. Hence, it is important to understand the built environment correlates of walking to provide an empirical basis for planning and urban design actions aimed at creating walkable environments. A growing body of research relates pedestrian-friendly neighbourhood design to measured walking behaviour [13,14]. The underlying idea is that environmental supports for physical activity will enable people to walk more and thereby be more active. Yet few neighbourhood studies actually include the micro-scale (i.e., the presence and continuity of sidewalks) and the macro-scale (i.e., spatial structure of urban networks) environmental features in the same model. Hence, the present research is designed to (a) identify the extent to which micro-scale (street-level urban design qualities) and macro-scale (street network configuration and land-use) environmental correlates are associated with pedestrian movement and (b) consider the implications of the findings for urban design and planning-policies aimed to design active built environments.

## 1.1. Built Environment Correlates of Walking

The past decade has witnessed a growing attention to the physical environmental correlates [15–18] of walking behaviour. Previous reviews on children, adolescents and adults have reported consistent relationships between physical environmental characteristics and physical activity, in particular walking [19–21]. Studies that examined associations between attributes of the built environment and walking have focused on the macro-scale (land-use patterns and street network design) and micro-scale (street design) environmental characteristics.

## 1.2. Macro-Scale Environmental Correlates

### 1.2.1. Land-Use Characteristics

The systematic reviews on studies investigating the empirical analysis of macro-scale environmental correlates of walking have demonstrated consistent positive relations between walking and land-use mix (proximity of homes and destinations such as shops) [22–24]. These reviews and more concluded that mixed land-use, which is due to the decreased distance between or intermingling among different types of land uses, such as residential and commercial uses, is associated with more walking. It is argued that mixing offices, shops, restaurants, residences and other activities influences the decision to walk by making it more convenient to walk to various destinations [25,26] while having destinations within walking distance from origins (homes, stations, schools, etc.) increases the odds of walking [27,28]. This finding is also related to compactness (or density) of land-uses. In areas with higher density of land-uses, destinations can be closer together, which is thought to shape pedestrian activity by bringing numerous activities closer together, thus increasing their accessibility from trip origins [13,29]. It is suggested that people are willing to use slower modes of travel, such as walking, for shorter distances, especially if many trips can be chained [30,31]. Although the literature has demonstrated a strong positive relationship between non-residential uses and walking in general, the conclusions regarding the impacts of recreational uses on pedestrian movement is ambiguous. While some studies could not identify public open space (e.g., parks) as a significant correlate of walking for leisure or transport [32,33], others demonstrated that open space was positively related to walking for transport but not walking for recreation [34].

### 1.2.2. Street Network Design

Researchers in transportation and planning have also reported consistent relationships between street network design and walking behaviour [22,35]. The extent to which different parts of a neighbourhood are linked to one another determines the level of street connectivity. Here street connectivity refers to how connectivity is measured in general, not limiting to how it is correlated with pedestrian movement. Street connectivity refers to the degree to which pedestrian movement can flow with ease and it provides multiple choices between any two locations [36]. It can be measured with percent of gridded streets in a buffer of a person's home [37,38], distance between intersections [39,40], directness of routes [41,42], the area-weighted average perimeter [43] or "network density" [44].

Some researchers have used walkable catchments or "pedsheds" to measure the accessible streets along the network [45–47]. After discussing the shortcomings of existing measures of permeability, which relate to the capacity to move and the potential to interact in an urban environment, Pafka and Dovey [48] introduced "area-weighted average perimeter" and "interface catchments" as more effective measures of permeability that can measure both walkable access and what one gets access to. The commonly used block length measure denotes the average street segment length within an area and that several variants of block size have been used including block perimeter, block area and block density [49–51]. Criticism of several popular connectivity measures, such as intersection density (number of intersections per given area) and block length (street segment length), have revealed significant flaws in these measures [43,52,53]. Stangl and Guinn [54] argue that intersection density measures fail to account for street pattern and its actual permeability and that movement may be completely obstructed in areas with good intersection density scores. Route directness, which is the ratio of the shortest distance between two points on a network to the straight-line distance between these points, has also been applied, though less frequently, to measure the ease of movement to a destination (i.e., school) [41,47,55]. To make this measure more applicable to area-wide connectivity assessment, Stangl and Guinn [54] and Stangl [56] adapted a modified route directness measure, which can directly assess permeability.

In order to encourage non-motorized travel, continuous non-motorized rights of way must be provided that allow pedestrians to reach various destinations within a city [57]. Continuous street pattern not only reduces trip length, but it also offers greater choice of travel routes and modes. Higher street connectivity related to increased walking is defined as increased number of intersections with fewer dead-end streets [58], more streets [59], high node-link ratio [60] and smaller block length [61]. Street patterns with gridded street networks, which tend to have relatively higher street connectivity and street network density, are associated with increased walking and biking [62]. The 1 km Euclidean buffer was determined as the easy-walking distance [63] and used by studies in order to capture pedestrian activity in neighbourhoods [64,65]. Higher intersection density and link-node ratio within 1 km Euclidean buffers of homes were found to be [66] related to increased frequency of walking. Similarly, studies measuring connectivity at the neighbourhood level, found a positive relationship with total walking [67,68].

Even though research investigating the influences of land-use and street connectivity on walking has proliferated in recent years, no conclusions emerge on the relationships between street network design and travel. Part of the reason is due to collinearity between land-use mix and street network design. Fairly compact neighbourhoods, particularly in US and Australian cities, generally have more varied land-uses, on average shorter block lengths with more grid-like street patterns. Thus, the effect of street network design on overall travel remains unclear. Another reason is that the above-described measures describe the average connectivity properties of street networks. However, they fall short in describing the spatial and structural pattern of street networks that define urban areas.

The significance of the spatial structure of street networks in explaining walking behaviour has been apparent in recent studies [69–71]. Spatial structure may be defined as the collection of streets and street segments through certain alignments and hierarchies. The significance of spatial structure as a crucial correlate of walking has been highlighted within space syntax theory. Space syntax is a set of techniques that is used to better understand the interaction between societies and the spaces [72]. The main idea in space syntax is that not the buildings but the spaces between buildings –not solids but voids– are important as these are the spaces where people interact [73]. At the urban scale, it is a tool to describe and quantitatively measure the spatial configuration of public spaces, that is, street systems. Evidence from studies applying space syntax methodology suggests that streets that are accessible from their surroundings with fewer direction changes (evaluated through the connectivity measure of Integration) tend to attract higher densities of pedestrian flows [74,75]. Drawing on the work of space syntax, some researchers have applied metric reach, which measures the amount of street length accessible within a specific walking distance from the centre of each street segment in an urban network [76], to show that the configuration of individual street elements within an area is significantly associated with walking [47,77]. Moreover, recent studies have also shown that the structure of an urban street network, as defined by the connectivity hierarchy measured by direction changes (through a recent connectivity measure of directional reach), has an important impact on pedestrian travel [77,78].

### 1.3. Micro-Scale Environmental Correlates

Studies investigating the environmental correlates of walking have sufficiently documented associations between micro-scale environmental attributes (pedestrian-friendly street design) and pedestrian activity. In fact, some researchers argue that in spite of the plethora of studies on macro-level urban form characteristics, studies focusing on micro-level attributes are limited [79,80]. In related literature, street-level walkability indicators that affect pedestrian experience include pedestrian-oriented design features, such as pedestrian crossings (e.g., pedestrian crossing coverage rate, signal coverage rate and crossing facility design index), sidewalks (e.g., sidewalk coverage rate, sidewalk width, length) as well as curb to curb roadways (e.g., number of traffic lanes). Indeed, surveys of the literature found sufficient evidence to conclude that the continuity and width of sidewalks [21,81,82], the presence and ease of street crossings [83], aesthetic qualities (the attractiveness of the environment, presence of tree-lined streets) [84] and signalization [39,85–88], as well as the presence of aesthetic or safety features, such as cleanliness, interesting sights and architecture [34,89,90], encourage walking among adults and children. For example, by conducting a Delphi study with experts, Pikora et al. [39] identified five factors among a list of potentially important environmental factors: safety, aesthetics, destination, functionality and subjective assessments. This study underlined the impact of micro-scale criteria, such as crossings, path continuity (for safety), presence of trees, parks, maintenance and cleanliness (for aesthetics) and attractiveness and difficulty of the environment (for subjective assessments), on walking. Wilcox and others [91] defined nine environmental factors in their study related to physical activity in the US. They mentioned the importance of the presence of sidewalks, effect of heavy traffic, hills, presence of streetlights, having an enjoyable scenery, crime rates, observing others exercising and accessibility of walking trails to analyse environmental characteristics. In their audit comparison chart, Lee and Talen [92] stated four key factors: land-uses, sidewalks, vehicle-pedestrian interactions and safety and appeal. In this study, researchers listed the quality of sidewalks (aesthetics), natural barriers (ditch or creeks), unique markers, enclosure as criteria, different from other research. Bentley et al. [93] showed that increasing proportion of segments with a walking/cycling path-design and proportion of streets with one or more crossings were associated with more time spent on walking. However, in their study, which included crossing aids and trees as part of the street-level attributes to calculate an Environmental Factor Score, Pikora et al. [94] did not find any significant relationship between these factors and walking behaviour. In some studies using mixed-methods, participants reported access to sidewalks as key characteristics that support their walking [95,96], while lack of pedestrian crossings were reported to be a barrier [97]. Effect of sidewalks, safety, lighting, recreational facilities was discussed by others researchers as well [98,99]. In accordance with the results demonstrated in literature, urban planning and transport policies employ several strategies, such as providing pedestrian crossing devices, to improve the safety of pedestrians and thus, to encourage walking [100–102].

Although there is much evidence documenting the relationship between the built environment and walking, their usefulness is limited for urban designers and planners working at the local, neighbourhood level. One of the underlying reasons is that most of the indicators applied in the literature account for relatively coarse-resolution data, such as census tract levels, which do not lend to any useful findings for local comparative analysis. Second, to help policy makers and planners/designers in the assessment of urban areas, these analyses need to be localised but related studies generally focus on a comparison between cities rather than within cities. Third, the indicators used in such studies fail to evaluate spatial structure of urban form. For example, although most studies aim to evaluate the built environment on the basis of land-use patterns and street-level attributes, they tend to omit qualities regarding the spatial configuration of street networks. Lastly, while there is substantial work on the relationship between urban form (land-use and street design) and walking, both the transportation and physical activity literatures largely ignore the micro-scale environmental correlates deemed so important by urban designers. More importantly, only few studies contain objective measures of streetscape design quality [103,104].

To address the above-mentioned limitations of current studies, we examined the relative associations of macro-scale (land-use patterns and street network configuration) and micro-scale (local qualities of street environment) built environment correlates of walking with the observed distribution of pedestrian flows in four peripheral neighbourhoods in İstanbul. In doing so, we were able to develop well-specified statistical models that allow researchers to accurately evaluate the individual effects of each variable. Additionally, the quantitative data applied in this study is based on a smaller unit of assessment (street segment). Hence, this study gauges the significance of fine-grained design features that are fundamental for urban designers. Finally, in order to localise the findings in a meaningful way, this study focuses on an intra-urban (within city) comparison. Thus, the present research relates one walking-friendly neighbourhood environmental indicator –quantitative evidence of pedestrian movement– to objective macro- and micro-scale measures of the built environment. Based on this quantitative comparison some practical design guidelines are suggested towards more pedestrian-friendly peripheral districts.

## 2. Design of the Study/Method

### 2.1. Case Context

Case studies of this paper are chosen from İstanbul's peripheral areas, which function as sub-centres for their surroundings. These neighbourhoods—Küçükçekmece, Avcılar, Büyükçekmece and Beylikdüzü—are located in districts which have grown towards the periphery after the 1980s, parallel to E-5 highway, and have dominated the macro-form of the city (Figure 1). The selected areas are directly related to E-5 highway, which served as pedestrian access for the integration of the increased populations agglomerated within peripheral neighbourhoods with the sub-centres. These neighbourhoods are also directly related to the existing Bus Rapid Transit (BRT) line and its stations along the E-5 highway. This transit network, which was integrated into the mass rapid transit system of the city in 2007, has generated significant transit links that help integrate the peripheral populations with the study areas. Each area varies in the spatial configuration of its surrounding urban fabric, differing in the layout of street networks, morphological characteristics and land-use compositions, while all of them have similar characteristics (socio-economic and demographic structure).

Avcılar consists of an urban fabric that is made up of low-rise (3-4 storeys) buildings built on the perimeter of the block. The buildings are vertically mixed-use (non-residential uses located on the ground floor, residences on the upper floors). The uniform urban grid is clear with regular urban blocks, with average size of 90 by 100 m. It includes a fine-grained land-use pattern, with small shops, cafes and so forth, spread evenly within the neighbourhood.

While Beylikdüzü has similar average number of retail activities on the ground-floor as Avcılar, the first encompasses coarse-grained active ground floor uses (i.e. large shopping malls). The urban fabric in Beylikdüzü comprises a mixed street layout pattern: partial grid-iron layout with relatively larger blocks (150 by 200 m) as well as a partial curvilinear pattern. Individual high-rise blocks are located sparsely within the urban blocks.

Küçükçekmece neighbourhood is characterized by a dominating curvilinear street network pattern, which partially turns into cul-de-sacs, with varied block sizes and lot patterns. The average block size is 100 by 200 m. As opposed to Beylikdüzü, the blocks in Küçükçekmece are relatively densified with buildings of relatively smaller plots (30 × 50 m). The urban fabric has relatively higher commercial street fronts.

Büyükçekmece neighbourhood is a predominantly residential neighbourhood at the ground-floor level. The urban fabric is characterized by partially a deformed urban grid-iron and partially a curvilinear street network pattern with varied block sizes and lot patterns. The average block size within the grid-iron part is 150 × 200 m whereas it is 100 × 100 m within the curvilinear system.

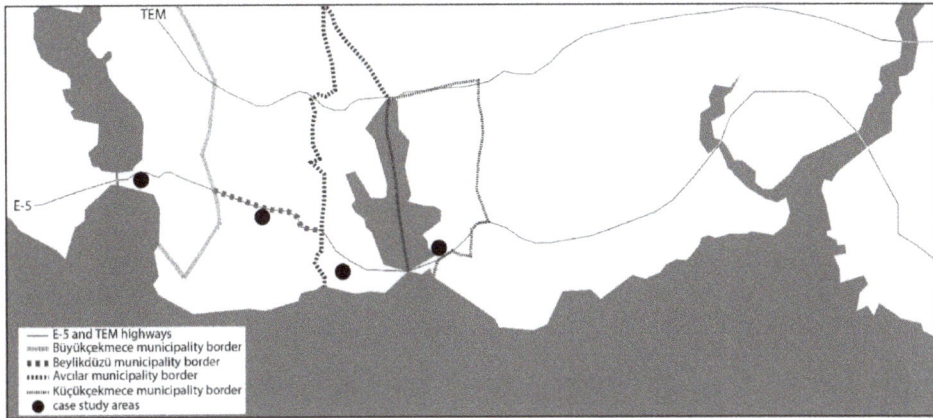

**Figure 1.** The location of case study areas within the city map.

## 2.2. Methodology

### 2.2.1. Pedestrian Observations

Pedestrian counts were collected on street segments within four neighbourhoods in İstanbul. The case context borders were designated as 800 m buffers surrounding the public square within each neighbourhood. 800 m distance was selected as the threshold since guidelines often use one-half mile (800 m) as a key distance in network planning [105,106]. Due to resource limitations, approximately 30 street segments were observed per area. These segments were selected to include a variety of connectivity levels, measured through Integration. Integration is a structural connectivity measure which calculates how close each segment is to all the others within a radius. Proportionate stratified random sampling was applied to select the segments. Street segments located within the study areas were grouped as low (bottom tercile), medium (middle tercile) and high (top tercile). Terciles are identified based on the Integration values for each street segment. Similar numbers of segments (~30) from each category was randomly selected to measure pedestrian flows. Pedestrian observations were conducted for 10-min intervals on two different weekdays distributed over two different time periods (morning and afternoon) per day. 10-min interval is used since this duration appears to be the length of manual count which is most commonly applied in literature [107–109]. Pedestrian counts were observed on weekdays only, since preliminary observations indicated no significant differences between weekday and weekend pedestrian activity rates within the areas. Figure 2 illustrates graphically the distribution of movement densities using circles of different diameters for the selected areas. Figure 3, which provides statistical information on pedestrian densities, shows how strongly the four areas differ. The median density of moving pedestrians per 100 m is 31.6, 23.9, 39.5 and 43.8 for Beylikdüzü, Küçükçekmece, Büyükçekmece and Avcılar respectively, while the corresponding means are 71.8, 52.0, 68.8 and 215.1. In total 124 street segments were observed.

Ethics approval was granted by Human Ethics Commission, Özyeğin University (Ethics ID 2015/01) and relevant permissions were granted by the İstanbul Metropolitan Municipality (ID 30872936-02-622.1-1768-42338).

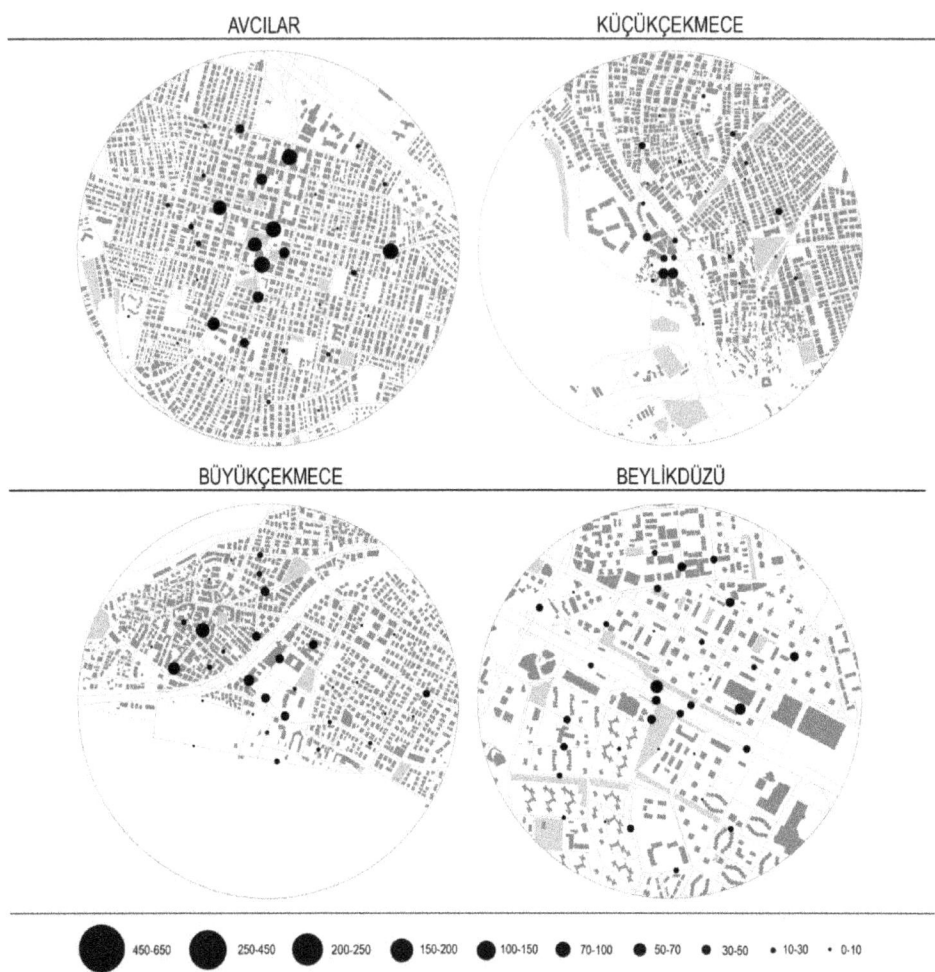

**Figure 2.** Graphic representation of observed pedestrian densities in four areas.

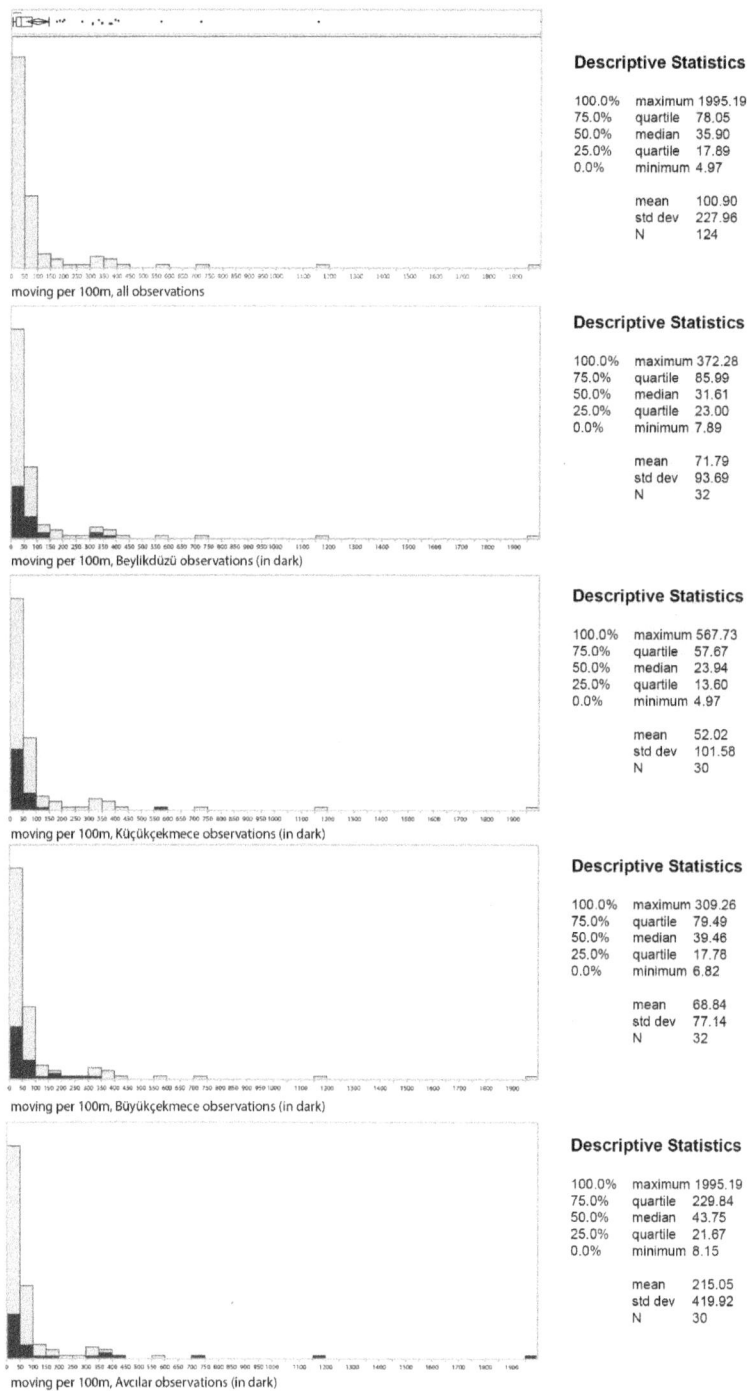

**Figure 3.** Statistical profile of observed pedestrian densities.

### 2.2.2. Street Design and Land-Use

The same street segments selected for pedestrian observations were characterised through detailed field surveys to document the street-level pedestrian environment. The pedestrian quality attributes to document were selected from local qualities of street environment that are shown to affect pedestrian movement behaviour via their impacts on people's perception on safety and aesthetics [39,110–114]. These include average sidewalk width as well as the presence of pedestrian crossings, traffic lights and trees. Where available, sidewalk width on both sides of the segment was measured and the average width is included in the analysis. Similarly, the presence of trees for both sidewalks is considered (i.e., coded "yes" if there were trees on either side of the audited segment). The selected segments were also surveyed in terms of the number of ground-floor frontages opening directly onto the street, relativized by street length. Land-use was categorised into residential, retail (including commercial and offices) and recreational (i.e., public parks and open areas for recreation such as playgrounds) to distinguish between the effects of each on the distribution of movement.

### 2.2.3. Street Network Configuration

To assess the street network configuration within the study areas, the entire street network of the European part of İstanbul Metropolitan area was evaluated using a standard space syntax measure, angular segment Integration and a more recent segment-based syntactic measure, Directional Reach. Integration measures how accessible each space is from all the others within the radius using the least angle measure of distance. Directional reach measures the total street length accessible within a specific number of direction changes from the centre of each street segment in an urban network. Directional reach was computed for 2 direction changes subject to a 20° angle threshold. Computing directional reach for two direction changes provides an estimate of how well a street segment is embedded in its surroundings from the point of view of directional distance. 20° was selected as the threshold since it reveals continuities that correspond to named streets and also in the sense that it helps identify stronger associations between street connectivity and non-residential land-uses, as well as stronger associations between street connectivity and vehicular traffic [115]. Figure 4 illustrates the street network configuration of each study area embedded within the surrounding 800 m radius buffer, coded according to Directional reach (2-direction changes, 20°) and Integration (n). Integration radius n, (n), is a global measure, which calculates the distance from each segment to all the others within the system. Hence, it represents the integration pattern of a system at the largest scale.

Integration was calculated using Depthmap software [116,117], while Directional Reach was calculated in Java. Figure 4 illustrates study area street networks using Integration and Directional Reach. Streetmap 2014 obtained from the İstanbul Metropolitan Municipality was used to calculate these different street connectivity measures. ArcGIS 10.2.2 (Geographic Information Systems) (ESRI, 2014, Redlands, CA, USA) was used to merge all these different data sets. Linear models were developed in JMP (JMP®, Version 13. SAS Institute Inc., Cary, NC, USA, 1989–2019) to investigate the relationships among street design, street network configuration, land-use and walking behaviour.

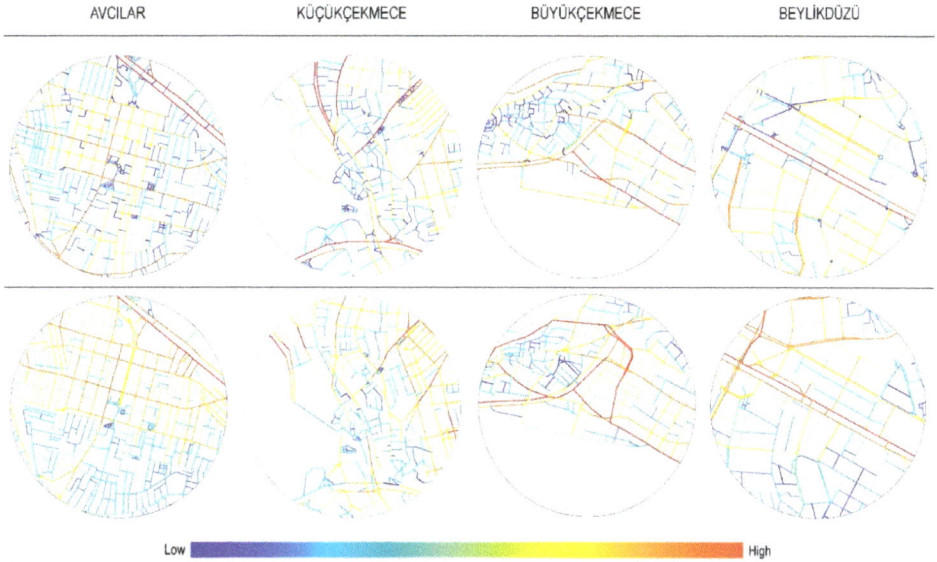

**Figure 4.** Street network configuration within study sites, coded according to: top) Directional reach (2-direction changes, 20°) and bottom) Integration (r:n).

## 3. Analysis

Two types of analyses were conducted to investigate the relative association of streetscape design –local qualities of street environment–, street network configuration –spatial structure of the urban grid– and land-use patterns with the distribution of flows. First, descriptive statistics were estimated for each area, summarising the averages of population/pedestrian densities, street network configuration, street-level attributes and land-uses. This allowed for illustrating the similarities and differences between the study areas as well as hinting to any existing general trend between the pedestrian densities and other attributes (e.g., land-use compositions). Second, multivariate regression analyses were conducted to examine the associations between street network configuration, streetscape design and street-level land-use characteristics in explaining the distribution of pedestrian densities. Linear models were developed both for all areas as considered as a single set and separately for individual areas. Three sets of models were constructed in the linear models. The first set of models includes land-use variables (land-use variables were entered into the regression first to allow for the evaluation of these variables in context relative to other factors affecting pedestrian behaviour). In the second and third sets of models, street network configuration and street-level design measures were entered respectively to understand the comparative effect and significance levels of each measure in explaining the distribution of pedestrian flows. Logarithmic transformation was applied to transform the distribution of flows into a normal distribution. Models were checked for multivariate regression assumptions (normality, constant variance and multi-collinearity) in JMP statistical software (SAS Institute, Cary, NC, USA). All results indicate that the models do not violate multivariate regression assumptions.

## 4. Findings

### 4.1. Gross Differences Between the Four Areas

Table 1 presents a quantitative profile of the selected areas in terms of population and pedestrian densities, configuration of street layouts, street-level pedestrian environments and land-uses at the ground-floor level. This preliminary benchmarking demonstrates notable differences between areas.

The population densities of the areas, calculated on the basis of the census blocks associated with the street segments for which pedestrian counts were taken, range from 15 to 204 per hectare with Avcılar and Beylikdüzü having similar densities. The average number of moving pedestrians per 100 m is 52.7, 44.5, 54.1 and 128.4 for Beylikdüzü, Küçükçekmece, Büyükçekmece and Avcılar respectively. The four areas also differ significantly in their street configuration. Average 2-directional reach is highest for Beylikdüzü and lowest for Küçükçekmece. While Küçükçekmece and Avcılar have the highest average Integration, Beylikdüzü and Büyükçekmece have similar lower averages. In terms of street-level pedestrian attributes, all areas have approximately similar average sidewalk width, with Büyükçekmece and Küçükçekmece having the highest and lowest averages respectively. While average number of streets with trees and crosswalks are consistently low for Küçükçekmece, this area has the highest average presence of traffic lights. Küçükçekmece has the highest average number of residential uses per 100m. Average number of recreational uses per 100m is similar for all areas, except for Beylikdüzü, which has the highest average. Similarly, the average number of retail uses is comparable across Beylikdüzü, Büyükçekmece and Avcılar, while Küçükçekmece has the highest retail ground-floor activities.

Overall, the initial tabulation suggests a correspondence between the average volume of pedestrian movement, street design and land development. However, since a sample of only four areas does not allow further statistical inference, linear models are developed in the next section to examine the associations further.

**Table 1.** Characteristics of selected areas summarised in terms of population and pedestrian densities, street network configuration, street design and land-use.

| Variable | Beylizdüzü | Küçükcekmece | Büyükçekmece | Avcılar | All |
|---|---|---|---|---|---|
| Densities of residential Population and pedestrians | | | | | |
| population density per hectare | 84.57 | 204.19 | 15.45 | 104.11 | 102.08 |
| average number of pedestrians per 100 m | 52.72 | 44.51 | 54.14 | 128.41 | 69.94 |
| Segment-level street configuration | | | | | |
| avg 2-Directional Reach (20°) | 480.92 | 192.77 | 241.85 | 317.16 | 307.25 |
| avg Integration (*n*) | 0.79 | 0.95 | 0.71 | 0.96 | 0.85 |
| Street-level pedestrian environment | | | | | |
| avg.sidewalk width | 165.12 | 109.62 | 196.3 | 167.06 | 160.2 |
| tree presence [yes] | 43% | 7% | 53% | 59% | 49% |
| crosswalk presence [yes] | 20% | 7% | 13% | 2% | 12% |
| traffic light presence [yes] | 7% | 10% | 4% | 3% | 6% |
| Street-level land-use | | | | | |
| avg # residential use per 100 m | 1.46 | 7.63 | 3.49 | 5.40 | 4.37 |
| avg # recreational use per 100 m | 0.62 | 0.36 | 0.37 | 0.36 | 0.44 |
| avg # retail use per 100 m | 0.90 | 2.91 | 1.16 | 1.20 | 1.36 |

*4.2. Analysis of the Four Areas as a Single Set*

Table 2 summarizes the results of regression models for three sets of models estimating the natural logarithm of pedestrians relativized by 100 m for all areas considered as a single set. Ground-floor land-use is found to explain more than $1/3$ of the variation in the distribution of flows. The inclusion of structural measures and streetscape attributes results in similar levels of increase in the predictive power of the model (adj $R^2$ change = 3–4%; $p < 0.001$) and the final urban form model can explain around 50% of the variation in pedestrian densities. By looking at the standardised Beta (std $\beta$) values, it can be argued that the number of recreational land-uses per 100 m is the most significant predictor of movement densities. In fact, the impact level and significance of this variable is quite consistent across the three sets of models. The effect levels of the number of retail activities per 100 m and 2-directional reach are similar (std $\beta$ = 0.25–26, 99% CI), both being positively and significantly associated with the variation in pedestrian flows. In other words, increased retail uses opening onto a street, which has relatively higher directional accessibility, draws pedestrians within the surrounding network. Number of residential uses per 100 m is negatively associated (95% CI) with the pedestrian densities, which indicates that decreasing residential frontages and in turn increasing retail activities on the ground-floor, would significantly increase pedestrian movement densities. This finding is in conformity with recent research suggesting that pedestrian movement levels decrease with increased residential density [68,118,119]. For street design measures, the only significant correlate of movement density is the average sidewalk width. Surprisingly, no significant associations were found between the presence of crosswalks, traffic lights and trees along the segments and distribution of flows. This may be due to the fact that there is not enough variability among the selected areas in terms of this safety and aesthetics attributes.

**Table 2.** Multivariate regression for three sets of models estimating the distribution of pedestrian flows for all areas considered as a single set. "Land-use" shows the effects of solely land-use variables on the distribution of flows. "Land-use+spatial structure" and "Urban Form" show the effects of adding street network configuration and street-level design measures into the model respectively.

| Variable | Land-Use | | | Land-Use+Spatial Structure | | | Urban Form | | |
|---|---|---|---|---|---|---|---|---|---|
| | β | t | std β | β | t | std β | β | t | std β |
| Street-level Land use (ground-floor) | | | | | | | | | |
| # residential-use per 100m | −0.07 *** | −3.53 | −0.28 | −0.06 ** | −3.16 | −0.24 | −0.05 * | −2.47 | −0.20 |
| # retail-use per 100m | 0.12 *** | 4.12 | 0.31 | 0.12 *** | 4.13 | 0.31 | 0.10 ** | 3.33 | 0.26 |
| # recreational-use per 100m | 0.57 *** | 6.14 | 0.46 | 0.62 *** | 6.82 | 0.50 | 0.67 *** | 7.32 | 0.54 |
| Street network configuration | | | | | | | | | |
| Integration (n) | | | | −0.00 * | −2.06 | −0.15 | −0.00 | −1.05 | −0.08 |
| 2-Directional Reach (20°) | | | | 0.00 ** | 3.15 | 0.23 | 0.00 *** | 3.40 | 0.25 |
| Street-level design | | | | | | | | | |
| crosswalk presence [yes] | | | | | | | −0.11 | 0.80 | −0.06 |
| traffic light presence [yes] | | | | | | | −0.24 | 1.27 | 0.10 |
| average sidewalk width | | | | | | | 0.00 ** | 2.96 | 0.23 |
| presence of trees [yes] | | | | | | | 0.07 | 0.86 | 0.06 |
| Number of observations: 120 | | | | | | | | | |
| Adj R-squared | 0.38 *** | | | 0.42 *** | | | 0.45 *** | | |

*** $p < 0.001$; ** $p < 0.01$; * $p < 0.05$ (two-tailed tests).

### 4.3. Analysis of Individual Areas

In order to better understand the distribution of pedestrians in each neighbourhood, multivariate regression models were estimated by considering individual areas separately. Tables 3–6 demonstrate the results of regression models estimating the distribution of pedestrian densities for individual areas.

In line with the previous overall model, the results suggest that the primary factors in explaining the distribution of pedestrian movement are the number of recreational land-uses at the street segment scale along with the configurational measure 2-directional reach. Even though Integration (r:n) does not appear as a significant variable, the inclusion of configurational measures, Integration and 2-directional reach, adds a considerable increase (adj $R^2$ change = 12–20%, $p < 0.001$) to the explanatory powers of the models for each individual area, except for Küçükçekmece.

Table 3 presents the individual impacts of land-use, street configuration and streetscape attributes on the distribution of movement in Avcılar. While street-level land-use explains 53% (99% CI) of the variation in pedestrian movement, the inclusion of spatial structural measures adds a 12% increase ($p < 0.001$) in the explanatory power of the model. Land-use and spatial structure variables together explain 65% (99% CI) of the variation in pedestrian movement. However, the inclusion of streetscape design measures does not add any significant improvement in the explanatory power of the overall model. In fact, none of the streetscape design attributes entered as significant measures.

Similarly, in Beylikdüzü (Table 4), the inclusion of street network measures adds a significant increase of 20% ($p < 0.001$) to the predictive power of the model, whereas, no significant increase in the explanatory power of the model is observed when streetscape design variables are added to the model. On the contrary, there was an inconsequential drop (2%, $p < 0.01$). Again, none of the street-level design attributes were found to be significantly correlated with pedestrian movement.

More interestingly, similar to the findings reported in section 'Analysis of the four areas as a single set', the coefficient of 2-directional reach is statistically significant in all models, except for Küçükçekmece. Put simply, street segments that give more direct access to more surrounding streets draw greater volumes of pedestrians. In other words, pedestrians choose to walk on streets with increased directional accessibility provided by the straightness of street alignment.

In Küçükçekmece, however, spatial variable 2-directional reach fails to correlate with pedestrian movement, as shown in Table 5. Land-use variables, on the other hand, are the strongest correlates of movement. Both the number of retail and recreational activities related with the street segment within this area is positively and significantly associated with the distribution of flows. This finding shows that the pedestrians in Küçükçekmece do not orient themselves according to the spatial structure of the network but are directed towards local attractors, such as various restaurants and shops. Hence, it appears that in Küçükçekmece land-use evolved in a manner that did not minimize travel distances from surrounding areas, and, as a result, street network configuration appears not to be a significant correlate of walking behaviour.

In Büyükçekmece (Table 6), which has an even pattern of land-use dominated by residences, there is a moderate relationship between land-use and pedestrian movement (44%, $p < 0.01$). By including spatial structural measures in the model, the explanatory role of land-use in predicting movement density is significantly attenuated (adj $R^2$ change = 17%; $p < 0.001$). Surprisingly, 2-directional reach is negatively correlated with movement. This contradictory result could be due to the fact that there is limited variability in the spectrum of this measure within the study area and that streets with increased directional accessibility are located in the outskirts of the neighbourhood, where observation points are few. Interestingly, when streetscape design variables are added, a modest increase of 9% ($p < 0.001$) is observed in the predictive power of the model. Average sidewalk width is the only variable that is significantly associated with the distribution of flows. In fact, in Büyükçekmece average sidewalk width has the highest effect level among all the variables. The weak correlation of this variable with movement in other areas might be due the fact that these neighbourhoods have more or less a uniform standard of sidewalk width.

In conclusion, results reporting analyses for all areas considered as a single set are quite consistent with those obtained from the analyses of areas separately. Two macro-scale environmental variables –number of recreational uses at the street segment-level and 2-directional reach– are the most significant correlates of movement. Consistent with theory, movement densities are strongly associated with the number of recreational (i.e., parks) uses related to the individual segment. The above-results suggest that the impact of recreational land-use on the distribution of flows is quite consistent across models. The model developed considering all areas as a single set demonstrates the number of residential and retail frontages as significant correlates of walking. However, in the analysis of individual areas, these land-use measures are less consistently correlated with the distribution of flows. The consistent relation of 2-directional reach with pedestrian movement across models indicates that the manner in which streets are aligned and the direction changes needed to navigate the network also affect movement. This is consistent with findings reported in recent studies [77]. In Küçükçekmece, the network plays a secondary role in explaining the distribution of pedestrians.

The evidence relating micro-scale environmental variables to walking is rather limited. While average sidewalk width is positively and significantly associated with pedestrian flows in the overall model (when all areas are analysed as a single set), a different picture emerges when areas are analysed separately. The significance of this variable is prevalent only in Büyükçekmece, which has a wider range of average sidewalk widths. On the other hand, no other consistent associations are found for the rest of the street design variables.

**Table 3.** Multivariate regression for three sets of models estimating the distribution of pedestrian flows in Avcılar. "Land-use" shows the effects of solely land-use variables on the distribution of flows. "Land-use+spatial structure" and "Urban Form" show the effects of adding street network configuration and street-level design measures into the model respectively.

| Variable | Land-Use | | | Land-Use+Spatial Structure | | | Urban Form | | |
|---|---|---|---|---|---|---|---|---|---|
| | β | t | std β | β | t | std β | β | t | std β |
| Street-level Land use (ground-floor) | | | | | | | | | |
| # residential-use per 100m | −0.23 *** | −3.85 | −0.54 | −0.17 ** | −2.79 | −0.40 | −0.15 * | −2.16 | −0.35 |
| # retail-use per 100m | 0.24 * | 2.39 | 0.33 | −0.14 | −0.94 | −0.19 | −0.15 | −0.94 | −0.20 |
| # recreational-use per 100m | 0.30 | 1.29 | 0.19 | 0.46 * | 2.04 | 0.29 | 0.58 * | 2.16 | 0.37 |
| Street network configuration | | | | | | | | | |
| Integration (n) | | | | 0.00 | 0.39 | 0.06 | 0.00 | 0.14 | 0.02 |
| 2-directional reach (20°) | | | | 0.00 ** | 2.93 | 0.58 | 0.00 ** | 3.04 | 0.63 |
| Street-level design | | | | | | | | | |
| traffic light presence [yes] | | | | | | | −0.23 | 0.43 | 0.06 |
| average sidewalk width | | | | | | | 0.00 | 1.22 | 0.17 |
| presence of trees [yes] | | | | | | | 0.11 | 0.52 | 0.08 |
| Number of observations: 30 | | | | | | | | | |
| Adj R-squared | 0.53 *** | | | 0.65 *** | | | 0.63 *** | | |

*** p < 0.001; ** p < 0.01; * p < 0.05 (two-tailed tests).

**Table 4.** Multivariate regression for three sets of models estimating the distribution of pedestrian flows in Beylizdüzü. "Land-use" shows the effects of solely land-use variables on the distribution of flows. "Land-use+spatial structure" and "Urban Form" show the effects of adding street network configuration and street-level design measures into the model respectively.

| Variable | Land-Use | | | Land-Use+Spatial Structure | | | Urban Form | | |
|---|---|---|---|---|---|---|---|---|---|
| | β | t | std β | β | t | std β | β | t | std β |
| Street-level Land use (ground-floor) | | | | | | | | | |
| # residential-use per 100m | −0.14 | −1.27 | −0.19 | −0.05 | −0.50 | −0.07 | 0.08 | 0.52 | 0.10 |
| # retail-use per 100m | 0.08 | 1.18 | 0.18 | 0.09 | 1.43 | 0.19 | 0.07 | 1.07 | 0.16 |
| # recreational-use per 100m | 0.54 *** | 3.75 | 0.58 | 0.57 *** | 4.14 | 0.61 | 0.51 ** | 3.21 | 0.55 |
| Street network configuration | | | | | | | | | |
| Integration (n) | | | | 0.00 | 0.68 | 0.12 | 0.00 | 1.02 | 0.24 |
| 2-directional reach (20°) | | | | 0.00 ** | 2.68 | 0.41 | 0.00 * | 2.21 | 0.38 |
| Street-level design | | | | | | | | | |
| crosswalk presence [yes] | | | | | | | 0.17 | 0.82 | 0.15 |
| traffic light presence [yes] | | | | | | | −0.34 | −1.07 | −0.17 |
| average sidewalk width | | | | | | | −0.00 | −0.60 | −0.12 |
| presence of trees [yes] | | | | | | | 0.05 | 0.31 | 0.05 |
| Number of observations: 31 | | | | | | | | | |
| Adj R-squared | 0.35 ** | | | 0.55 *** | | | 0.53 ** | | |

*** p < 0.001; ** p < 0.01 (two-tailed tests).

**Table 5.** Multivariate regression for three sets of models estimating the distribution of pedestrian flows in Küçükçekmece. "Land-use" shows the effects of solely land-use variables on the distribution of flows. "Land-use+spatial structure" and "Urban Form" show the effects of adding street network configuration and street-level design measures into the model respectively.

| Variable | Land-Use | | | Land-Use+Spatial Structure | | | Urban Form | | |
|---|---|---|---|---|---|---|---|---|---|
| | β | t | std β | β | t | std β | β | t | std β |
| Street-level Land use (ground-floor) | | | | | | | | | |
| # residential-use per 100m | −0.01 | −0.66 | −0.08 | −0.03 | −1.38 | −0.21 | −0.01 | −0.49 | −0.08 |
| # retail-use per 100m | 0.09 *** | 3.91 | 0.43 | 0.12 *** | 3.79 | 0.57 | 0.13 ** | 3.61 | 0.64 |
| # recreational-use per 100m | 0.91 *** | 7.24 | 0.78 | 0.86 *** | 6.36 | 0.74 | 0.92 *** | 6.28 | 0.78 |
| Street network configuration | | | | | | | | | |
| Integration (n) | | | | 0.00 | −1.11 | −0.17 | −0.00 | −1.09 | −0.17 |
| 2-directional reach (20°) | | | | −0.00 | −0.40 | −0.05 | −0.00 | −0.17 | −0.03 |
| Street-level design | | | | | | | | | |
| crosswalk presence [yes] | | | | | | | −0.37 | −1.31 | −0.18 |
| traffic light presence [yes] | | | | | | | 0.36 | 1.76 | 0.24 |
| average sidewalk width | | | | | | | −0.00 | −0.46 | −0.07 |
| presence of trees [yes] | | | | | | | −0.10 | −0.76 | −0.09 |
| Number of observations: 29 | | | | | | | | | |
| Adj R-squared | 0.71 *** | | | 0.71 *** | | | 0.71 *** | | |

*** p < 0.001; ** p < 0.01 (two-tailed tests).

**Table 6.** Multivariate regression for three sets of models estimating the distribution of pedestrian flows in Büyükçekmece. "Land-use" shows the effects of solely land-use variables on the distribution of flows. "Land-use+spatial structure" and "Urban Form" show the effects of adding street network configuration and street-level design measures into the model respectively.

| Variable | Land-Use | | | Land-Use+Spatial Structure | | | Urban Form | | |
|---|---|---|---|---|---|---|---|---|---|
| | $\beta$ | $t$ | std $\beta$ | $\beta$ | $t$ | std $\beta$ | $\beta$ | $t$ | std $\beta$ |
| Street-level Land use (ground-floor) | | | | | | | | | |
| # residential-use per 100m | −0.14 ** | −2.81 | −0.40 | −0.13 ** | −3.02 | −0.37 | −0.14 ** | −3.58 | −0.39 |
| # retail-use per 100m | 0.20 ** | 2.88 | 0.40 | 0.23 ** | 3.48 | 0.45 | 0.15 | 1.97 | 0.29 |
| # recreational-use per 100m | 0.35 * | 2.15 | 0.31 | 0.23 | 1.66 | 0.21 | 0.26 * | 2.05 | 0.23 |
| Street network configuration | | | | | | | | | |
| Integration (n) | | | | 0.01 ** | 2.76 | 0.36 | 0.01 | 1.56 | 0.20 |
| 2-directional reach (20°) | | | | −0.00 ** | −2.93 | −0.38 | −0.00B * | −2.10 | −0.26 |
| Street-level design | | | | | | | | | |
| crosswalk presence [yes] | | | | | | | 0.21 | 1.07 | 0.14 |
| traffic light presence [yes] | | | | | | | – | – | – |
| average sidewalk width | | | | | | | 0.00 * | 2.38 | 0.33 |
| presence of trees [yes] | | | | | | | −0.05 | −0.42 | 0.04 |
| Number of observations: 31 | | | | | | | | | |
| Adj R-squared | 0.44 ** | | | 0.61 *** | | | 0.70 *** | | |

*** $p < 0.001$; ** $p < 0.01$; * $p < 0.05$ (two-tailed tests).

## 5. Discussion

In this research, linear models were developed to determine the extent to which streetscape design –local qualities of street environment–, street network configuration –spatial structure of the urban grid– and land-use patterns are associated with the distribution of walking within four peripheral neighbourhoods in İstanbul. Overall, the analyses presented suggest that local conditions within peripheral neighbourhoods are significantly related to walking behaviour.

The results of this study emphasize the importance of including measures of street connectivity in physical activity and walkability studies. The results indicate that street connectivity is significantly associated with the distribution of pedestrian density over an area. This suggests that even after controlling for land-use and street-level design attributes, street layout plays a significant role in the way movement densities of pedestrians are distributed in the city. Street connectivity is measured through two syntactic measures, Integration and directional reach, which can capture the structural qualities of the street network. In all models, the standardized coefficient (std $\beta$) for directional reach, which measures the extent of streets captured within fewer direction changes, is positive and statistically significant (at a 95–99% level of confidence). This finding underscores the significance of the spatial structure of street networks, specifically the alignment of streets and the directional distance hierarchy engendered by the street network. This supports earlier findings arguing that street segments that give more direct access to more surrounding streets (accessible with fewer direction changes from the surroundings) tend to attract higher pedestrian flows [70,120].

In terms of local qualities of street environment, findings of this study are consistent with earlier findings arguing that sidewalk design provisions seem to be strong predictors of walking behaviour [121]. The models developed indicate that average sidewalk width is significantly and positively associated with movement densities over and above other urban design features. While street-level pedestrian indicators, such as the presence of crosswalks/traffic lights and tree-lined streets, are found to be significantly associated with walking [122], our data showed no significant relationships between these factors and pedestrian movement.

The present study confirms past research findings that land-use is often associated with pedestrian movement. The regression models developed suggest that increased number of retail frontages is significantly associated with increased pedestrian volumes. This finding extends those of previous studies reporting that ease of pedestrian access to relatively higher nearby destinations is related particularly to walking [24]. Hence, it can be concluded that streets with increased retail fronts, such as cafes, banks, shops and other services, are usually more stimulating to the passer-by, attracting pedestrians from the immediate surroundings as well as further away areas. Particularly in peripheral areas characterised by pedestrian-oriented retail development on ground-floors (such as Küçükçekmece), retail use out-performs the effects of street network configuration. It is important to note that Küçükçekmece neighbourhood, which dates back to the end of the 19th century, evolved over time (as opposed to the other study sites, which were fully or partially planned). This is partly apparent in its street network layout, which is dominated by a curvilinear street network pattern that partially turns into cul-de-sacs. Therefore, it appears that in Küçükçekmece land-use evolved along the streets with relatively lower connectivity levels (in a manner that did not minimize travel distances from surrounding areas), and, as a result, street network configuration is no longer a significant correlate of walking behaviour in this area (i.e. notwithstanding the adverse location of shops, people still have to access these). Although this finding is opposed to the arguments of Space Syntax theory, it is indicative of the fact that history does not always follow regular rules.

The negative coefficients of the number of residences on the street segment indicate that movement levels decrease with higher residential frontages. The findings are somewhat in contrast to those indicating positive significant correlations between residential land-uses and walking behaviour [123,124]. This contrast among studies might be due in part to scale of measurement (e.g., most studies investigating the physical activity correlates of built environment measure residential activities in terms of densities or as a component of mixed land-use entropy index) or to the specific nature of İstanbul (e.g., in contrast to studies reporting on the US, where single zoning is dominant, in İstanbul the prevailing pattern consists of non-residential land-uses such as shops, cafes and banks located on the ground-floors of residences). In fact, recent studies conducted in different parts of İstanbul have reported similar results [113]. Thus, it can be suggested that in peripheral neighbourhoods walking behaviour can be enhanced by increasing retail activities and reducing residential uses on the ground-floors, thus increasing local attractors within the area.

In addition, stronger relationships are observed between the number of recreational land-uses and movement, suggesting public open space (e.g., playground, public parks) as a significant correlate of walking. In fact, the consistent positive effects of this indicator across the models (both all areas considered as a single set and four areas considered individually) contributes to past research, which presented ambiguous findings with regard to the associations of recreational land-uses and walking behaviour. Having greater number of recreational activities within peripheral districts might lead to increased densities of pedestrian movement, leading to greater levels of physical activity.

*5.1. Study Limitations*

Our conclusions are tempered by several study limitations. First, the explanatory power of the linear model considering all areas as a single set (Table 2) displays a moderate degree of correlation, which indicates that there might be other factors (e.g., pedestrian perceptions regarding safety) influencing the distribution of pedestrian densities within the peripheral districts. However, it should be noted that the coefficients of correlations for all models considering individual areas separately (Tables 3–6) show high correlations, ranging from 53% to 71%. Second, land-use is measured based on the number of frontages at the segment-level. Other studies have shown land-use density at the segment scale to be a significant correlate of movement as well [77]. Thus, future research needs to consider land-use at different measurement scales. However, recent research has also shown number of frontages on ground-floors to be more significantly correlated with pedestrian movement than land-use densities at the segment scale [113]. Third, the sample is based on four areas with similar peripheral characteristics in a single city. Hence, these results need to be tested in other peripheral areas of various metropolitan areas to see whether these results are generalizable to other peripheral urban conditions. Fourth, the study areas lacked heterogeneity across some of the measures used, such as the sidewalk widths. This might be one of the reasons why no significant relationships are identified between street-scale attributes and walking. More research conducted within more heterogeneous urban environments is needed to shed more light into this association. Furthermore, pedestrian observations were conducted for a limited duration (10-min intervals on two different weekdays on mornings and afternoons) on a limited number of segments (~30 per area), which might have tempered the results. Since the use of advanced data collection technologies, such as video cameras and position sensors, is not yet prevalent in Turkey, a limited amount of data could be captured manually. Further research that includes pedestrian counts taken at varying times, various durations and along an increased number of segments through automated systems might more clearly detect relationships with walking. In addition, because the analysis is cross-sectional, the relationships observed do not necessarily indicate causality. Future work is needed to develop an understanding of how micro- and macro-scale street-level attributes are interrelated and how they are associated with walking relative to other environmental (e.g., aesthetics and comfort such as tree-aligned streets) and social features (e.g., future research should include both perceived and objective measures, particularly for characteristics such as safety [23,125–127]. Finally, there is an inherent limitation to this research and similar studies: they do not consider whether people enjoy walking or not. For example, through observation and surveys Mehta [128] found that some attributes of the street environment, such as the presence of other people, multiple activities and street width, added to the sensory pleasure of the street. The activity of walking is definitely important for public health professionals, yet the pleasure of walking is also important for city planners and urban designers. Thus, future research, such as Mehta's [129] and Darker et al.'s [130], should also take into account the perceptions of pedestrians in different neighbourhoods.

Research in these areas is fairly limited; hence, this study contributes to the literature by investigating the comparative roles of macro-scale (land-use and street design) and micro-scale (pedestrian-friendly street design) environmental correlates of walking. The results of the present study also demonstrate the significance of a more recent walkability indicator, directional reach, which can provide alternative means to quantify street design and capture a subtler relationship between movement patterns and urban systems.

### 5.2. Practical Implications

Important implications arise from the findings on the significance of street network design, average sidewalk width and ground-floor frontages in explaining the distribution of walking within peripheral areas. These findings also add support to calls for policy initiatives to create more-walkable neighbourhoods at the periphery [23,131]. One practical implication of these findings would be the provision of more generous sidewalks on spatially more prominent streets (i.e. streets with higher directional accessibility provided by the straightness of street alignments) in the light of the association between measures of the built environment and movement densities. The consistent association of land-use patterns with the distribution of movement shown in this study is critical for urban designers since it points to the fact that the strategic design of the ground-floor at the road segment scale is essential in designing for urban vitality and enhanced physical activity. Findings from this study also suggest that public health, urban design and planning strategies and intervention programmes to promote walking need to consider the contribution of street-level (both micro- and macro-scale) built environment factors to facilitate physical activity among communities.

### 6. Conclusions

City planning and healthy policy agendas to promote physical activity or walking need to emphasize the crucial role of micro- and macro-level environmental attributes that facilitate opportunities for people to be more active. In this respect, findings from this study suggest that peripheral neighbourhoods containing more direct and linear streets with extensive sidewalks, greater amounts of open green spaces for recreation and increased numbers of retail frontages, are likely to be supportive of walkable neighbourhoods. Since the results show the relative contribution of each of these environmental characteristics to walking, the results can lead to evidence-based policies and programs aimed at increasing walking and hence physical activity. For example, urban designers presume that pedestrian-oriented street-level features are important for active street life but they have little empirical evidence to back their claim. Hence, the results of this study underlie the argument that the layout of suburbs and traditional urban neighbourhoods is insufficient to encourage walking over automobile use and that a number of factors, including the location of retail stores and pedestrian-oriented commercial buildings, are required [132,133].

**Author Contributions:** Conceptualization, A.O.; Data curation, T.G., D.Y. and E.Z.; Formal analysis, A.O.; Funding acquisition, A.O.; Methodology, A.O.; Project administration, A.O.; Visualization, T.G. and D.Y.; Writing—review & editing, A.O., T.G. and D.Y.

**Funding:** This research was funded by The Scientific and Technological Research Council of Turkey (TUBITAK), grant number 113K796 and The APC was funded by Northumbria University.

**Conflicts of Interest:** The authors declare no conflict of interest.

## References

1.  Pate, R.R.; Pratt, M.; Blair, S.N.; Haskell, W.L.; Macera, C.A.; Bouchard, C.; Buchner, D.; Ettinger, W.; Heath, G.W.; King, A.C.; et al. Physical activity and public health: A recommendation from the centers for disease control and prevention and the american college of sports medicine. *JAMA* **1995**, *273*, 402–407. [CrossRef]
2.  U.S. Department of Health and Human Services. *Physical Activity and Health: A Report of the Surgeon General*; Department of Health and Human Services, Centers for Disease Control and Prevention, National Center for Chronic Disease Prevention and Health Promotion: Washington, DC, USA, 1996; ISBN 9780763706364.
3.  Ahern, S.M.; Arnott, B.; Chatterton, T.; de Nazelle, A.; Kellar, I.; McEachan, R.R.C. Understanding parents' school travel choices: A qualitative study using the theoretical domains framework. *J. Transp. Health* **2017**, *4*, 278–293. [CrossRef]
4.  Lorenc, T.; Brunton, G.; Oliver, S.; Oliver, K.; Oakley, A. Attitudes to walking and cycling among children, young people and parents: A systematic review. *J. Epidemiol. Community Health* **2008**, *62*, 852–857. [CrossRef]
5.  Sport England. *Active Lives Children and Young People Survey Academic Year 2017/18*; Sport England: London, UK, 2018.
6.  National Institute for Health and Care Excellence (NICE). *Public Health Guideline: Physical Activity: Walking and Cycling*; National Institute for Health and Care Excellence (NICE): London, UK, 2012.
7.  Johansson, M.; Hartig, T.; Staats, H. Psychological benefits of walking: Moderation by company and outdoor environment. *Appl. Psychol. Health Well-Being* **2011**, *3*, 261–280. [CrossRef]
8.  Barton, J.; Hine, R.; Pretty, J. The health benefits of walking in greenspaces of high natural and heritage value. *J. Integr. Environ. Sci.* **2009**, *6*, 261–278. [CrossRef]
9.  Oppezzo, M.; Schwartz, D.L. Give your ideas some legs: The positive effect of walking. *J. Exp. Psychol. Learn. Mem. Cogn.* **2014**, *40*, 1142–1152. [CrossRef]
10. Sælensminde, K. Cost–benefit analyses of walking and cycling track networks taking into account insecurity, health effects and external costs of motorized traffic. *Transp. Res. Part A Policy Pract.* **2004**, *38*, 593–606. [CrossRef]
11. Azmi, D.I.; Karim, H.A. Implications of walkability towards promoting sustainable urban neighbourhood. *Procedia Soc. Behav. Sci.* **2012**, *50*, 204–213. [CrossRef]
12. Choguill, C.L. Developing sustainable neighbourhoods. *Habitat Int.* **2008**, *32*, 41–48. [CrossRef]
13. Cervero, R.; Kockelman, K. Travel demand and the 3Ds: Density, diversity and design. *Transp. Res. Part D Transp. Environ.* **1997**, *2*, 199–219. [CrossRef]
14. Ewing, R.; Handy, S.; Brownson, R.; Clemente, O.; Winston, E. Identifying and measuring urban design qualities related to walkability. *J. Phys. Act. Health* **2006**, *3*, 223–240. [CrossRef]
15. Brownson, R.C.; Hoehner, C.M.; Day, K.; Forsyth, A.; Sallis, J.F. Measuring the built environment for physical activity: State of the science. *Am. J. Prev. Med.* **2009**, *36*, S99–S123. [CrossRef]
16. Brug, J.; van Lenthe, F.J.; Kremers, S.P.J. Revisiting Kurt Lewin: How to gain insight into environmental correlates of obesogenic behaviors. *Am. J. Prev. Med.* **2006**, *31*, 525–529. [CrossRef]

17. Santos, M.S.R.; Vale, M.S.S.; Miranda, L.; Mota, J. Socio-demographic and perceived environmental correlates of walking in Portuguese adults—A multilevel analysis. *Health Place* **2009**, *15*, 1094–1099. [CrossRef]

18. Trost, S.G.; Owen, N.; Bauman, A.E.; Sallis, J.F.; Brown, W. Correlates of adults' participation in physical activity: Review and update. *Med. Sci. Sports Exerc.* **2002**, *34*, 1996–2001. [CrossRef]

19. Bauman, A.E.; Bull, F.C. *Environmental Correlates of Physical Activity and Walking in Adults and Children: A Review of Reviews*; National Institute for Health and Care Excellence (NICE): London, UK, 2007.

20. Pont, K.; Ziviani, J.; Bennett, S.; Abbott, R. Environmental correlates of children's active transportation: A systematic literature review. *Health Place* **2009**, *15*, 849–862. [CrossRef]

21. Saelens, B.E.; Handy, S.L. Built environment correlates of walking: A review. *Med. Sci. Sports Exerc.* **2008**, *40*, 550. [CrossRef]

22. Badland, H.; Schofield, G. Transport, urban design and physical activity: An evidence-based update. *Transp. Res. Part D Transp. Environ.* **2005**, *10*, 177–196. [CrossRef]

23. Heath, G.W.; Brownson, R.C.; Kruger, J.; Miles, R.; Powell, K.E.; Ramsey, L.T. The effectiveness of urban design and land use and transport policies and practices to increase physical activity: A systematic review. *J. Phys. Act. Health* **2006**, *3*, S55–S76. [CrossRef]

24. Saelens, B.E.; Sallis, J.F.; Frank, L.D. Environmental correlates of walking and cycling: Findings from the transportation, urban design and planning literatures. *Ann. Behav. Med.* **2003**, *25*, 80–91. [CrossRef]

25. Rodríguez, D.A.; Joo, J. The relationship between non-motorized mode choice and the local physical environment. *Transp. Res. Part D Transp. Environ.* **2004**, *9*, 151–173. [CrossRef]

26. Cervero, R. Built environments and mode choice: Toward a normative framework. *Transp. Res. Part D Transp. Environ.* **2002**, *7*, 265–284. [CrossRef]

27. Frank, L.D.; Engleke, P. *How Land Use and Transportation Systems Impact Public Health: A Literature Review of the Relationship between Physical Activity and Built Form*; Georgia Institute of Technology: Atlanta, GA, USA, 2000.

28. Handy, S.; Clifton, K. Evaluating neighborhood accessibility: Possibilities and practicalities. *J. Transp. Stat.* **2001**, *4*, 67–78.

29. Krizek, K.J. Operationalizing neighborhood accessibility for land use-travel behavior research and regional modeling. *J. Plan. Educ. Res.* **2003**, *22*, 270–287. [CrossRef]

30. Frank, L.D.; Pivo, G. *Relationship between Land Use and Travel Behavior in the Puget Sound Region*; The National Academies of Sciences, Engineering, and Medicine: Washington, DC, USA, 1994.

31. Marshall, N.; Grady, B. Travel demand modeling for regional visioning and scenario analysis. *Transp. Res. Rec. J. Transp. Res. Board* **2005**, *1921*, 44–52. [CrossRef]

32. Cerin, E.; Leslie, E.; du Toit, L.; Owen, N.; Frank, L.D. Destinations that matter: Associations with walking for transport. *Health Place* **2007**, *13*, 713–724. [CrossRef]

33. Ball, K.; Timperio, A.; Salmon, J.; Giles-Corti, B.; Roberts, R.; Crawford, D. Personal, social and environmental determinants of educational inequalities in walking: A multilevel study. *J. Epidemiol. Community Health* **2007**, *61*, 108–114. [CrossRef]

34. Giles-Corti, B.; Donovan, R.J. Socioeconomic status differences in recreational physical activity levels and real and perceived access to a supportive physical environment. *Prev. Med.* **2002**, *35*, 601–611. [CrossRef]

35. Frank, L.D.; Engelke, P.O. The built environment and human activity patterns: Exploring the impacts of urban form on public health. *J. Plan. Lit.* **2001**, *16*, 202–218. [CrossRef]

36. Peimani, N. Transit-Oriented Morphologies and Forms of Urban Life. Available online: http://contour.epfl.ch/?p=1137&lang=en (accessed on 24 May 2019).

37. Boarnet, M.; Sarmiento, S. Can Land-use policy really affect travel behaviour? A study of the link between non-work travel and land-use characteristics. *Urban Stud.* **1998**, *35*, 1155–1169. [CrossRef]

38. Boarnet, M.G.; Greenwald, M.J. Land use, urban design and nonwork travel: Reproducing other urban areas' empirical test results in Portland, Oregon. *Transp. Res. Rec.* **2000**, *1722*, 27–37. [CrossRef]

39. Pikora, T.; Giles-Corti, B.; Bull, F.; Jamrozik, K.; Donovan, R. Developing a framework for assessment of the environmental determinants of walking and cycling. *Soc. Sci. Med.* **2003**, *56*, 1693–1703. [CrossRef]

40. Pikora, T.J.; Bull, F.C.L.; Jamrozik, K.; Knuiman, M.; Giles-Corti, B.; Donovan, R.J. Developing a reliable audit instrument to measure the physical environment for physical activity. *Am. J. Prev. Med.* **2002**, *23*, 187–194. [CrossRef]

41. Randall, T.A.; Baetz, B.W. Evaluating Pedestrian Connectivity for Suburban Sustainability. *J. Urban Plan. Dev.* **2001**, *127*, 1–15. [CrossRef]

42. Stangl, P. The pedestrian route directness test: A new level-of-service model. *Urban Des. Int.* **2012**, *17*, 228–238. [CrossRef]

43. Pafka, E.; Dovey, K. Permeability and interface catchment: Measuring and mapping walkable access. *J. Urban. Int. Res. Placemaking Urban Sustain.* **2017**, *10*, 150–162. [CrossRef]

44. Berghauser Pont, M.; Haupt, P. *Spacematrix: Space, Density and Urban Form*; NAi Publishers: Rotterdam, The Netherlands, 2010.

45. Schlossberg, M. From TIGER to audit instruments: Measuring neighborhood walkability with street data based on geographic information systems. *Transp. Res. Rec.* **2006**, *1982*, 48–56. [CrossRef]

46. Sevtsuk, A.; Mekonnen, M. Urban network analysis: A new toolbox for ArcGIS. *Rev. Int. Géomat.* **2012**, *22*, 287–305. [CrossRef]

47. Ellis, G.; Hunter, R.; Tully, M.A.; Donnelly, M.; Kelleher, L. Connectivity and physical activity: Using footpath networks to measure the walkability of built environments. *Environ. Plan. B Plan. Des.* **2016**, *43*, 130–151. [CrossRef]

48. Dovey, K.; Pafka, E. The science of urban design? *Urban Des. Int.* **2016**, *21*, 1–10. [CrossRef]

49. Hooper, P.; Knuiman, M.; Foster, S.; Giles-Corti, B. The building blocks of a 'Liveable Neighbourhood': Identifying the key performance indicators for walking of an operational planning policy in Perth, Western Australia. *Health Place* **2015**, *36*, 173–183. [CrossRef]

50. McDonald, K.N.; Oakes, J.M.; Forsyth, A. Effect of street connectivity and density on adult BMI: Results from the Twin Cities Walking Study. *J. Epidemiol. Community Health* **2012**, *66*, 636–640. [CrossRef]

51. Oakes, J.M.; Forsyth, A.; Schmitz, K.H. The effects of neighborhood density and street connectivity on walking behavior: The Twin Cities walking study. *Epidemiol. Perspect. Innov.* **2007**, *4*, 16. [CrossRef]

52. Knight, P.L.; Marshall, W.E. The metrics of street network connectivity: Their inconsistencies. *J. Urban. Int. Res. Placemaking Urban Sustain.* **2015**, *8*, 241–259. [CrossRef]

53. Stangl, P. Block size-based measures of street connectivity: A critical assessment and new approach. *Urban Des. Int.* **2015**, *20*, 44–55. [CrossRef]

54. Stangl, P.; Guinn, J.M. Neighborhood design, connectivity assessment and obstruction. *Urban Des. Int.* **2011**, *16*, 285–296. [CrossRef]

55. Hess, P. Measures of connectivity. *Places* **1997**, *11*, 217–220.

56. Stangl, P. Overcoming flaws in permeability measures: Modified route directness. *J. Urban. Int. Res. Placemaking Urban Sustain.* **2019**, *12*, 1–14. [CrossRef]

57. Owens, P.M. Neighborhood form and pedestrian life: Taking a closer look. *Landsc. Urban Plan.* **1993**, *26*, 115–135. [CrossRef]

58. Lee, C.; Moudon, A.V. The 3Ds+R: Quantifying land use and urban form correlates of walking. *Transp. Res. Part D Transp. Environ.* **2006**, *11*, 204–215. [CrossRef]

59. Matley, T.M.; Goldman, L.M.; Fineman, B.J. Pedestrian travel potential in northern New Jersey: A metropolitan planning organization's approach to identifying investment priorities. *Transp. Res. Rec.* **2000**, *1705*, 1–8. [CrossRef]

60. Rodrigue, J.-P.; Comtois, C.; Slack, B. *The Geography of Transport Systems*, 2nd ed.; Routledge: London, UK, 2006.

61. Berrigan, D.; Pickle, L.; Dill, J. Associations between street connectivity and active transportation. *Int. J. Health Geogr.* **2010**, *9*, 1. [CrossRef]

62. Marshall, W.E.; Garrick, N.W. Effect of street network design on walking and biking. *Transp. Res. Rec.* **2010**, *2198*, 103–115. [CrossRef]

63. Timperio, A.; Ball, K.; Salmon, J.; Roberts, R.; Giles-Corti, B.; Simmons, D.; Baur, L.A.; Crawford, D. Personal, family, social and environmental correlates of active commuting to school. *Am. J. Prev. Med.* **2006**, *30*, 45–51. [CrossRef]

64. Lee, C.; Moudon, A.V. Physical activity and environment research in the health field: Implications for urban and transportation planning practice and research. *J. Plan. Lit.* **2004**, *19*, 147–181. [CrossRef]

65. Hoehner, C.M.; Brennan, L.K.; Brownson, R.C.; Handy, S.L.; Killingsworth, R. Opportunities for integrating public health and urban planning approaches to promote active community environments. *Am. J. Health Promot.* **2003**, *18*, 14–20. [CrossRef]

66. Hou, N.; Popkin, B.M.; Jacobs, D.R.; Song, Y.; Guilkey, D.; Lewis, C.E.; Gordon-Larsen, P. Longitudinal associations between neighborhood-level street network with walking, bicycling and jogging: The CARDIA study. *Health Place* **2010**, *16*, 1206–1215. [CrossRef]

67. Li, F.; Fisher, J.K.; Brownson, R.C.; Bosworth, M. Multilevel modelling of built environment characteristics related to neighbourhood walking activity in older adults. *J. Epidemiol. Community Health* **2005**, *59*, 558–564. [CrossRef] [PubMed]

68. Nagel, C.L.; Carlson, N.E.; Bosworth, M.; Michael, Y.L. The relation between neighborhood built environment and walking activity among older adults. *Am. J. Epidemiol.* **2008**, *168*, 461–468. [CrossRef] [PubMed]

69. Baran, P.K.; Rodríguez, D.A.; Khattak, A.J. Space Syntax and walking in a new urbanist and suburban neighbourhoods. *J. Urban Des.* **2008**, *13*, 5–28. [CrossRef]

70. Koohsari, M.J.; Sugiyama, T.; Mavoa, S.; Villanueva, K.; Badland, H.; Giles-Corti, B.; Owen, N. Street network measures and adults' walking for transport: Application of space syntax. *Health Place* **2016**, *38*, 89–95. [CrossRef]

71. Lamiquiz, P.J.; Lopez-Dominguez, J. Effects of built environment on walking at the neighbourhood scale. A new role for street networks by modelling their configurational accessibility? *Transp. Res. Part A Policy Pract.* **2015**, *74*, 148–163. [CrossRef]

72. Bafna, S. Space syntax: A brief introduction to its logic and analytical techniques. *Environ. Behav.* **2003**, *35*, 17–29. [CrossRef]

73. Hillier, B.; Hanson, J. *The Social Logic of Space*; Cambridge University Press: Cambridge, UK, 1984.

74. Hillier, B.; Penn, A.; Hanson, J.; Grajewski, T.; Xu, J. Natural movement: Or, configuration and attraction in urban pedestrian movement. *Environ. Plan. B Plan. Des.* **1993**, *20*, 29–66. [CrossRef]

75. Peponis, J.; Ross, C.; Rashid, M. The structure of urban space, movement and co-presence: The case of Atlanta. *Geoforum* **1997**, *28*, 341–358. [CrossRef]

76. Peponis, J.; Bafna, S.; Zhang, Z. The connectivity of streets: Reach and directional distance. *Environ. Plan. B Plan. Des.* **2008**, *35*, 881–901. [CrossRef]

77. Ozbil, A.; Peponis, J.; Stone, B. Understanding the link between street connectivity, land use and pedestrian flows. *Urban Des. Int.* **2011**, *16*, 125–141. [CrossRef]

78. Hillier, B.; Iida, S. Network effects and psychological effects: A theory of urban movement. In Proceedings of the 5th International Space Syntax Symposium, Delft, The Netherlands, 13–17 June 2005; pp. 553–564.

79. Park, S.; Deakin, E.; Lee, J.S. Perception-based walkability index to test impact of microlevel walkability on sustainable mode choice decisions. *Transp. Res. Rec.* **2014**, *2464*, 126–134. [CrossRef]

80. Aghaabbasi, M.; Moeinaddini, M.; Shah, M.Z.; Asadi-Shekari, Z. A new assessment model to evaluate the microscale sidewalk design factors at the neighbourhood level. *J. Transp. Health* **2017**, *5*, 97–112. [CrossRef]

81. Troped, P.J.; Saunders, R.P.; Pate, R.R.; Reininger, B.; Addy, C.L. Correlates of recreational and transportation physical activity among adults in a New England community. *Prev. Med.* **2003**, *37*, 304–310. [CrossRef]

82. Duncan, M.J.; Spence, J.C.; Mummery, W.K. Perceived environment and physical activity: A meta-analysis of selected environmental characteristics. *Int. J. Behav. Nutr. Phys. Act.* **2005**, *2*, 11. [CrossRef]

83. Van Cauwenberg, J.; Van Holle, V.; Simons, D.; Deridder, R.; Clarys, P.; Goubert, L.; Nasar, J.; Salmon, J.; De Bourdeaudhuij, I.; Deforche, B. Environmental factors influencing older adults' walking for transportation: A study using walk-along interviews. *Int. J. Behav. Nutr. Phys. Act.* **2012**, *9*, 85. [CrossRef]

84. Mitra, R.; Siva, H.; Kehler, M. Walk-friendly suburbs for older adults? Exploring the enablers and barriers to walking in a large suburban municipality in Canada. *J. Aging Stud.* **2015**, *35*, 10–19. [CrossRef]

85. Sallis, J.F.; Saelens, B.E.; Frank, L.D.; Conway, T.L.; Slymen, D.J.; Cain, K.L.; Chapman, J.E.; Kerr, J. Neighborhood built environment and income: Examining multiple health outcomes. *Soc. Sci. Med.* **2009**, *68*, 1285–1293. [CrossRef]

86. Salon, D.; Boarnet, M.G.; Handy, S.; Spears, S.; Tal, G. How do local actions affect VMT? A critical review of the empirical evidence. *Transp. Res. Part D Transp. Environ.* **2012**, *17*, 495–508. [CrossRef]

87. Agrawal, A.W.; Schlossberg, M.; Irvin, K. How far, by which route and why? A spatial analysis of pedestrian preference. *J. Urban Des.* **2008**, *13*, 81–98. [CrossRef]

88. Cao, X.; Mokhtarian, P.L.; Handy, S.L. Do changes in neighborhood characteristics lead to changes in travel behavior? A structural equations modeling approach. *Transportation* **2007**, *34*, 535–556. [CrossRef]

89. Carnegie, M.A.; Bauman, A.; Marshall, A.L.; Mohsin, M.; Westley-Wise, V.; Booth, M.L. Perceptions of the physical environment, stage of change for physical activity and walking among Australian adults. *Res. Q. Exerc. Sport* **2002**, *73*, 146–155. [CrossRef]

90. Humpel, N.; Owen, N.; Leslie, E. Environmental factors associated with adults' participation in physical activity: A review. *Am. J. Prev. Med.* **2002**, *22*, 188–199. [CrossRef]

91. Wilcox, S.; Castro, C.; King, A.C.; Housemann, R.; Brownson, R.C. Determinants of leisure time physical activity in rural compared with urban older and ethnically diverse women in the United States. *J. Epidemiol. Community Health* **2000**, *54*, 667–672. [CrossRef] [PubMed]

92. Lee, S.; Talen, E. Measuring walkability: A note on auditing methods. *J. Urban Des.* **2014**, *19*, 368–388. [CrossRef]

93. Bentley, R.; Jolley, D.; Kavanagh, A.M. Local environments as determinants of walking in Melbourne, Australia. *Soc. Sci. Med.* **2010**, *70*, 1806–1815. [CrossRef]

94. Pikora, T.J.; Giles-Corti, B.; Knuiman, M.W.; Bull, F.C.; Jamrozik, K.; Donovan, R.J. Neighborhood environmental factors correlated with walking near home: Using SPACES. *Med. Sci. Sports Exerc.* **2006**, *38*, 708–714. [CrossRef]

95. Stathi, A.; Gilbert, H.; Fox, K.R.; Coulson, J.; Davis, M.; Thompson, J.L. Determinants of neighborhood activity of adults age 70 and over: A mixed-methods study. *J. Aging Phys. Act.* **2012**, *20*, 148–170. [CrossRef] [PubMed]

96. Belon, A.P.; Nieuwendyk, L.M.; Vallianatos, H.; Nykiforuk, C.I.J. How community environment shapes physical activity: Perceptions revealed through the PhotoVoice method. *Soc. Sci. Med.* **2014**, *116*, 10–21. [CrossRef]

97. Mahmood, A.; Chaudhury, H.; Michael, Y.L.; Campo, M.; Hay, K.; Sarte, A. A photovoice documentation of the role of neighborhood physical and social environments in older adults' physical activity in two metropolitan areas in North America. *Soc. Sci. Med.* **2012**, *74*, 1180–1192. [CrossRef]

98. Maghelal, P.K.; Capp, C.J. Walkability: A review of existing pedestrian indices. *J. Urban Reg. Inf. Syst. Assoc.* **2011**, *23*, 5–19.

99. Brownson, R.C.; Baker, E.A.; Housemann, R.A.; Brennan, L.K.; Bacak, S.J. Environmental and policy determinants of physical activity in the United States. *Am. J. Public Health* **2001**, *91*, 1995–2003. [CrossRef] [PubMed]

100. Pucher, J.; Dijkstra, L. Making walking and cycling safer: Lessons from Europe. *Transp. Q.* **2000**, *54*, 25–50.

101. Forsyth, A. What is a walkable place? The walkability debate in urban design. *URBAN Des. Int.* **2015**, *20*, 274–292. [CrossRef]

102. Burden, D.; Wallwork, M.; Sides, K.; Trias, R.; Rue, H. *Street Design Guidelines for Healthy Neighbourhoods*; Center for Livable Communities: Sacramento, CA, USA, 1999.

103. Wells, N.M.; Yang, Y. Neighborhood design and walking: A quasi-experimental longitudinal study. *Am. J. Prev. Med.* **2008**, *34*, 313–319. [CrossRef] [PubMed]

104. Sarkar, C.; Webster, C.; Pryor, M.; Tang, D.; Melbourne, S.; Zhang, X.; Jianzheng, L. Exploring associations between urban green, street design and walking: Results from the Greater London boroughs. *Landsc. Urban Plan.* **2015**, *143*, 112–125. [CrossRef]

105. NSW Ministry of Transport. *Service Planning Guidelines for Sydney Contract Regions*; NSW Ministry of Transport: Sydney, Australia, 2006.

106. Daniels, R.; Mulley, C. Explaining walking distance to public transport: The dominance of public transport supply. *J. Transp. Land Use* **2013**, *6*, 5. [CrossRef]

107. Diogenes, M.C.; Greene-Roesel, R.; Arnold, L.S.; Ragland, D.R. Pedestrian counting methods at intersections: A comparative study. *Transp. Res. Rec.* **2007**, *2002*, 26–30. [CrossRef]

108. Turvey, I.G.; May, A.D.; Hopkinson, P.G. *Counting Methods and Sampling Strategies Determining Pedestrian Numbers*; University of Leeds: Leeds, UK, 1987.

109. Mooney, S.J.; DiMaggio, C.J.; Lovasi, G.S.; Neckerman, K.M.; Bader, M.D.M.; Teitler, J.O.; Sheehan, D.M.; Jack, D.W.; Rundle, A.G. Use of google street view to assess environmental contributions to pedestrian injury. *Am. J. Public Health* **2016**, *106*, 462–469. [CrossRef]

110. Rodríguez, D.A.; Brisson, E.M.; Estupiñán, N. The relationship between segment-level built environment attributes and pedestrian activity around Bogota's BRT stations. *Transp. Res. Part D Transp. Environ.* **2009**, *14*, 470–478. [CrossRef]

111. Borst, H.C.; Miedema, H.M.E.; de Vries, S.I.; Graham, J.M.A.; van Dongen, J.E.F. Relationships between street characteristics and perceived attractiveness for walking reported by elderly people. *J. Environ. Psychol.* **2008**, *28*, 353–361. [CrossRef]

112. McGinn, A.P.; Evenson, K.R.; Herring, A.H.; Huston, S.L. The relationship between leisure, walking and transportation activity with the natural environment. *Health Place* **2007**, *13*, 588–602. [CrossRef] [PubMed]

113. Ozbil, A.; Yesiltepe, D.; Argin, G. Modeling walkability: The effects of street design, street-network configuration and land-use on pedestrian movement. *A Z ITU J. Fac. Archit.* **2015**, *12*, 189–207.

114. Forsyth, A.; Hearst, M.; Oakes, J.M.; Schmitz, K.H. Design and destinations: Factors influencing walking and total physical activity. *Urban Stud.* **2008**, *45*, 1973–1996. [CrossRef]

115. Ozbil, A.; Argin, G.; Yesiltepe, D. Pedestrian route choice by elementary school students: The role of street network configuration and pedestrian quality attributes in walking to school. *Int. J. Des. Creat. Innov.* **2016**, *4*, 67–84. [CrossRef]

116. Turner, A.; Friedrich, E. *Depthmap Software*; University College London: London, UK, 2011.

117. Turner, A.; Friedrich, E. *Depthmap Software, Version 10.14.00b*; University College London: London, UK, 2010.

118. Forsyth, A.; Oakes, M.J.; Schmitz, K.H.; Hearst, M.O. Does residential density increase walking and other physical activity. *Urban Stud.* **2007**, *44*, 679–697. [CrossRef]

119. Kang, C.-D. The effects of spatial accessibility and centrality to land use on walking in Seoul, Korea. *Cities* **2015**, *46*, 94–103. [CrossRef]

120. Ozbil, A. Modeling walking behavior in cities based on street network and land-use characteristics: The case of İstanbul. *METU J. Fac. Archit.* **2013**, *30*, 17–33.

121. Alfonzo, M.; Boarnet, M.G.; Day, K.; Mcmillan, T.; Anderson, C.L. The relationship of neighbourhood built environment features and adult parents' walking. *J. Urban Des.* **2008**, *13*, 29–51. [CrossRef]

122. Doescher, M.P.; Lee, C.; Saelens, B.E.; Lee, C.; Berke, E.M.; Adachi-Mejia, A.M.; Patterson, D.G.; Moudon, A.V. Utilitarian and recreational walking among spanish-and english-speaking latino adults in micropolitan US towns. *J. Immigr. Minor. Health* **2017**, *19*, 237–245. [CrossRef] [PubMed]

123. Vojnovic, I.; Jackson-Elmoore, C.; Holtrop, J.; Bruch, S. The renewed interest in urban form and public health: Promoting increased physical activity in Michigan. *Cities* **2006**, *23*, 1–17. [CrossRef]

124. Carr, L.J.; Dunsiger, S.I.; Marcus, B.H. Walk score$^{tm}$ as a global estimate of neighborhood walkability. *Am. J. Prev. Med.* **2010**, *39*, 460–463. [CrossRef]

125. Cunningham, G.O.; Michael, Y.L. Concepts guiding the study of the impact of the built environment on physical activity for older adults: A review of the literature. *Am. J. Health Promot.* **2004**, *18*, 435–443. [CrossRef]

126. McCormack, G.; Giles-Corti, B.; Lange, A.; Smith, T.; Martin, K.; Pikora, T.J. An update of recent evidence of the relationship between objective and self-report measures of the physical environment and physical activity behaviours. *J. Sci. Med. Sport* **2004**, *7*, 81–92. [CrossRef]

127. Brown, B.B.; Werner, C.M.; Amburgey, J.W.; Szalay, C. Walkable route perceptions and physical features: Converging evidence for en route walking experiences. *Environ. Behav.* **2007**, *39*, 34–61. [CrossRef]

128. Mehta, V. Lively streets: Determining environmental characteristics to support social behavior. *J. Plan. Educ. Res.* **2007**, *27*, 165–187. [CrossRef]

129. Mehta, V. *Lively Streets: Exploring the Relationship Between Built Environment and Social Behavior*; University of Maryland: College Park, MD, USA, 2006.

130. Darker, C.D.; Larkin, M.; French, D.P. An exploration of walking behaviour—An interpretative phenomenological approach. *Soc. Sci. Med.* **2007**, *65*, 2172–2183. [CrossRef] [PubMed]

131. Transportation Research Board and Institute of Medicine. *Does the Built Environment Influence Physical Activity: Examining the Evidence*; Special Report 282; The National Academies Press: Washington, DC, USA, 2005.

132. Corbett, J.; Velasquez, J. *The Ahwahnee Principles: Toward more Livable Communities, Center for Livable Communities*; Local Government Commission: Sacramento, CA, USA, 1994.

133. Berman, M.A. The transportation effects of neo-traditional development. *J. Plan. Lit.* **1996**, *10*, 347–363. [CrossRef]

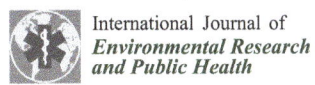

Article

# Associations of Neighborhood Walkability with Sedentary Time in Nigerian Older Adults

**Adewale L. Oyeyemi [1,*], Sanda M. Kolo [1], Adamu A. Rufai [1], Adetoyeje Y. Oyeyemi [1], Babatunji A. Omotara [2] and James F. Sallis [3,4]**

[1]   Department of Physiotherapy, College of Medical Sciences, University of Maiduguri, Maiduguri 600243, Nigeria; kolosanda@gmail.com (S.M.K.); adamuarufai@gmail.com (A.A.R.); adeoyeyemi@aol.com (A.Y.O.)
[2]   Department of Community Medicine, College of Medical Sciences, University of Maiduguri, Maiduguri 600243, Nigeria; atunjeba@yahoo.com
[3]   Department of Family Medicine and Public Health, University of California, San Diego, CA 92093-0631, USA; jsallis@ucsd.edu
[4]   Mary MacKillop Institute for Health Research, Australian Catholic University, Melbourne 3000, Australia
*   Correspondence: alaoyeyemi@yahoo.com; Tel.: +234-802-945-8230

Received: 27 April 2019; Accepted: 27 May 2019; Published: 28 May 2019

**Abstract:** Previous studies have investigated the potential role of neighborhood walkability in reducing sedentary behavior. However, the majority of this research has been conducted in adults and Western developed countries. The purpose of the present study was to examine associations of neighborhood environmental attributes with sedentary time among older adults in Nigeria. Data from 353 randomly-selected community-dwelling older adults (60 years and above) in Maiduguri, Nigeria were analyzed. Perceived attributes of neighborhood environments and self-reported sedentary time were assessed using Nigerian-validated and reliable measures. Outcomes were weekly minutes of total sedentary time, minutes of sitting on a typical weekday, and minutes of sitting on a typical weekend day. In multivariate regression analyses, higher walkability index, proximity to destinations, access to services, traffic safety, and safety from crime were associated with less total sedentary time and sedentary time on both a weekday and a weekend day. Moderation analysis showed that only in men was higher walking infrastructure and safety found to be associated with less sedentary time, and higher street connectivity was associated with more sedentary time. The findings suggest that improving neighborhood walkability may be a mechanism for reducing sedentary time among older adults in Nigeria.

**Keywords:** walkable neighborhood; sitting; elderly; built environment; non-communicable diseases; Africa

## 1. Introduction

The global population of older adults (aged 60 years and above) has increased substantially in recent years and is expected to double by 2050 when it is projected to reach about 2 billion [1]. The number of older adults is expected to grow fastest in Africa, where it is projected to increase more than threefold, from 69 to 226 million between the years 2017 and 2050 [2]. Due to weak health care systems in sub-Saharan Africa [3], the cost and burden of age-related non-communicable diseases (NCDs) is expected to be unsustainable in the region if urgent actions are not taken. Reducing population levels of physical inactivity and sedentary behavior is one of the recommended strategies for stemming the growing epidemics of NCDs worldwide [4]. Yet, there is little research to drive evidence-based intervention in most of the developing African countries [5].

Sedentary time (too much sitting), which is distinct from physical inactivity (too little physical activity) [6], is highly prevalent among older adults [7–9] and is a strong risk factor for many NCDs and all-cause mortality [6,10,11]. Among older adults, high levels of sedentary time have been associated with frailty, disablement, social isolation [12], and less successful aging [13]. Yet, very few studies of sedentary time as a distinct health behavior, distinct from physical inactivity, have been conducted among older adults in Africa [14,15]. The few available African studies suggest that sedentary behavior is highly prevalent and may be associated with low socioeconomic status and adverse clinical conditions in African older adults [14,15]. Because older adults may concurrently be at risk of high sedentary time and physical inactivity, developing effective population-wide strategies to improve both behaviors is a public health priority for African countries. However, to develop effective strategies for such interventions, it is important to first identify modifiable factors that can be targeted for reducing the prevalence of high sedentary time among older adults in Africa.

Built environment and related policy approaches are promising interventions that have been advocated internationally for improving behavioral risk factors, including physical inactivity and excessive sedentary time [4]. The theoretical framework for understanding such interventions is ecological models of health behaviors [16]. These models have also provided the conceptual basis for guiding studies on the neighborhood environmental correlates and determinants of sedentary behavior in older adults [17]. Generally, the presence of favorable built environment attributes like high residential density, well-connected streets, a mixture of land uses, and pedestrian facilities that support active transportation have been used to describe the 'walkability' of a neighborhood [18–21]. However, most of the studies regarding how neighborhood built environmental characteristics may contribute to sedentary behavior have been conducted among adults than older adults [21–23]. Yet, evidence from the studies of adults have been mostly inconsistent [24–26].

The few studies of associations of neighborhood built environments with sedentary behavior of older adults have also produced some mixed results [21–23]. For example, perceived safety and presence of street lightning were associated with lower levels of TV viewing among Belgian [22] and Hong Kong older adults [23], but no direct association was found between neighborhood social environment and overall sedentary time of older adults in Belgium [21]. Only among residents of highly-walkable neighborhoods were higher social environmental factors related to less TV viewing and overall sedentary time among Belgian older adults [21]. Since adults and older adults may interact differently with their neighborhood environments [18,27], more studies of older adults are needed to identify the environmental correlates of sedentary time that can be targeted for effective health promotion strategies addressing less sedentary time in this age group.

The few available studies of older adults on environmental correlates of sedentary behavior were conducted in Western developed countries, and findings may not directly apply to African countries. Many cities in Africa have different environmental features (e.g., presence of slums and very densely packed small housing patterns and absence of walkways and pedestrian crossings), transportation systems (e.g., use of tricycles and motor bikes as modes of public transportation) and urban developmental patterns (e.g., organic and unplanned urbanization) compared to those in Western countries [28]. Thus, there is need for more context-specific research in African settings. A recent African study demonstrated the relevance of neighborhood built environment attributes, like availability of roads and walking paths, to sedentary time among people with mental illness in Uganda [29]. Understanding the role of neighborhood built environments on sedentary time among the apparently healthy population is particularly relevant in African countries because chronic disease rates are rising in the region [3,4]. Africa-specific studies can provide more targeted evidence for environmental and urban design policy initiatives aimed at promoting less sitting time and more active living in the African region. Until now, no study has focused on neighborhood environmental correlates of sedentary time of older adults in Africa. Therefore, the primary aim of the present study was to examine associations of perceived neighborhood environmental attributes with self-reported sedentary time among older adults in Nigeria. Because patterns of sedentary time can be different between men and women [30], we also investigated the interaction effect of sex on the association between neighborhood environment variables and sedentary time. Based on positive associations found between neighborhood environmental attributes and physical activity of older adults in our previous analysis [31], we hypothesized that positive perceptions of the neighborhood environments would be negatively associated with sedentary time among older adults in Nigeria.

## 2. Materials and Methods

### 2.1. Sampling and Procedure

This study represents secondary analyses of cross-sectional data from the Maiduguri study of neighborhood environmental correlates of older adults' physical activity conducted in 2012 [31]. Maiduguri is the capital city of the state of Borno in North-Eastern Nigeria. The city consists of the inner city and Government Reserve Areas (GRA) or new layout areas that have a diversity of housing types, land use mix, and access and street connectivity. Similar to typical African cities [28], localities (e.g., neighborhoods) in the inner city of Maiduguri have a high concentration of multiple family and densely packed houses, non-residential land uses (small retail stores, shops, local markets, and many places of worship) and streets with short block length with many alternative unofficial routes to destinations (street connectivity). Neighborhoods in the GRA/new layout areas of Maiduguri are characterized by predominantly single-family homes, few non-residential land-uses, and streets with longer block-length with fewer alternative unofficial routes to destinations [28].

Data were collected among community-dwelling older adults (60 years and older) who were recruited from 2 high-SES/low walkable and 3 low-SES/high walkable neighborhoods in five localities (e.g., neighborhoods) that were randomly selected from 15 available localities in Maiduguri. A locality (e.g., neighborhood) in Maiduguri is an administrative unit that is made up of clusters of enumeration areas with a minimum of 45 households, and determined for this study as all the areas that the participants can walk to from home between 20 and 30 min. Power calculation conducted using Cohen's formula determined that 385 participants (77 from each of the five localities) were needed to detect a moderate to large effect size with more than 80% power [32]. A detailed description of the methodology including the setting, neighborhood selection procedure, participant recruitment and measures can be found elsewhere [31].

Four hundred and twenty-seven older adults (163 in high-SES/low walkable and 264 in low-SES/high walkable neighborhoods) were invited in person to participate in the study. In total, 353 older adults in all neighborhoods provided complete surveys and were included in the analyses (353/427, 83% response rate). Participants who were unwilling ($n = 51$), did not provide complete survey information ($n = 9$), or had a disability ($n = 14$) were excluded from the study. The participants gave written informed consent and completed the survey through interview by trained interviewers in their homes. The study protocol was approved by the Human Research Ethics Committee of the University of Maiduguri Teaching Hospital in Nigeria.

### 2.2. Measures

#### 2.2.1. Neighborhood Environment Attributes

Perception of neighborhood environment attributes was assessed using the 54-item Neighborhood Environment Walkability Scale-Abbreviated (NEWS-A) whose items have been adapted for use in Africa [28]. NEWS-A assessed perceived neighborhood environmental attributes related to walking and physical activity of older adults [33,34]. It gauged perceived neighborhood environmental attributes in eight domains: (1) residential density; (2) land-use mix—diversity (proximity to non-residential destinations); (3) land-use mix—access (ease of access to services and places); (4) street/road connectivity; (5) infrastructure and safety for walking; (6) aesthetics; (7) traffic safety; and (8) safety from crime. With the exception of residential density and land use mix-diversity domains, all items were rated by using Likert-type response options ranging from 1 (strongly disagree) to 4 (strongly agree). Residential density subscale was a weighted sum of six items that reflected common housing patterns in Africa ranging from predominantly few-residential buildings/dwellings (lowest density) to densely packed multiple-family dwellings/houses (highest density). Land use mix-diversity/proximity was assessed by the reported time it takes to walk from one's home to 26 various types of destinations, with responses ranging from 1- to 5-min walking distance (coded as 5) to >30-min walking distance (coded as 1). All NEWS-A domains were computed as the mean of responses to items in the domain, with responses coded (or reverse-coded) such that higher values indicated higher walkability of the neighborhood. In addition, a total NEWS-A score (called 'Walkability Index') was constructed by computing the mean of the standardized scores of the eight NEWS-A domains. The domains and individual items of the NEWS-A demonstrated "good" (Intraclass Correlation Coefficient (ICC) range = 0.60–0.74) to "excellent" (ICCs > 0.75%) test-retest reliability [28] and acceptable construct validity among adults (18–85 years) in seven African countries, including Nigeria [35].

### 2.2.2. Sedentary Time

Self-reported sedentary time was assessed using the adapted Nigerian version of the International Physical Activity Questionnaire (Hausa-IPAQ; long form (LF), assessing past 7 days) [36]. The sedentary domain of the Hausa-IPAQ LF assessed the duration (minutes/day) of time spent sitting while at home, work, and during leisure time on a typical weekday and a weekend day. The minutes of sitting on weekday, weekend day, and total sitting minutes in a week were the three outcomes examined in the present study. Total sitting minutes/week was computed as: weekday sitting minutes × 5 weekdays + weekend day sitting minutes × 2 weekend days [37]. Test-retest reliability (ICC = 0.62, 95% CI = 0.42–0.75) and construct validity (rho = 0.16; compared to biological variable) of the sedentary domain of the Hausa-IPAQ LF among Nigerian adults (including older people) were acceptable [36].

### 2.2.3. Covariates

Participants self-reported their sociodemographics including age, sex, marital status (married/living with a partner versus not married or not living with a partner i.e., widowed/widower), education attainment ('greater than secondary school', 'at least secondary school', 'at least primary school', and 'never attended school), and employment status ('formal employment i.e., government/office work', 'self-employed i.e., traders, business men/women, farmers', and 'retired' or 'unemployed'). Self-reported information on time spent (minutes/week) in total moderate-to-vigorous physical activity (MVPA) by the participants was measured with the Hausa IPAQ-LF and included as a covariate.

### 2.3. Statistical Analyses

Descriptive statistics (e.g., means, standard deviations, medians, interquartile ranges, frequencies, and percentages), stratified by sex, were computed as appropriate for the sociodemographic characteristics, sedentary time outcomes, and neighborhood environmental attributes. Multivariable linear regression analyses were used to examine the direct associations between neighborhood environmental attributes (eight scales; independent variables) and each of the sedentary time outcomes (weekday sitting time, weekend day sitting time, and total weekly sitting time; dependent variables), as well as the moderating effects of sex (women versus men). All covariates including neighborhood strata (high-SES/low walkable and low-SES/high walkable) were entered in the first block of the regression models. The environmental variables were added as a second block. The cross-product terms of sedentary time (separately for weekday, weekend day, and total weekly sitting) × each environmental variable was entered as a third block to examine the potential moderating effects of sedentary time. Since pattern of neighborhood environment features has been found to be more strongly related to health behaviors than individual items [24,38], additional models were run, separately, for each outcome and the overall 'Walkability index'. Multicollinearity was not a concern because only one neighborhood environment variable was included per model plus the covariates and the interaction term. Statistical significance was set at $p = 0.05$ for interpreting main effect and at $p < 0.10$ for interpreting the moderating effects [39]. When there was a significant interaction effect, separate sex-specific models were run to interpret the direction of the moderating effects. All analyses were conducted using SPSS version 18 (Armonk, NY, USA).

## 3. Results

### 3.1. Sample Characteristics

Table 1 shows the sociodemographic characteristics of the sample, as well as the descriptive statistics of the neighborhood environment variables and sedentary time outcomes. A total of 353 Nigerian older adults (39.9% women) with a mean age (± standard deviation) of 68.9 ± 9.1 years were included in the analysis. More than two-thirds of the final sample were married or living with a partner (71.4%), and more than half had never attended school (51.6%) and were unemployed (55.8%). Significantly more women than men were unemployed (72.4% vs. 44.8%), had less than secondary school education (69.5% vs. 57.5%) and were not married or living with a partner (41.1% vs. 20.3%). The perception of neighborhood environment attributes was not significantly different between women and men (all $p > 0.05$). As a group, the mean overall walkability index, proximity to destinations and traffic safety was −0.01 ± 3.21 (range = −7.19 to 13.86), 3.02 ± 0.47 (range = 2.04 to 4.69), and 2.32 ± 0.53 (range = 1.00 to 4.00), respectively. The participants spent an average of 1960.7 min/week (median of 31 h/week) in sedentary time. The average sedentary time on a typical weekday was 284.8 ± 125.4 min/day with a median of 5 h/day (IQR = 3–6 h/day). On a weekend day, participants reported daily sitting time of 268.2 ± 118.6 min/day (median = 4 h/day; IQR = 3– 6 h/day). Men marginally accumulated about 1 h median sedentary time more than the women on a typical weekday ($p = 0.05$).

**Table 1.** Participants' sociodemographic characteristics and descriptive information of neighborhood environmental attributes and sedentary time ($n$ = 353).

| Variables | Total Sample | Men ($n$ = 212) | Women ($n$ = 141) | $p$ * |
|---|---|---|---|---|
| socio-demographics | | | | |
| Age (years) [a] | 68.9 ± 9.1 | 69.0 ± 9.4 | 68.8 ± 8.6 | NS |
| Marital status ($n$, %) | | | | |
| Married | 252 (71.4) | 169 (79.7) | 83 (58.9) | <0.01 |
| Not married | 101 (28.6) | 43 (20.3) | 58 (41.1) | |
| Education ($n$, %) | | | | |
| > Secondary school | 88 (24.9) | 64 (30.2) | 24 (17.0) | <0.05 |
| Secondary school | 45 (12.7) | 26 (12.3) | 19 (13.5) | |
| Primary school | 38 (10.8) | 23 (10.8) | 15 (10.6) | |
| Never attended school | 182(51.6) | 99 (46.7) | 83 (58.9) | |
| Employment ($n$, %) | | | | <0.01 |
| Formal (office work) | 47 (13.3) | 36 (17.0) | 11 (7.8) | |
| Self-employed | 109 (30.9) | 81 (38.2) | 28 (19.9) | |
| Unemployed | 197 (55.8) | 95 (44.8) | 102 (72.4) | |
| Neighborhood type ($n$, %) | | | | NS |
| Low-SES/high walkable | 181 (51.3) | 115 (54.2) | 66 (46.8) | |
| High-SES/low walkable | 172 (48.7) | 97 (45.8) | 75 (53.2) | |
| Environmental attributes [a] | | | | |
| Overall walkability index | −0.01 ± 3.21 | 0.03 ± 3.25 | -0.08 ± 3.15 | NS |
| Residential density | 235.66 ± 84.79 | 232.37 ± 80.87 | 240.59 ± 90.43 | NS |
| Proximity to destinations | 3.02 ± 0.47 | 2.99±0.46 | 3.08 ± 0.48 | NS |
| Access to services and places | 1.19 ± 0.47 | 1.16±0.41 | 1.23 ± 0.54 | NS |
| Street connectivity | 2.94 ± 0.52 | 2.97±0.50 | 2.88 ± 0.55 | NS |
| Walking infrastructure and safety | 3.03 ± 0.43 | 3.04±0.40 | 3.01 ± 0.43 | NS |
| Aesthetics | 2.51 ± 0.59 | 2.55 ± 0.56 | 2.46 ± 0.62 | NS |
| Traffic safety | 2.32 ± 0.53 | 2.34 ± 0.52 | 2.29 ± 0.55 | NS |
| Safety from crime | 2.85 ± 1.02 | 2.89 ± 1.05 | 2.79 ± 0.99 | NS |

**Table 1.** *Cont.*

| Variables | Total Sample | Men (n = 212) | Women (n = 141) | p * |
|---|---|---|---|---|
| Sedentary time outcomes [b] | | | | |
| Weekday (min/day) | 300 (180–360) | 300 (240–360) | 240 (180–360) | 0.05 |
| Weekend (min/day) | 240 (180–360) | 240 (180–360) | 240 (180–360) | NS |
| Total weekly (min/week) | 1860 (1380–2520) | 1980 (1560–540) | 1680 (1260–2520) | NS |

* = Based on independent t-tests statistics for continuous variables and chi-square statistics for categorical variables; [a] = values for age and environmental attributes are mean ± standard deviation; [b] = values for sedentary time outcomes are median and inter quartile range (25th and 75th percentile values); SES = socioeconomic status; NS = not significant.

## 3.2. Associations of Neighborhood Environmental Attributes with Total Weekly Sedentary Time

The overall walkability index and four of eight neighborhood environment attributes were significantly related to lower weekly minutes in total sedentary time (Table 2). The estimated difference in total sedentary time between those with minimum ($-7.19$) and maximum (13.86) values on the overall walkability index was 1140 min/week (19 h/week) of sedentary time. A one unit increase in the overall walkability index was associated with about 71 min/week decrease in total sedentary time (B = $-70.573$; 95% CI = $-109.204$, $-31.947$). Each unit increase in proximity to destinations (B = $-695.745$; 95% CI = $-980.781$, $-410.705$) and access to services (B = $-480.703$; 95% CI = $-802.161$, $-159.245$) was associated with about an 11 h/week and 8 h/week, respectively, decrease in total sedentary time. Traffic safety (B = $-597.377$; 95% CI = $-865.533$, $-329.221$) and safety from crime (B = $-303.065$; 95% CI = $-489.786$, $-116.344$) were related to lower sedentary time for about 10 h/week and 5 h/week, respectively. The estimated difference in total sedentary time between those with minimum (2.04) and highest (4.69) values on proximity to destinations was 1260 min/week of sedentary time. While the estimated difference in total sedentary time between those with minimum (1.0) and maximum (4.0) values on access to services was 1075.8 min/week of sedentary time, it was 340.8 min/week of sedentary time for traffic safety and 272 min/week for safety from crime. The associations between total sedentary time and proximity to destinations and traffic safety was stronger in men than women. In contrast, higher street connectivity (B = 305.128, 95% CI = 14.622, 595.634) was associated with higher levels of sedentary time in men only (Table 2).

**Table 2.** Associations between perceived neighborhood environmental attributes and total sedentary time (min/week).

| Environmental Attributes | B | 95% CI | p-Value |
|---|---|---|---|
| Main effects | | | |
| Residential density | −1.791 | −3.730, 0.147 | 0.070 |
| Proximity to destinations | −695.745 | −980.781, −410.705 | <0.001 ** |
| Access to services and places | −480.703 | −802.161, −159.245 | 0.004 * |
| Street connectivity | −45.740 | −299.299, 207.819 | 0.722 |
| Walking infrastructure and safety | −223.886 | −513.865, 66.092 | 0.129 |
| Aesthetics | −78.829 | −333.024, 175.366 | 0.541 |
| Traffic safety | −597.377 | −865.533, −329.221 | <0.001 ** |
| Safety from crime | −303.065 | −489.786, −116.344 | 0.002 * |
| Overall walkability index | −70.575 | −109.204, −31.947 | <0.001 ** |

Table 2. *Cont.*

| Environmental Attributes | B | 95% CI | *p*-Value |
|---|---|---|---|
| Interaction effects of sex | | | |
| Residential density | | | |
| Women-specific | - | - | - |
| Men-specific | - | - | - |
| Proximity to destinations | 62.841 | −11.493, 137.175 | 0.097 |
| Women-specific | −578.101 | −1042.425, 113.777 | 0.015 * |
| Men-specific | −644.242 | −1008.793, −279.692 | 0.001 * |
| Access to services and places | | | |
| Women-specific | - | - | - |
| Men-specific | - | - | - |
| Street connectivity | 100.352 | 18.272, 182.433 | 0.017 * |
| Women-specific | −51.756 | −369.023, 265.511 | 0.746 |
| Men-specific | 305.128 | 14.622, 595.634 | 0.040 * |
| Walking infrastructure and safety | | | |
| Women-specific | - | - | - |
| Men-specific | - | - | - |
| Aesthetics | | | |
| Women-specific | - | - | - |
| Men-specific | - | - | - |
| Traffic safety | 118.674 | 22.975, 214,374 | 0.015 * |
| Women-specific | −376.580 | −678.416, −74.744 | 0.015 * |
| Men-Specific | −521.107 | −832.816, −209.398 | 0.001 * |
| Safety from crime | | | |
| Women-Specific | - | - | - |
| Men-specific | - | - | - |
| Overall walkability index | | | |
| Women-Specific | - | - | - |
| Men-specific | - | - | - |

B = regression coefficient; 95% CI = 95% confidence intervals; - = not applicable because no significant moderating effect of sex was found. For environmental attributes with significant sex moderating effects, sex-specific associations (men- and women-specific) are reported. All regression coefficients are adjusted for participants' age, sex, marital status, education, employment, neighborhood types, and moderate-to-vigorous physical activity. ** = *p*-value significant at <0.001; * = *p*-value significant at <0.05.

### 3.3. Associations of Neighborhood Environmental Attributes with Sedentary Time on Weekday and Weekend

Multivariable results for sedentary time outcomes on weekday and weekend can be retrieved from supplementary materials (Table S1). The estimated difference in sedentary time on a weekday and a weekend between those with minimum (−7.19) and maximum (13.86) values on the overall walkability index was 180 min/day and 120 min/day of sedentary time, respectively. Higher walkability index, proximity to destinations, traffic safety, and safety from crime were associated with less sedentary time on both a weekday and a weekend day among the older adults. The associations were stronger on a weekday than the weekend. Access to services and places was associated with less sedentary time only on a weekday (B = −85.679, 95% CI = −134.507, −36.851). Each additional unit on the overall walkability index was associated with about 11 min/day decrease in sedentary time on a weekday (B = −10.981, 95% CI = −16.897, −5.065) but with about 8 min/day decrease in sedentary time on a weekend day (B = −7.836, 95% CI = −13.540, −2.135). Proximity to destinations was associated with about 2 h/day decrease in sedentary time on a weekday (B = −116.558, 95% CI = −159.697, −74.421) and with less than 1 h/day of sedentary time on a weekend day (B = −56.478, 95% CI = −99.889, 13.070). Traffic safety was associated with about 1.5 h/day decrease in sedentary time on a weekday (B = −89.813, 95% CI = −131.063, −48.571) but with 74 min/day decrease in sedentary time on a weekend day. Safety from crime was associated with about 25 min/day more decrease in sedentary time on a weekday (B = −50.339, 95% CI = −78.826, −21.853) than on a weekend day (B = −25.684, 95% CI = −53.398,

2.029). On a weekday, higher walking infrastructure and safety was found to be associated with less sedentary time (B = −39.178, 95% CI = −77.598, −0.758) in men only, while higher street connectivity was found to be unexpectedly associated with higher sedentary time (B = 46.555, 95% CI = 2.575, 90.536) in men only.

## 4. Discussion

To our knowledge, this was the first study to examine the associations of neighborhood environments with older adults' sedentary behavior in Africa. Compared to the few previous studies of older adults conducted in high-income countries [21–23], we found more consistent associations of neighborhood environmental attributes with sedentary time among older Nigerian adults. The overall walkability index and five of eight independent neighborhood environment attributes were significantly associated with less weekly total sedentary time, and weekday and weekend day sedentary time in our sample.

Higher overall walkability was associated with about 71 min/week less total sedentary time and by 11 min/day and 8 min/day during a weekday and a weekend day, respectively. No moderation effect of sex was found for the association between the walkability index and sedentary time, suggesting that overall walkability of the neighborhood could be important for reducing sedentary time in older Nigerian men and women. This finding confirmed a previous multi-country study documenting the international importance of an overall pattern of activity-supportive neighborhood environment design for lower sedentary time among adults [24]. However, compared to the overall walkability index, we found much stronger effect sizes for the inverse associations of sedentary time with some individual neighborhood environmental attributes. This is explainable because the overall walkability index was constructed by combining the mean of the standardized scores (z-scores) of all the environmental variables, while the association of each environmental domain with sedentary time was based on the unstandardized mean score of individual environmental attributes. Thus, the index and individual scores were on different scales. However, the difference in total sedentary time between the older adults with the lowest and highest scores on the overall walkability index was about 19 h/week, suggesting that substantial sedentary behavior change could be possible for Nigerian older adults if the overall walkability of the environment is improved.

Interestingly, two destination-related attributes (proximity to destinations and ease of access to places and services) that reflect mixed land use, which is a key component of the construct of neighborhood walkability internationally [18–21], were consistently related to less sedentary time in the present study. Previous studies of older adults did not find direct associations of diversity and proximity of destinations with sedentary behavior of older adults in Belgium [22] and Hong Kong [23]. Thus, our finding extended evidence about the potential of land use mix for controlling excessive sedentary time among older adults in the African context. It is behaviorally plausible that older adults who perceive destinations to be closer to home and easy access to places and services engage in more neighborhood-based active living that could account for reduced sitting time. It is not clear why such results would be stronger among the African sample, but it may be related to less access to motor vehicles leading to more walking trips to nearby destinations.

Traffic safety and safety from crime were related to less sedentary time, suggesting that improved safety conditions are important for reducing sedentary time among older adults in Nigeria. Perceived crime safety has consistently emerged as a negative correlate of physical activity in the Nigerian population [40–42], so it is interesting that lack of safety from crime is also an important concern that has the potential to increase sedentary time among older adults in Nigeria. Similarly, neighborhood safety has been related to less sitting time among Belgian older adults [22] and older adults in Hong Kong [23]. Possibly, a neighborhood that is safe from crime and traffic creates a more conducive environment that facilitate engagement in greater levels of outdoor physical activity and lower levels of sedentary time among older adults. Moreover, a neighborhood that is unsafe from crime and traffic may lead older adults to sit more at home to avoid being a victim of crime or road injury.

Better walking infrastructure and safety was associated with lower levels of sedentary time on a weekday among men only. This is interesting because men in the present study were more sedentary than women during the weekday. Perhaps, older Nigerian men are more conscious of walking infrastructure as an avenue for engaging in more recreational and transportation walking and reducing sedentary time during the weekday. Somewhat related, pedestrian safety was found to be associated with lower daily minutes and frequency of motorized transport among older adults in Hong Kong [23]. This finding together with ours, support the importance of improvements in pedestrian infrastructure and safety as a means of decreasing sedentary time in older adults.

Street connectivity, which is also a major component of neighborhood walkability, was unexpectedly related to higher sedentary time among older men in our study. This finding was the only evidence of an unfavorable association in the present study, and it was contrary to a recent study which reported higher street connectivity to be related to less sedentary time among adults in 10 countries [24]. It has been espoused in our previous studies that the concept of street connectivity (e.g., many four-way intersections, cross-junctions, and distance between official routes/roads) may connote different meaning to African residents compared with residents of the developed countries [35,40]. Another analysis using same data found higher street connectivity to be related to lower walking for transport [31], which also is inconsistent with international evidence supporting the importance of higher street connectivity to increased physical activity for transportation [18–20]. Perhaps, a qualitative study is needed to further explore the meaning of street connectivity in the African context.

*Strengths and Limitations*

An important strength was the utilization of valid and internationally recognized questionnaires to measure sitting time and neighborhood environments that allowed for comparison with previous studies. However, the study also had some limitations. The cross-sectional design means that causal relationships cannot be determined. The use of self-report measures of sedentary time and neighborhood environment may increase the chance of measurement bias, recall problems, and inaccurate estimates of the outcomes. The use of GIS could have provided a more objective assessment of the walkability index of the neighborhood environment. However, perceptions of environmental attributes may also have greater influence on physical activity behaviors than objective environmental characteristics, even if they may not correspond to reality [43]. Thus, it is equally important as objective assessment, to examine perceived aspects of the neighborhood environment in research of built environmental correlates of health behaviors. Only overall sitting time was assessed in the present study, but specific sedentary behaviors like TV viewing and motorized transport may be more strongly related to neighborhood environmental attributes. Future studies should use objective measures and/or more detailed contextually-specific measures of sedentary behavior (e.g., TV watching, listening to radio, or chatting with friends and families while sitting) to identify whether environmental attributes are more related to some sedentary behaviors than others among Nigerian older adults. However, our findings are similar to those of previous studies in Belgium [21,22] and Hong Kong [23], supporting the assertion that some aspects of neighborhood walkability encouraging less sitting time in older adults in these countries may be similar for Nigeria.

## 5. Conclusions

The overall perceived walkability index and five of eight individual perceived neighborhood environment attributes were related to less sedentary time in Nigerian older adults, and there were few instances of sex-specific results. Some of the effect sizes were large; up to 10 h per week less sitting. The findings of potential protective effects of neighborhood environment design on sedentary behavior in this sample of Nigerian older adults were more consistent than previous studies conducted in high-income countries. An important implication of the study is that the same neighborhood environment attributes shown to be associated with more physical activity [31] had an apparent additional benefit of being related to lower sedentary time. The present study uniquely contributes to the literature by providing scarce evidence on the relationships of neighborhood environments with older adults' sedentary time from an understudied region of the world.

**Supplementary Materials:** The following are available online at http://www.mdpi.com/1660-4601/16/11/1879/s1, Table S1: title. Associations between perceived neighborhood environment attributes with sedentary time (min/day) on a weekday and a weekend day

**Author Contributions:** Conceptualization, A.L.O., A.Y.O., and J.F.S.; Data curation, A.L.O. and S.M.K.; Formal analysis, A.L.O.; Investigation, A.L.O., S.M.K., and A.Y.O.; Methodology, A.L.O., S.M.K., A.A.R., A.Y.O., B.A.O., and J.F.S.; Project administration, A.L.O., S.M.K., A.A.R., A.Y.O., B.A.O., and J.F.S.; Supervision, A.L.O.; Writing—original draft, A.L.O.; Writing—review and editing, S.M.K., A.A.R., A.Y.O., B.A.O., and J.F.S.. All authors (A.L.O., S.M.K., A.A.R., A.Y.O., B.A.O., and J.F.S.) revised the manuscript for important intellectual content, and all authors read and approved the final version.

**Funding:** This research received no external funding.

**Conflicts of Interest:** The authors declare no conflict of interest.

## References

1. World Health Organization. Ageing and Health. Geneva: World Health Organization; 2019. Available online: https://www.who.int/news-room/fact-sheets/detail/ageing-and-health (accessed on 27 May 2019).
2. United Nations, Department of Economic and Social Affairs, Population Division. World Population Ageing 2017 Highlights. Available online: https://www.un.org/en/development/desa/population/publications/pdf/ageing/WPA2017_Highlights.pdf (accessed on 27 May 2019).
3. Chikafu, H.; Chimbari, M.J. Cardiovascular disease healthcare utilization in Sub-Saharan Africa: A scoping review. *Int. J. Environ. Res. Public Health* **2019**, *16*, 419. [CrossRef]
4. World Health Organization. *Global Action Plan for the Prevention and Control of Noncommunicable Diseases, 2013–2020*; World Health Organization: Geneva, Switzerland, 2013; pp. 21–27.
5. Sallis, J.F.; Bull, F.C.; Guthold, R.; Heath, G.W.; Inoue, S.; Kelly, P.; Oyeyemi, A.L.; Perez, L.G.; Richards, J.; Hallal, P.C. Progress in physical activity over the Olympic quadrennium. *Lancet* **2016**, *388*, 1325–1336. [CrossRef]
6. Owen, N.; Healy, G.N.; Matthews, C.E.; Dunstan, D.W. Too much sitting: The population health science of sedentary behavior. *Exerc. Sport Sci. Rev.* **2010**, *38*, 105–113. [CrossRef] [PubMed]
7. Shiroma, E.J.; Freedson, P.S.; Trost, S.G.; Lee, I.M. Patterns of accelerometer-assessed sedentary behavior in older women. *JAMA* **2013**, *310*, 2562–2563. [CrossRef]
8. Bellettiere, J.; Carlson, J.A.; Rosenberg, D.; Singhania, A.; Natarajan, L.; Berardi, V.; LaCroix, A.Z.; Sears, D.D.; Moran, K.; Crist, K.; et al. Gender and age differences in hourly and daily patterns of sedentary time in older adults living in retirement communities. *PLoS ONE* **2015**, *10*, e0136161. [CrossRef]
9. Arnardottir, N.Y.; Koster, A.; Van Domelen, D.R.; Brychta, R.J.; Caserotti, P.; Eiriksdottir, G.; Syerrisdottir, J.E.; Lanner, L.J.; Gudnason, V.; Johnnsson, E.; et al. Objective measurements of daily physical activity patterns and sedentary behaviour in older adults: Age, Gene = Environment Susceptibility – Reykjavik Study. *Age Ageing* **2013**, *42*, 222–229. [CrossRef]
10. Ekelund, U.; Steene-Johannessen, J.; Brown, W.J.; Fagerland, M.W.; Owen, N.; Powell, K.E.; Bauman, A.; Lee, I.M. Does physical activity attenuate, or even eliminate, the detrimental association of sitting time with mortality? A harmonised meta-analysis of data from more than 1 million men and women. *Lancet* **2016**, *388*, 1302–1310. [CrossRef]
11. Vallance, J.K.; Gardiner, P.A.; Lynch, B.M.; D'Silva, A.; Boyle, T.; Taylor, L.M.; Johnson, S.T.; Buman, M.P.; Owen., N. Evaluating the evidence on sitting, smoking, and health: Is sitting really the new smoking? *Am. J. Public Health* **2018**. [CrossRef]
12. De Rezende, L.F.M.; Rey-López, J.P.; Matsudo, V.K.R.; Do Carmo Luiz, O. Sedentary behavior and health outcomes among older adults: A systematic review. *BMC Public Health* **2014**, *14*, 333. [CrossRef] [PubMed]
13. Dogra, S.; Stathokostas, L. Sedentary behavior and physical activity are independent predictors of successful aging in middle-aged and older adults. *J. Aging Res.* **2012**, *2012*, 190654. [CrossRef]
14. Koyanagi, A.; Stubbs, B.; Vancampfort, D. Correlates of sedentary behavior in the general population: A cross-sectional study using nationally representative data from six low- and middle-income countries. *PLoS ONE* **2018**, *13*, e0202222. [CrossRef] [PubMed]

15. Peltzer, K.; Phaswana-Mafuya, N.; Pengpid, S. Prevalence and correlates of sedentary behaviour among a national sample of 15-98 years old individuals in South Africa. *Afr. J. Phys. Act. Health Sci.* **2018**, *24*, 286–298.

16. Sallis, J.F.; Owen, N. Ecological models of health behavior. In *Health Behavior: Theory, Research and Practice*, 5th ed.; Glanz, K., Rimer, B., Viswanath, V., Eds.; Jossey-Bass/Pfeiffer: San Francisco, CA, USA, 2015; pp. 43–64.

17. Chastin, S.F.M.; Buck, C.; Freiberger, E.; Murphy, M.; Brug, J.; Cardon, G.; O'Donoghue, G.; Pigeot, I.; Oppert, J.M. Systematic literature review of determinants of sedentary behaviour in older adults: A DEDIPAC study. *Int. J. Behav. Nutr. Phys. Act.* **2015**, *12*, 127. [CrossRef]

18. Cerin, E.; Nathan, A.; Van Cauwenberg, J.; Barnett, D.W.; Barnett, A. The neighbourhood physical environment and active travel in older adults: A systematic review and meta-analysis. *Int. J. Behav. Nutr. Phys. Act.* **2017**, *14*, 15. [CrossRef] [PubMed]

19. Van Cauwenberg, J.; De Bourdeaudhuij, I.; De Meester, F.; Van Dyck, D.; Salmon, J.; Clarys, P.; Deforche, B. Relationship between the physical environment and physical activity in older adults: A systematic review. *Health Place* **2011**, *17*, 458–469. [CrossRef]

20. Van Holle, V.; Van Cauwenberg, J.; Van Dyck, D.; Deforche, B.; Van de Weghe, N.; De Bourdeaudhuij, I. Relationship between neighborhood walkability and older adults' physical activity: Results from the Belgian Environmental Physical Activity Study in Seniors (BEPAS Seniors). *Int. J. Behav. Nutr Phys. Act.* **2014**, *11*, 110. [CrossRef]

21. Van Holle, V.; Van Cauwenberg, J.; De Bourdeaudhuij, I.; Deforche, B.; Van de Weghe, N.; Van Dyck, D. Interactions between neighborhood social environment and walkability to explain Belgian older adults' physical activity and sedentary time. *Int J. Environ. Res. Public Health* **2016**, *13*, 569. [CrossRef] [PubMed]

22. Van Cauwenberg, J.; De Donder, L.; Clarys, P.; De Bourdeaudhuij, I.; Owen, N.; Dury, S.; De Witte, N.; Buffel, T.; Verte, D.; Deforche, B. Relationships of individual, social, and physical environmental factors with older adults' television viewing time. *J. Aging Phys. Act.* **2014**, *22*, 508–517. [CrossRef]

23. Barnett, A.; Cerin, E.; Ching, C.S.; Johnston, J.M.; Lee, R.S. Neighbourhood environment, sitting time and motorised transport in older adults: A cross-sectional study in Hong Kong. *BMJ Open* **2015**, *5*, e007557. [CrossRef]

24. Owen, N.; Sugiyama, T.; Koohsari, M.J.; De Bourdeaudhuij, I.; Hadgraft, N.; Oyeyemi, A.L.; Aguinaga-Ontoso, I.; Mitáš, J.; Troelsen, J.; Davey, R.; et al. Associations of neighborhood environmental attributes with adults' objectively-assessed sedentary time: IPEN adults multi-country study. *Prev. Med.* **2018**, *115*, 126–133. [CrossRef]

25. Foster, S.; Pereira, G.; Christian, H.; Knuiman, M.; Bull, F.; Giles-Corti, B. Neighborhood correlates of sitting time for Australian adults in new suburbs: Results from ReSide. *Environ. Behav.* **2015**, *47*, 902–922. [CrossRef]

26. Koohsari, M.J.; Sugiyama, T.; Sahlqvist, S.; Mavoa, S.; Hadgraft, N.; Owen, N. Neighborhood environmental attributes and adults' sedentary behaviors: Review and research agenda. *Prev. Med.* **2015**, *77*, 141–149. [CrossRef] [PubMed]

27. Clarke, P.; Nieuwenhuijsen, E.R. Environments for healthy ageing a critical review. *Maturitas* **2009**, *64*, 14–19. [CrossRef]

28. Oyeyemi, A.L.; Kasoma, S.S.; Onywera, V.O.; Assah, F.; Adedoyin, R.A.; Conway, T.L.; Moss, S.J.; Ocansey, R.; Kolbe-Alexander, T.L.; Akinroye, K.K.; et al. NEWS for Africa: Adaptation and reliability of a built environment questionnaire for physical activity in seven African countries. *Int. J. Behav. Nutr. Phys. Act.* **2016**, *13*, 33. [CrossRef]

29. Vancampfort, D.; Stubbs, B.; Sallis, J.F.; Nabanoba, J.; Basangwa, D.; Oyeyemi, A.L.; Kasoma, S.S.; De Hert, M.; Myin-Germeys, I.; Mugisha, J. Associations of the built environment with physical activity and sedentary time in Ugandan outpatients with mental health problems. *J. Phys. Act. Health* **2019**. [CrossRef]

30. Shibata, A.; Oka, K.; Ishii, K.; Miyawaki, R.; Inoue, S.; Sugiyama, T.; Owen, N. Objectively-assessed patterns and reported domains of sedentary behavior among Japanese older adults. *J. Epidemiol.* **2018**. [CrossRef]

31. Oyeyemi, A.L.; Kolo, S.M.; Oyeyemi, A.Y.; Omotara, B.A. Neighborhood environmental factors are related to health-enhancing physical activity and walking among community dwelling older adults in Nigeria. *Physiother. Theory Pract.* **2019**, *35*, 288–297. [CrossRef]

32. Cohen, J.A. *Statistical Power Analysis for the Behavioural Sciences*, 2nd ed.; Lawrence Erlbaum Associates: Hillsdale, NJ, USA, 1988.

33. Cerin, E.; Sit, C.H.P.; Cheung, M.; Ho, S.; Lee, L.J.; Chan, W. Reliable and valid NEWS for Chinese seniors: Measuring perceived neighborhood attributes related to walking. *Int. J. Behav. Nutr. Phys. Act.* **2010**, *7*, 84. [CrossRef] [PubMed]

34. Ding, D.; Sallis, J.F.; Norman, G.J.; Frank, L.D.; Saelens, B.E.; Kerr, J.; Conway, T.L.; Cain, K.; Hovll, M.F.; Hofstetter, C.R.; et al. Neighborhood environment and physical activity among older adults: Do the relationships differ by driving status? *J. Aging Phys. Act.* **2014**, *22*, 421–431. [CrossRef]

35. Oyeyemi, A.L.; Conway, T.L.; Adedoyin, R.A.; Akinroye, K.K.; Aryeetey, R.; Assah, F.; Cain, K.L.; Gavand, K.A.; Kasoma, S.S.; Kolbe-Alexander, T.L.; et al. Construct validity of the neighbourhood environment walkability scale for Africa. *Med. Sci. Sports Exerc.* **2017**, *49*, 482–491. [CrossRef]

36. Oyeyemi, A.L.; Bello, U.M.; Philemon, S.T.; Aliyu, H.N.; Majidadi, R.W.; Oyeyemi, A.Y. Examining the reliability and validity of a modified version of the International Physical Activity Questionnaire, long form (IPAQ-LF) in Nigeria: A cross-sectional study. *BMJ Open* **2014**, *4*, e005820. [CrossRef]

37. International Physical Activity Questionnaire. Guidelines for Data Processing and Analysis of the International Physical Activity Questionnaire (IPAQ)—Short and Long Forms. Available online: http://www.ipaq.ki.se/scoring.pdf (accessed on 21 March 2019).

38. Cain, K.L.; Millstein, R.A.; Sallis, J.F.; Conway, T.L.; Gavand, K.A.; Frank, L.D.; Saelens, B.E.; Geremia, C.M.; Chapman, J.; Adams, M.A.; et al. Contribution of streetscape audits to explanation of physical activity in four age groups based on the microscale audit of pedestrian streetscapes (MAPS). *Soc. Sci. Med.* **2014**, *116*, 82–92. [CrossRef] [PubMed]

39. Twisk, J.W.R. *Applied Multilevel Analysis*; Cambridge University Press: Cambridge, UK, 2006.

40. Oyeyemi, A.L.; Sallis, J.F.; Deforche, B.; Oyeyemi, A.Y.; De Bourdeaudhuij, I.; Van Dyck, D. Evaluation of the Neighborhood Environment Walkability Scale in Nigeria. *Int. J. Health Geogr.* **2013**, *12*, 16. [CrossRef]

41. Oyeyemi, A.L.; Adegoke, B.O.; Sallis, J.F.; Oyeyemi, A.Y.; De Bourdeaudhuij, I. Perceived crime and traffic safety is related to physical activity among adults in Nigeria. *Bmc Pub. Health* **2012**, *12*, 294. [CrossRef]

42. Oyeyemi, A.L.; Adegoke, B.O.A.; Oyeyemi, A.Y.; Sallis, J.F. Perceived environmental correlates of physical activity and walking in African young adults. *Am. J. Health Promot.* **2011**, *25*, e10–e19. [CrossRef]

43. Kirtland, K.A.; Porter, D.E.; Addy, C.L.; Neet, M.J.; Williams, J.E.; Sharpe, P.A.; Neff, L.J.; Kimsey, C.D.; Ainsworth, B.E. Environmental measures of physical activity supports: Perception versus reality. *Am. J. Prev. Med.* **2003**, *24*, 323–331. [CrossRef]

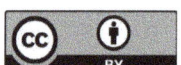

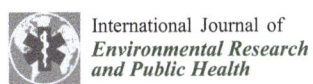

International Journal of
*Environmental Research
and Public Health*

*Article*

# Test-Retest Reliability and Walk Score® Neighbourhood Walkability Comparison of an Online Perceived Neighbourhood-Specific Adaptation of the International Physical Activity Questionnaire (IPAQ)

**Levi Frehlich \*, Anita Blackstaffe and Gavin R. McCormack**

Department of Community Health Sciences, Cumming School of Medicine, University of Calgary, Calgary,
AB T2N 4Z6, Canada; ambortni@ucalgary.ca (A.B.); Gavin.McCormack@ucalgary.ca (G.R.M.)
\* Correspondence: lcfrehli@ucalgary.ca

Received: 10 April 2019; Accepted: 28 May 2019; Published: 30 May 2019

**Abstract:** There is a growing public health interest in the contributions of the built environment in enabling and supporting physical activity. However, few tools measuring neighbourhood-specific physical activity exist. This study assessed the reliability of an established physical activity tool (International Physical Activity Questionnaire: IPAQ) adapted to capture perceived neighbourhood-specific physical activity (N-IPAQ) administered via the internet and compared N-IPAQ outcomes to differences in neighbourhood Walk Score®. A sample of $n = 261$ adults completed an online questionnaire on two occasions at least seven days apart. Questionnaire items captured walking, cycling, moderate-intensity, and vigorous-intensity physical activity, undertaken inside the participant's perceived neighbourhood in the past week. Intraclass correlations, Spearman's rank correlation, and Cohen's Kappa coefficients estimated item test-retest reliability. Regression estimated the associations between self-reported perceived neighbourhood-specific physical activity and Walk Score®. With the exception of moderate physical activity duration, participation and duration for all physical activities demonstrated moderate reliability. Transportation walking participation and duration was higher ($p < 0.05$) in more walkable neighbourhoods. The N-IPAQ administered online found differences in neighbourhoods that vary in their walkability. Future studies investigating built environments and self-reported physical activity may consider using the online version of the N-IPAQ.

**Keywords:** walkable environment; physical activity; sedentary behaviour; neighbourhood; walkability; active living; survey; questionnaire

---

## 1. Introduction

There is a growing public health interest in the contributions of the built environment in enabling and supporting physical activity. Several systematic reviews provide consistent evidence for an association between neighbourhood built characteristics and physical activity [1–3]. While this evidence is encouraging, the accuracy of estimated associations between the built environment and physical activity have been limited by the use of non-context specific physical activity measures; that is, measures of physical activity associated with built environment characteristics have not been specific to the neighbourhood, rather capturing behaviour regardless of the location. There have been previous calls for the development and use of context-specific physical activity measures [3]; however, few context-specific self-report measures of neighbourhood-specific physical activity, in particular, exist [4,5]. Ideally, the use of objective measures of physical activity are preferable; however, these approaches for physical activity measurement are not always feasible, especially in large population-based studies or for research teams with limited financial resources and technical expertise to purchase and use accelerometers and global positioning system (GPS) monitors.

Several studies have captured neighbourhood-specific physical activity via self-report questionnaires [4–7]. To date, psychometric testing of items capturing self-reported neighbourhood-specific physical activity have included primarily assessments of test-retest reliability [4,7,8]. For instance, the Neighbourhood Physical Activity Questionnaire (NPAQ) that captures transportation and recreational walking and cycling (i.e., traveling to and from work, doing errands, or going from place to place) inside the neighbourhood (within a 15-min walking distance from home) during a usual week has been demonstrated to have adequate reliability in Australian adults [4]. Furthermore, a modified version of the NPAQ has also been found to be reliable in Canadian adults [8]. Physical activity estimates derived from the NPAQ have been associated with neighbourhood built characteristics in Australian [4], Canadian [8], and Chinese [7] populations. However, available options of tools capturing neighbourhood-specific physical activity are limited, and of those that exist, most capture "usual" week behaviour that may overestimate physical activity undertaken in the past week. Although not providing a habitual measure of behaviour, the latter recall type might be more sensitive to immediate changes in the neighbourhood built environment or other neighbourhood-level interventions on physical activity [9]. However, while items for capturing self-reported neighbourhood-specific physical activity in the "last" week have been used in previous built environment–physical activity studies [5,6], none to the best of our knowledge have undergone a thorough assessment of reliability.

Studies using internet-administered questionnaires to capture physical activity are becoming more frequent [10–13]. Internet questionnaires, despite some limitations, have several advantages over "paper-and-pencil" questionnaires, such as being low cost, allowing the researcher more control over the sequence in which questions and response options are presented, as well as offering skip patterns, allowing the researcher to embed procedures for reducing incomplete data, to instantaneously monitor questionnaire completion and survey participation, and to incorporate visual and audio prompts within the questionnaire to aid comprehension [14]. Internet-based questionnaires are being used more often in population surveys [14–16], which has been facilitated by the continued growth in internet access and availability in relation to signal coverage, increased number of internet connected devices or devices offering internet connection, and social and cultural shifts in relation to the perceived importance and expectation of being continually connected to the internet or having internet access [17,18]. It is estimated that globally approximately 52% of households have access to the internet, while in developed countries about 83% have internet access [19].

The International Physical Activity Questionnaire (IPAQ) is widely used in physical activity research and has demonstrated reliability and validity [20]. The IPAQ has also been shown to be reliable when used in an online format to measure physical activity in Danish [11] and UK [13] populations. The IPAQ has been adapted to capture perceived neighbourhood-specific physical activity (N-IPAQ) [21,22]. The aim of this study was to adapt, administer, and test the N-IPAQ via the internet in a Canadian population. Specifically, we aimed to assess the reliability of the N-IPAQ and compare differences in self-reported perceived neighbourhood-specific physical activity found from the N-IPAQ by neighbourhood walkability measured with Walk Score®. Our goal was to provide researchers interested in capturing neighbourhood-specific physical activity with a reliable online self-report option, capturing past week physical activity undertaken within perceived residential neighbourhoods.

## 2. Materials and Methods

### 2.1. Study and Sample Design

The sample list for the current methods study was derived from a database of participants from a larger study (i.e., *Pathways to Health*) investigating the relations between neighbourhoods, physical activity, diet, and weight status. The methods for the *Pathways to Health* study have been described in detail elsewhere [23,24]; however, briefly, in April 2014 $n = 173$ established Calgary (Alberta, Canada) neighbourhoods were stratified into 12 strata. Strata were based on the neighbourhood street pattern (grid, warped grid, and curvilinear) and socioeconomic status (advantaged, somewhat advantaged, somewhat disadvantaged, and disadvantaged). Following computer automation, a random sample of $n = 10,500$ households were sent recruitment postcards. A total of $n = 1023$ participants completed a physical activity, health, and demographic questionnaire (PAHDQ). Within the Calgary context, neighbourhoods with grid street patterns were more supportive of walking (high walkability) compared to neighbourhoods with warped-grid (medium walkability) and curvilinear street patterns (low walkability) [25]. Grid street pattern neighbourhoods, typically found centrally in urban areas, have higher land use or destination mix, more street and pedestrian connectivity, and higher population or residential density than those curvilinear street pattern neighbourhoods that are typically found in suburban areas. Land use mix, connectivity, and density are consistent correlates of physical activity [26] and considered to be important built characteristics for determining the walkability of a neighbourhood [27]. Furthermore, walking for transportation has been consistently linked to neighbourhoods with higher population density, distance to non-residential destinations, and proximal non-residential destinations [1]. These relationships have been tested in different countries, such as Canada [28], Australia [29], France [30], Sweden [6], and the United States [31], with studies finding an increased likelihood of transportation walking with increasing access to services and street connectivity. The estimation of neighbourhood socioeconomic status, described elsewhere [23,24], was based on 2006 Canadian census data and included the proportion of those 25–64 years of age who obtained less than a high school diploma; the proportion of single-parent families and the proportion of divorced, separated, or widowed among those ≥15 years of age; the proportion of individuals renting private dwellings and the average value of dwellings; the proportion of unemployment among those ≥25 years of age, and median gross household income.

The *Pathways to Health* participants also noted their willingness (and contact details) to participate in follow-up research. Thus, in January 2017 we approached all participants who were willing to participate in follow-up research and who did not complete the reliability and validity testing of the paper N-IPAQ ($n = 515$). Of those approached, $n = 151$ did not respond, $n = 65$ refused to participate, $n = 18$ emails returned undeliverable, and $n = 281$ consented to participate in the study. Those consenting were sent instructions and a web-link for completing the online N-IPAQ on two occasions (i.e., Time 1 and Time 2) at least seven days apart. The Time 1 and Time 2 questionnaires were identical with respect to physical activity variables; however, sociodemographic variables were only collected at Time 1. SurveyMonkey® (SurveyMonkey Inc, San Mateo, California, USA) was used for creating and delivering the questionnaire and for collecting responses. Completion of all questions was mandatory in order to progress through the questionnaire (i.e., from page to page) and to submit the questionnaire. Participants who completed both Time 1 and Time 2 questionnaires were entered into a prize draw with a 1 in 40 chance to win a gift card ($50 value). Data collection occurred between January and March 2017. The University of Calgary Conjoint Health Research Ethics Board approved this study (Ethics ID: REB15-2940).

## 2.2. Variables

### 2.2.1. Neighbourhood Adapted International Physical Activity Questionnaire (N-IPAQ)

We modified items from the IPAQ (long-form) capturing frequency (number of days) and usual minutes (on one of the reported days) of perceived neighbourhood-specific walking for transportation, bicycling for transportation, walking for leisure, moderate-intensity physical activity, and vigorous-intensity physical activity during the last seven days. The original questionnaire item wording was modified to reflect our focus on capturing neighbourhood-specific physical activity by inserting the phrase " ... inside your neighbourhood". For example, "During the last 7 days, on how many days did you walk to go from place to place inside your neighbourhood?". Within the questionnaire, participants were provided with fixed response options for physical activity frequency (i.e., 0 to 7 days) and duration (i.e., 5 to 480 min/day, in 5-min increments). Participants were instructed to think about activities undertaken inside their residential neighbourhood; however, we did not provide an operational definition for neighbourhood, and instead we permitted the participant to interpret "residential neighbourhood" in their own way. By not placing limits on the neighbourhood geographical area (e.g., 400 m or 5 min walk) or boundary (e.g., administrative boundary), we may have obtained a better understanding on how residents perceive their neighbourhood in terms of a context for physical activity behaviour. Previous research has found a paper administrated version of the N-IPAQ to be reliable [22] and valid compared with accelerometers and GPS monitors [21]. Furthermore, our intention was to go beyond the current assessment of online reliability in future research by comparing self-reported neighbourhood physical activity (using the online N-IPAQ) with context-specific physical activity captured using accelerometers and GPS monitors. The N-IPAQ can be found online under Supplementary Material (Questionnaire S1: N-IPAQ).

### 2.2.2. Sociodemographic Characteristics

Sociodemographic characteristics collected at Time 1 included participants' sex and age, the number of dependents living at home, the number of dogs living in the household, their access to a motor vehicle for personal use, their access to a bicycle for personal use, and if they had post-secondary school education.

### 2.2.3. Neighbourhood Walkability

We linked participants' six-digit residential postal code to Walk Score® to estimate walkability (www.walkscore.com). In the Canadian urban context, a six-digit postal code corresponds to a relatively small geographical unit, which maintains participant confidentiality [32]. Walk Score® has been validated in both the United States [33,34] and Canada [35]. Furthermore, Walk Score® is positively associated with other objective indicators of neighbourhood walkability [36] and walking behaviour [37]. Walk Score® was broken up into tertiles to define low, medium, and high neighbourhood walkability. Walk Score® uses a proprietary algorithm in which amenities located close to home are assigned higher scores and amenities located farther away are assigned a lower score using a distance decay function. Maximum points are received for amenities located within 400 m (a 5 min walk) and a zero score is assigned to amenities located farther than a 30 min walk from home.

## 2.3. Statistical Analysis

Descriptive statistics including means, standard deviations, and frequencies were calculated for sociodemographic variables for the overall sample and stratified by neighbourhood walkability. We calculated weekly minutes of physical activity by multiplying the reported frequency (in days per week) by the duration of activity (in minutes on a usual day). Participation variables were created by recoding each physical activity into "participation" (at least 1 day/week) versus "no participation" (0 days/week). Similar to previous studies using the IPAQ, to address outliers all variables were truncated at the 99th percentile and weekly physical activity (days × daily duration) was truncated to 1680 min [38–40].

The reliability of the online N-IPAQ participation variables was assessed using Cohen's Kappa coefficients (κ) and proportion of overall agreement, while the reliability of the online N-IPAQ continuous variables was assessed using intraclass correlations (ICC) and Spearman's rank correlations ($\rho$). Furthermore, we estimated ICC and $\rho$ among: (1) All participants regardless of participation, and; (2) all participants excluding those who reported zero minutes/week. We used published cut-points for describing our estimates (i.e., ICC, $\rho$, and Kappa correlations: Poor < 0.40, moderate ≥ 0.40 to 0.75, and excellent > 0.75, and proportion of overall agreement ≥75% was considered acceptable) [41].

The online N-IPAQ captured perceived neighbourhood-specific differences in physical activity. Highly walkable neighbourhoods have been consistently shown to be associated with more physical activity, especially walking [1,2,30,42]. Notably, several studies have found a higher Walk Score® to be associated with more transportation walking [32,36,37]. We used binary logistic regression to estimate the associations (odds ratios: (OR) and 95% confidence intervals (CI)) between participation in neighbourhood-specific walking for transportation, walking for leisure, bicycling for transport, moderate-intensity and vigorous-intensity physical activity, and neighbourhood walkability. In separate linear regression models, we estimated differences for Walk Score® in relation to weekly minutes of neighbourhood-specific walking for transportation, walking for leisure, bicycling for transport, moderate-intensity and vigorous-intensity physical activity. All models were adjusted for covariates (sex, age, number of dependents, dog ownership, motor vehicle access, bicycle access, and education) and included data from Time 1 only. All statistical analyses were undertaken using STATA version 14.2 (StataCorp, College Station, TX, USA). Statistical significance was set at $\alpha \le 0.05$.

## 3. Results

### 3.1. Sample Characteristics

In total, $n = 261$ participants provided complete data at Time 1 and Time 2 and were included in the analysis. The mean (SD) age of our sample was 53.9 (13.2) years. The sample consisted of 69.4% women, 68.6% with university education, 40.6% dog-owners, 99.7% with access to a motor vehicle, and 82.0% with access to a bicycle. Participants were evenly distributed by neighbourhood walkability (low (35.2%), medium (32.6%), and high (32.2%)). The mean (SD) Walk Score® was 60.8 (14.7); Walk Score® differed significantly for all neighbourhood walkability comparisons ($p < 0.05$ ANOVA: Bonferroni). The average Walk Score® among participants from high walkable neighbourhoods (78.7 (5.5)) was significantly ($p < 0.05$) higher compared with participants from medium (59.8 (5.7)) and low walkable (45.4 (4.8)) neighbourhoods. Participants from low walkable neighbourhoods were on average older than those from medium walkable and high walkable neighbourhoods ($p < 0.05$ ANOVA, Bonferroni: Table 1).

### 3.2. Self-Reported Participation in Perceived Neighbourhood-Specific Physical Activity

The proportion of overall agreement in participation of neighbourhood-specific physical activity between Time 1 and Time 2 ranged from 72.8% for moderate physical activity to 94.6% for bicycling for transport. With the exception of moderate physical activity (72.8%) and walking for recreation (73.2%), the proportion of overall agreement for other physical activities was acceptable (≥75%). Kappa estimated agreement for participation in neighbourhood-specific physical activities was considered moderate (κ = 0.41 to 0.58) (Table 2).

### 3.3. Self-Reported Days and Minutes of Perceived Neighbourhood-Specific Physical Activity

The correlations in self-reported perceived neighbourhood-specific physical activities between Time 1 and Time 2 were moderate for days per week (ICC = 0.50 to 0.66), poor to moderate for usual minutes per day (ICC = 0.37 to 0.57), and moderate for calculated minutes per week (ICC = 0.49 to 0.69) (Table 3). All Spearman's rank correlations when all participants were included were moderate and ranged from $\rho$ = 0.41 for minutes per week of moderate physical activity to $\rho$ = 0.75 for computed total minutes active per week (Table 3). After excluding participants who reported zero minutes (no participation), the ICC magnitude increased for all bicycling (days/week: From 0.52 to 0.70, and min/day: From 0.40 to 0.81, min/week: From 0.60 to 0.85) and walking for leisure variables (days/week: From 0.60 to 0.75, min/day: From 0.50 to 0.55, and min/week: From 0.69 to 0.71) (Table 4). After excluding participants who reported no participation, the majority (11/16) of the Spearman's rank correlations increased in magnitude, with computed total minutes active per week ($\rho$ = 0.76) and minutes per week of bicycling for transportation ($\rho$ = 0.87) displaying excellent correlations (Table 4).

### 3.4. Relations between Perceived Neighbourhood-Specific Physical Activity and Neighbourhood Built Environment

After adjusting for all covariates, compared with participants in low walkable neighbourhoods, those in high walkable neighbourhoods were more likely to report participation in perceived neighbourhood-specific walking for transportation (OR = 3.02, 95% CI: 1.39 to 6.56) and undertook on average 41.08 (95% CI: 2.87 to 79.30) more minutes per week of walking for transportation. Participants in medium walkable neighbourhoods were more likely to report participation in perceived neighbourhood-specific moderate-intensity physical activity (OR = 2.02, 95% CI: 1.06 to 3.86) than those in low walkable neighbourhoods (Table 5). After adjusting for all covariates, a 1-unit increase in Walk Score® was linearly associated ($p < 0.05$) with a 1.4 min per week increase in perceived neighbourhood-specific walking for transportation (Table 5). Neighbourhood walkability and Walk Score® were not statistically associated with any other physical activity outcomes.

**Table 1.** Sample demographic characteristics by neighbourhood walkability.

| Demographic Characteristic | Low Walkable (n = 92) Estimate | Medium Walkable (n = 85) Estimate | High Walkable (n = 84) Estimate | Total (n = 261) Estimate |
|---|---|---|---|---|
| Age in years, mean (SD) * | 57.1 (12.5) | 52.5 (13.4) | 52.0 (13.2) | 53.9 (13.2) |
| Female, n (%) | 61 (66.3) | 63 (74.2) | 57 (67.9) | 181 (69.4) |
| Dependents living in the home, n (%) | | | | |
| One or more aged <6 years | 8 (8.7) | 15 (17.7) | 17 (20.2) | 40 (15.3) |
| One or more aged 6–18 years | 17 (18.5) | 25 (29.4) | 19 (22.6) | 61 (23.4) |
| Dogs living in the home, n (%) | 38 (41.3) | 36 (42.4) | 32 (38.1) | 106 (40.6) |
| Had access to a motor vehicle for personal use, n (%) | 92 (100.0) | 82 (96.5) | 81 (96.4) | 255 (97.7) |
| Had access to a bicycle for personal use, n (%) | 74 (80.4) | 67 (78.8) | 73 (86.9) | 214 (82.0) |
| Highest level of education, n (%) | | | | |
| Lower than University | 35 (38.0) | 22 (25.9) | 25 (29.8) | 82 (31.4) |
| University | 57 (62.0) | 63 (74.1) | 59 (70.2) | 179 (68.6) |

* $p < 0.05$. One-Way ANOVA: Bonferroni (continuous variable), Low walkable older than medium and high walkable neighbourhoods. Chi$^2$ (categorical variables).

**Table 2.** Proportion (%) of Overall Agreement ($p_0$) and Kappa ($\kappa$) coefficients for self-reported physical activity between Time 1 and Time 2.

| Physical Activity | Time 1 % (n) | Time 2 % (n) | $P_0$ | $\kappa$ (95% CI) |
|---|---|---|---|---|
| Bicycled for transportation in perceived neighbourhood | 4.2 (11) | 6.5 (17) | 94.6 | 0.47 (0.24 to 0.71) * |
| Walked for transportation in perceived neighbourhood | 73.2 (191) | 67.8 (177) | 82.4 | 0.58 (0.47 to 0.69) * |
| Walked for recreation in perceived neighbourhood | 57.9 (151) | 54.0 (141) | 73.2 | 0.46 (0.35 to 0.57) * |
| Vigorous physical activity in perceived neighbourhood | 44.1 (115) | 41.4 (108) | 76.6 | 0.52 (0.42 to 0.63) * |
| Moderate physical activity in perceived neighbourhood | 35.3 (92) | 37.9 (99) | 72.8 | 0.41 (0.30 to 0.53) * |

* $p < 0.05$. $n = 261$ completed the Time 1 and Time 2 surveys. Seven days elapsed between the Time 1 and Time 2 survey.

**Table 3.** Intraclass Correlations (ICC) # and Spearman's rank correlation (ρ) for self-reported perceived neighbourhood physical activity between Time 1 and Time 2 for all participants (*n* = 261).

| Physical Activity Measure | Time 1 Mean (SD), Median | Time 2 Mean (SD), Median | ICC (95% CI) | ρ (95% CI) |
|---|---|---|---|---|
| Bicycling for transportation during the last 7 days (in days) | 0.13 (0.73), 0 | 0.15 (0.70), 0 | 0.52 (0.43 to 0.60) * | 0.50 (0.40 to 0.58) * |
| Usual time spent bicycling for transportation on one of those days (in minutes) | 0.77 (4.64), 0 | 1.78 (7.78), 0 | 0.40 (0.29 to 0.49) * | 0.48 (0.39 to 0.57) * |
| *Computed: Total transportation minutes/week by bicycle* | 2.38 (15.41), 0 | 4.27 (22.02), 0 | 0.60 (0.52 to 0.68) * | 0.49 (0.40 to 0.58) * |
| Walking for transportation during the last 7 days (in days) | 2.60 (2.39), 2 | 2.27 (2.30), 2 | 0.66 (0.58 to 0.72) * | 0.67 (0.60 to 0.73) * |
| Usual time spent walking for transportation on one of those days (in minutes) | 23.72 (23.67), 20 | 20.90 (21.50), 20 | 0.57 (0.48 to 0.65) * | 0.63 (0.55 to 0.70) * |
| *Computed: Total transportation minutes/week by walking* | 92.84 (131.59), 50 | 77.13 (109.51), 40 | 0.64 (0.56 to 0.71) * | 0.69 (0.62 to 0.75) * |
| Walking for leisure during the last 7 days (in days) | 2.01 (2.39), 1 | 1.95 (2.44), 1 | 0.60 (0.52 to 0.67) * | 0.55 (0.46 to 0.63) * |
| Usual time spent walking for leisure on one of those days (in minutes) | 26.36 (33.06), 20 | 25.23 (31.36), 20 | 0.50 (0.40 to 0.58) * | 0.56 (0.47 to 0.64) * |
| *Computed: Total minutes/week spent walking for recreation, leisure, or exercise* | 95.69 (156.25), 30 | 93.91 (144.50), 25 | 0.69 (0.61 to 0.74) * | 0.58 (0.49 to 0.66) * |
| Undertaking vigorous physical activity for leisure during the last 7 days (in days) | 1.21 (1.67), 0 | 1.13 (1.69), 0 | 0.55 (0.46 to 0.63) * | 0.55 (0.46 to 0.63) * |
| Usual time spent in vigorous physical activity for leisure on one of those days (in minutes) | 20.67 (28.63), 0 | 19.27 (33.32), 0 | 0.55 (0.46 to 0.63) * | 0.58 (0.49 to 0.65) * |
| *Computed: Total minutes/week spent in vigorous physical activity* | 59.18 (98.11), 0 | 56.74 (137.46), 0 | 0.49 (0.39 to 0.57) * | 0.58 (0.49 to 0.66) * |
| Undertaking moderate physical activity for leisure during the last 7 days (in days) | 0.98 (1.67), 0 | 1.08 (1.78), 0 | 0.50 (0.41 to 0.59) * | 0.48 (0.38 to 0.56) * |
| Usual time spent in moderate physical activity for leisure on one of those days (in minutes) | 13.60 (21.43), 0 | 16.49 (25.07), 0 | 0.37 (0.26 to 0.47) * | 0.41 (0.31 to 0.51) * |
| *Computed: Total minutes/week spent in moderate physical activity* | 39.18 (76.43), 0 | 48.54 (94.02), 0 | 0.49 (0.39 to 0.57) * | 0.47 (0.37 to 0.56) * |
| *Computed: Total minutes/week active* ^ | 289.25 (298.65), 210 | 280.59 (295.80), 210 | 0.70 (0.63 to 0.76) * | 0.75 (0.69 to 0.80) * |

# Two-way mixed model. * *p* < 0.05. ^ Sum of: Computed: Total transportation minutes/week by bicycle; Computed: Total transportation minutes/week by walking; Computed: Total minutes/week walking for recreation, leisure, or exercise; Computed: Total minutes/week spent in vigorous physical activity; and, Computed: Total minutes/week spent in moderate physical activity. Seven days elapsed between the Time 1 and Time 2 survey. SD: Standard deviation. CI: Confidence interval.

**Table 4.** Intraclass Correlations (ICC) # and Spearman's rank correlation (ρ) for self-reported perceived neighbourhood physical activity between Time 1 and Time 2 for participants reporting activity.

| Physical Activity Measure | n | Time 1 Mean (SD), Median | n | Time 2 Mean (SD), Median | n | ICC (95% CI) | n | ρ (95% CI) |
|---|---|---|---|---|---|---|---|---|
| Bicycling for transportation during the last 7 days (in days) | 11 | 3.09 (1.92), 2 | 17 | 2.29 (1.65), 1 | 7 | 0.70 (0.00 to 0.94) * | 7 | 0.74 (−0.03 to 0.96) |
| Usual time spent bicycling for transportation on one of those days (in minutes) | 11 | 18.18 (14.54), 15 | 17 | 27.35 (15.52), 25 | 7 | 0.81 (0.25 to 0.97) * | 7 | 0.87 (0.35 to 0.98) * |
| *Computed: Total transportation minutes/week by bicycle* | 11 | 56.36 (53.16), 40 | 17 | 65.59 (60.08), 45 | 7 | 0.85 (0.37 to 0.97) * | 7 | 0.75 (−0.01 to 0.96) |
| Walking for transportation during the last 7 days (in days) | 191 | 3.55 (2.10), 3 | 177 | 3.35 (2.05), 3 | 161 | 0.60 (0.49 to 0.69) * | 161 | 0.59 (0.48 to 0.68) * |
| Usual time spent walking for transportation on one of those days (in minutes) | 191 | 32.41 (21.99), 30 | 177 | 30.82 (19.38), 30 | 161 | 0.44 (0.31 to 0.56) * | 161 | 0.52 (0.39 to 0.62) * |
| *Computed: Total transportation minutes/week by walking* | 191 | 126.86 (139.12), 75 | 177 | 113.73 (116.32), 60 | 161 | 0.59 (0.48 to 0.68) * | 161 | 0.62 (0.52 to 0.71) * |
| Walking for leisure during the last 7 days (in days) | 151 | 3.48 (2.18), 3 | 141 | 3.62 (2.24), 3 | 111 | 0.75 (0.65 to 0.82) * | 111 | 0.73 (0.63 to 0.81) * |
| Usual time spent walking for leisure on one of those days (in minutes) | 151 | 45.56 (31.83), 40 | 141 | 46.70 (28.57), 40 | 111 | 0.55 (0.40 to 0.67) * | 111 | 0.66 (0.54 to 0.75) * |
| *Computed: Total minutes/week spent walking for recreation, leisure, or exercise* | 151 | 165.40 (175.24), 120 | 141 | 173.83 (157.44), 120 | 111 | 0.71 (0.61 to 0.79) * | 111 | 0.72 (0.62 to 0.80) * |
| Undertaking vigorous physical activity for leisure during the last 7 days (in days) | 115 | 2.76 (1.44), 3 | 108 | 2.74 (1.57), 2 | 81 | 0.49 (0.30 to 0.64) * | 81 | 0.47 (0.28 to 0.62) * |
| Usual time spent in vigorous physical activity for leisure on one of those days (in minutes) | 115 | 46.91 (25.05), 45 | 108 | 46.57 (37.60), 40 | 81 | 0.44 (0.24 to 0.60) * | 81 | 0.66 (0.51 to 0.77) * |
| *Computed: Total minutes/week spent in vigorous physical activity* | 115 | 134.30 (108.50), 100 | 108 | 137.13 (186.51), 100 | 81 | 0.37 (0.17 to 0.54) * | 81 | 0.49 (0.30 to 0.64) * |
| Undertaking moderate physical activity for leisure during the last 7 days (in days) | 92 | 2.77 (1.71), 2 | 99 | 2.85 (1.82), 2 | 60 | 0.45 (0.22 to 0.63) * | 60 | 0.50 (0.29 to 0.67) * |
| Usual time spent in moderate physical activity for leisure on one of those days (in minutes) | 92 | 38.59 (18.36), 30 | 99 | 43.48 (21.95), 40 | 60 | 0.34 (0.09 to 0.54) * | 60 | 0.46 (0.23 to 0.64) * |
| *Computed: Total minutes/week spent in moderate physical activity* | 92 | 111.14 (92.77), 90 | 99 | 127.98 (114.80), 90 | 60 | 0.46 (0.23 to 0.64) * | 60 | 0.48 (0.26 to 0.65) * |
| *Computed: Total minutes/week active ^* | 235 | 321.26 (297.96), 230 | 227 | 322.62 (295.03), 240 | 217 | 0.68 (0.60 to 0.74) * | 217 | 0.76 (0.69 to 0.81) * |

# Two-way mixed model. * $p < 0.05$. ^ Sum of: Computed: Total transportation minutes/week by bicycle; Computed: Total minutes/week spent walking for recreation, leisure, or exercise; Computed: Total minutes/week spent in vigorous physical activity; and; Computed: Total minutes/week spent in moderate physical activity. Seven days elapsed between the Time 1 and Time 2 survey. SD: Standard deviation. CI: Confidence interval.

**Table 5.** Associations between self-reported participation in and duration of perceived neighbourhood-based physical activity and Walk Score® measured neighbourhood walkability at Time 1 only (*n* = 261).

| Adjusted Logistic Regression Odds Ratios (OR) for the Association between Participation and Neighbourhood Walkability | | | | | |
|---|---|---|---|---|---|
| Walkability | Cycled for Transportation OR (95% CI) | Walked for Transportation OR (95% CI) | Walked for Recreation OR (95% CI) | Vigorous Physical Activity OR (95% CI) | Moderate Physical Activity OR (95% CI) |
| Low | Reference Group | Reference Group | Reference Group | Reference Group | Reference Group |
| Medium | 0.69 (0.14 to 3.32) | 1.20 (0.61 to 2.34) | 1.17 (0.62 to 2.21) | 1.42 (0.75 to 2.66) | 2.02 (1.06 to 3.86)* |
| High | 0.87 (0.20 to 3.81) | 3.02 (1.39 to 6.56)* | 0.78 (0.42 to 1.47) | 1.32 (0.70 to 2.49) | 1.61 (0.83 to 3.12) |

| Adjusted Linear Regression Unstandardized Regression Coefficients (b) for the Association between Duration and Neighbourhood Walkability | | | | | | |
|---|---|---|---|---|---|---|
| Walkability | Min/week Cycling for Transportation b (95% CI) | Min/week Walking for Transportation b (95% CI) | Min/week Walking for Recreation b (95% CI) | Min/week Vigorous Physical Activity b (95% CI) | Min/week Moderate Physical Activity b (95% CI) | Min/week Total Activity^ b (95% CI) |
| Low | Reference Group | Reference Group | Reference Group | Reference Group | Reference Group | Reference Group |
| Medium | −0.76 (−5.44 to 3.92) | 7.75 (−30.38 to 45.89) | −6.80 (−52.08 to 38.48) | −8.17 (−37.34 to 20.99) | 0.63 (−22.29 to 23.54) | −7.35 (−91.91 to 77.20) |
| High | −1.20 (−5.89 to 3.50) | 41.08 (2.87 to 79.30)* | −14.57 (−59.94 to 30.81) | 17.64 (−11.59 to 46.87) | 9.10 (−13.87 to 32.06) | 52.05 (−32.69 to 136.79) |

| Adjusted Linear Regression Unstandardized Regression Coefficients (b) for the Association between Duration and Neighbourhood Walk Score® | | | | | | |
|---|---|---|---|---|---|---|
| Walkability | Min/week Cycling for Transportation b (95% CI) | Min/week Walking for Transportation b (95% CI) | Min/week Walking for Recreation b (95% CI) | Min/week Vigorous Physical Activity b (95% CI) | Min/week Moderate Physical Activity b (95% CI) | Min/week Total Activity^ b (95% CI) |
| Walk Score | −0.03 (−0.17 to 0.10) | 1.40 (0.32 to 2.47)* | −0.32 (−1.59 to 0.96) | 0.50 (−0.32 to 1.33) | 0.12 (−0.53 to 0.76) | 1.67 (−0.72 to 4.06) |

* $p < 0.05$. ^ Sum of: Total of weekly transportation bicycling, transportation walking, recreation walking, vigorous physical activity, and moderate physical activity minutes. Logistic and linear regression models adjusted for age, sex, presence of dependent children under 6 and 6–18 years, dogs living in the household, access to a motor vehicle, access to a bicycle, and education. (b) Unstandardized regression coefficient. OR: Odds ratio. CI: Confidence interval. Min/week: Minutes per week.

## 4. Discussion

Our findings suggest that IPAQ items, that are adapted to capture self–reported perceived neighbourhood-specific physical activity and are administered via the internet, provide reliable estimates of behaviour. Notably, we also found that self–reported participation and minutes in perceived neighbourhood-specific walking for transportation differed by level of neighbourhood walkability, supporting previous findings showing consistent associations between the built environment and walking [1,5,6]. Although further assessment of the online N-IPAQs measurement validity is needed, our preliminary findings might suggest that this tool is suitable for use in studies investigating relationships between neighbourhood built environments and physical activity, and in particular transportation walking, in adult populations.

With the exception of daily minutes of moderate physical activity (ICC = 0.37), all of our measures had at least moderate test-retest reliability, with the highest test-retest reliability found for total minutes of perceived neighbourhood-specific physical activity during the last week ($\rho = 0.75$). It was not surprising that moderate physical activity outcomes had the lowest reliability statistics as moderate physical activity is often accumulated via many different types of non-walking behaviour that may not be easily recalled. Lower reliability for moderate physical activities captured using the IPAQ has been reported elsewhere [20], including when the IPAQ was administered online [13]. Nonetheless, future research may implement strategies to overcome this limitation, such as researcher-assisted administration, or better clarification and more examples about what constitutes moderate physical activity. The reliability of total physical activity in our study is congruent with previous studies whereby the estimated IPAQ test-retest correlations across 21 studies ranged from 0.46 to 0.96 [20], depending on the lapsed time between administrations (between three and seven days), the data collection mode (self-reported versus telephone interview), the number of administrations (between one and three), and if "usual week" or "last 7 days" was used in the questions. Of the 21 test-retest IPAQ studies, only two closely resembled our data collection procedure (i.e., used the long-form IPAQ, captured physical activity undertaken in the last seven days, and asked participants to complete two administrations); these studies had correlations of 0.72 and 0.79 [20]. However, the days between administrations were "up to" seven days later [20]; as time between our administrations was a "minimum" of seven days, these discrepancies in correlation may be due to participants being better able to recall their responses during the shorter time frame. Furthermore, other research using online administrations of the IPAQ showed a test-retest of total physical activity energy expenditure ICC = 0.58 [11] and total moderate–vigorous physical activity ICC = 0.70 [13]. Moreover, results from research undertaken in Canada produced similar reliability for weekly minutes of moderate physical activity inside the neighbourhood (ICC = 0.38) [8]. These results indicate that an online version of the N-IPAQ is a reliable tool for capturing self-reported perceived neighbourhood-specific physical activity.

Built environment characteristics have been consistently associated with physical activity [2,42] and in particular walking [1,30]. Furthermore, walking for transportation has been consistently linked to neighbourhoods with higher population density, distance to non-residential destinations, and proximal non-residential destinations [1]. These relationships have been tested in different countries, such as Canada [28], Australia [29], France [30], Sweden [6], and the United States [31], with studies finding an increased likelihood of transportation walking with increasing access to services and street connectivity. These findings are consistent with our results; that is, compared to lower walkable neighbourhoods, residents living in high walkable neighbourhoods had higher odds of walking for transportation. Our results also showed that residents from high walkable neighbourhoods undertook an average of 41 more total minutes a week of transportation walking compared to residents in low walkable neighbourhoods. This result is further supported by our finding of a statistically significant linear increase in minutes of transportation walking and Walk Score®. An association with Walk Score® and transportation walking was excepted as higher scores are linked with a closer proximity to services and amenities [28,36,37]. Importantly, the online N-IPAQ found associations between the neighbourhood environment and transportation walking in the expected direction.

The definition of neighbourhood may impact validity as residents and researchers may not have the same operational definition or perception of neighbourhood, leading to the modifiable areal unit problem [43,44]. Adams et al. [45] demonstrated that residents' neighbourhood perception of a 20-min "time to walk to a destination" produced stronger correlations with objective measures than a 10 or 30-min cut-point did. Furthermore, research using GPS devices found GPS points captured by varying buffers ranged from 28.6 to 97.9%, indicating some buffers may not accurately represent a resident's exposure to their neighbourhood built environment [43]. In our adaptation of the IPAQ, we did not explicitly define the size of the neighbourhood, thus allowing the tool to capture residents' physical activity within their perceived residential neighbourhood. A paper administration of the N-IPAQ found that perceived neighbourhood-specific physical activity provided strong agreement with physical activity captured with an accelerometer and GPS at a 400m buffer around the participant's home [21]; however, similar research is needed to test if these results would be found in the online administration of the N-IPAQ.

Our study has several limitations. Levels of self-reported physical activity are often over-reported [46]. Moreover, there may have been a learning effect of the questionnaire, whereby after the respondent completed Time 1, they were more cognizant to their physical activity for Time 2; thus, this could have attenuated our reliability results. The use of objective measures for capturing physical activity, such as GPS combined with accelerometers, may provide a better option for measuring context-specific physical activity; therefore, as was done with the paper version of the N–IPAQ [21], accelerometers synchronized with GPS monitors may be used in future research with smaller samples as a criterion measure to further validate the online N-IPAQ. We did not find statistical differences in education between levels of neighbourhood walkability; however, we did not measure other proxies of socioeconomic status or variables such as health status; therefore, our comparisons with Walk Score® walkability may have been confounded by other measures that may affect physical activity. Although Walk Score® has been validated against objective built environment characteristics [33–35], we did not measure these characteristics directly or measure residents' perceived neighbourhood environment; therefore, this may have introduced some measurement error. Moreover, Walk Score® measures are for a distinct location; therefore, if our participants perceived their neighbourhood as one outside of the Walk Score® buffer, our estimates would be discordant. Moreover, while our adapted tool was reliable and was sufficiently sensitive to detect changes in physical activity (i.e., transportation walking) based on differences in neighbourhood walkability, other approaches of validation, such as comparing self-reported physical activity captured by this tool against objective measures of physical activity are still required. Compared to the 2014 Calgary Census for our study neighbourhoods, our sample had similar education (68.6 vs. 63.0% in the 2014 Calgary Census obtained postsecondary education), had a higher proportion of women (69.4 vs. 49.7% in the 2014 Calgary Census), was older on average (53.9 vs. 39.0 in the 2014 Calgary Census) [24], and may have been more motivated—recruited from a pool of recent study participants who were willing to be contacted for future research—thus limiting generalizability of our findings. Moreover, participation in bicycling was low in our sample which influenced our estimate ICC for bicycling duration. For example, ICC and $\rho$ for usual time spent bicycling for transportation increased from 0.40 to 0.81 and 0.48 to 0.87, respectively, when only looking at participants reporting ($n = 7$) bicycling in the last week. Caution may be needed in using this tool to capture neighbourhood bicycling. More pilot testing of this tool in a sample consisting of a larger number of bicyclists is warranted. Lastly, although the use of an internet-based survey mode is convenient, offers more control over survey response patterns, and is low cost relative to other survey modes [14], some participants may have experienced technical difficulties, whether it be due to software, hardware, or personal computer skills resulting in loss of data and or study drop-out.

## 5. Conclusions

The online N-IPAQ has similar test-retest reliability as the non-modified IPAQ. The online N-IPAQ found differences in neighbourhoods that vary in their walkability. Future studies investigating built environment and physical activity may consider using the online version of the N–IPAQ for capturing perceived neighbourhood-specific physical activity.

**Supplementary Materials:** The following are available online at http://www.mdpi.com/1660-4601/16/11/1917/s1, Questionnaire S1: N-IPAQ.

**Author Contributions:** Conceptualization, L.F. and G.R.M.; methodology, L.F. and G.R.M.; software, A.B.; validation, L.F., G.R.M. and A.B.; formal analysis, A.B.; investigation, L.F.; resources, G.R.M.; data curation, A.B.; writing—original draft preparation, L.F.; writing—review and editing, L.F., G.R.M. and A.B.; visualization, A.B.; supervision, G.R.M.; project administration, L.F. and G.R.M.; funding acquisition, G.R.M.

**Funding:** This study was part of the Pathways to Health project funded by the Canadian Institutes of Health Research (CIHR; MOP-126133). Additional funding support was provided by an O'Brien Centre for Public Health Catalyst Grant, a University Research Grant Committee Seed Grant, and a CIHR Foundations Scheme Grant (FDN-154331).

**Acknowledgments:** The contributions of the co-investigators and collaborators on the Pathways to Health Study are greatly appreciated.

**Conflicts of Interest:** The authors declare no conflict of interest. The funders had no role in the design of the study; in the collection, analyses, or interpretation of data; in the writing of the manuscript, or in the decision to publish the results.

## References

1.  Saelens, B.E.; Handy, S.L. Built environment correlates of walking: A review. *Med. Sci. Sports Exerc.* **2008**, *40*, S550–S566. [CrossRef]
2.  Wendel-Vos, W.; Droomers, M.; Kremers, S.; Brug, J.; van Lenthe, F. Potential environmental determinants of physical activity in adults: A systematic review. *Obes. Rev.* **2007**, *8*, 425–440. [CrossRef] [PubMed]
3.  McCormack, G.R.; Shiell, A. In search of causality: A systematic review of the relationship between the built environment and physical activity among adults. *Int. J. Behav. Nutr. Phys. Act.* **2011**, *8*, 125. [CrossRef]
4.  Giles–Corti, B.; Timperio, A.; Cutt, H.; Pikora, T.J.; Bull, F.C.; Knuiman, M.; Bulsara, M.; Van Niel, K.; Shilton, T. Development of a reliable measure of walking within and outside the local neighborhood: Reside's neighborhood physical activity questionnaire. *Prev. Med.* **2006**, *42*, 455–459. [CrossRef] [PubMed]
5.  Owen, N.; Cerin, E.; Leslie, E.; duToit, L.; Coffee, N.; Frank, L.D.; Bauman, A.E.; Hugo, G.; Saelens, B.E.; Sallis, J.F. Neighborhood walkability and the walking behavior of australian adults. *Am. J. Prev. Med.* **2007**, *33*, 387–395. [CrossRef] [PubMed]
6.  Sundquist, K.; Eriksson, U.; Kawakami, N.; Skog, L.; Ohlsson, H.; Arvidsson, D. Neighborhood walkability, physical activity, and walking behavior: The swedish neighborhood and physical activity (snap) study. *Soc. Sci. Med.* **2011**, *72*, 1266–1273. [CrossRef]
7.  Cerin, E.; Barnett, A.; Sit, C.H.; Cheung, M.C.; Lee, L.C.; Ho, S.Y.; Chan, W.M. Measuring walking within and outside the neighborhood in chinese elders: Reliability and validity. *BMC Public Health* **2011**, *11*, 851. [CrossRef]
8.  McCormack, G.R.; Shiell, A.; Doyle-Baker, P.K.; Friedenreich, C.; Sandalack, B.; Giles-Corti, B. Testing the reliability of neighborhood-specific measures of physical activity among canadian adults. *J. Phys. Act. Health* **2009**, *6*, 367–373. [CrossRef] [PubMed]
9.  Doma, K.; Speyer, R.; Leicht, A.S.; Cordier, R. Comparison of psychometric properties between usual-week and past-week self-reported physical activity questionnaires: A systematic review. *Int. J. Behav. Nutr. Phys. Act.* **2017**, *14*, 10. [CrossRef]
10.  Anderson, D.; Seib, C.; Tjondronegoro, D.; Turner, J.; Monterosso, L.; McGuire, A.; Porter-Steele, J.; Song, W.; Yates, P.; King, N.; et al. The women's wellness after cancer program: A multisite, single-blinded, randomised controlled trial protocol. *BMC Cancer* **2017**, *17*, 98.
11.  Hansen, A.W.; Dahl-Petersen, I.; Helge, J.W.; Brage, S.; Gronbaek, M.; Flensborg-Madsen, T. Validation of an internet-based long version of the international physical activity questionnaire in danish adults using combined accelerometry and heart rate monitoring. *J. Phys. Act. Health* **2014**, *11*, 654–664.

12. Wong, F.Y. Influence of pokemon go on physical activity levels of university players: A cross-sectional study. *Int. J. Health Geogr.* **2017**, *16*, 8. [CrossRef]

13. Taylor, N.J.; Crouter, S.E.; Lawton, R.J.; Conner, M.T.; Prestwich, A. Development and validation of the online self-reported walking and exercise questionnaire (osweq). *J. Phys. Act. Health* **2013**, *10*, 1091–1101. [CrossRef]

14. Jones, T.L.; Baxter, M.A.; Khanduja, V. A quick guide to survey research. *Ann. Roy. Coll. Surg.* **2013**, *95*, 5–7. [CrossRef]

15. Statistics Canada. *List of Surveys in Collection*; Statistics Canada: Ottawa, ON, Canada, 2017.

16. Firestone, K.A.; Carson, J.W.; Mist, S.D.; Carson, K.M.; Jones, K.D. Interest in yoga among fibromyalgia patients: An international internet survey. *Int. J. Yoga Therap.* **2014**, *24*, 117–124.

17. Kuss, D.J.; Lopez-Fernandez, O. Internet addiction and problematic internet use: A systematic review of clinical research. *World J. Psychiatry* **2016**, *6*, 143–176. [CrossRef]

18. CRTC. *Telecom Regulatory Policy CRTC 2016-496. Modern Telecommunications Services—The Path Forward for Canada's Digital Economy*; CRTC: Ottawa, ON, Canada, 2016.

19. ITU. *Statistics*; International Telecommunication Union: Geneva, Switzerland, 2017.

20. Craig, C.L.; Marshall, A.L.; Sjostrom, M.; Bauman, A.E.; Booth, M.L.; Ainsworth, B.E.; Pratt, M.; Ekelund, U.; Yngve, A.; Sallis, J.F.; et al. International physical activity questionnaire: 12-Country reliability and validity. *Med. Sci. Sports Exerc.* **2003**, *35*, 1381–1395. [CrossRef]

21. Frehlich, L.; Friedenreich, C.; Nettel-Aguirre, A.; Schipperijn, J.; McCormack, G.R. Using accelerometer/gps data to validate a neighborhood-adapted version of the international physical activity questionnaire (ipaq). *J. Meas. Phys. Behav.* **2018**, *1*, 181–190. [CrossRef]

22. Frehlich, L.; Friedenreich, C.; Nettel-Aguirre, A.; McCormack, G.R. Test-retest reliability of a modified international physical activity questionnaire (ipaq) to capture neighbourhood physical activity. *J. Hum. Sport Exerc.* **2018**, *13*, 174–187. [CrossRef]

23. McInerney, M.; Csizmadi, I.; Friedenreich, C.M.; Uribe, F.A.; Nettel-Aguirre, A.; McLaren, L.; Potestio, M.; Sandalack, B.; McCormack, G.R. Associations between the neighbourhood food environment, neighbourhood socioeconomic status, and diet quality: An observational study. *BMC Public Health* **2016**, *16*, 984. [CrossRef]

24. McCormack, G.R.; Friedenreich, C.; McLaren, L.; Potestio, M.; Sandalack, B.; Csizmadi, I. Interactions between neighbourhood urban form and socioeconomic status and their associations with anthropometric measurements in canadian adults. *J. Environ. Public Health* **2017**, *2017*, 5042614. [CrossRef] [PubMed]

25. McCormack, G.R.; Friedenreich, C.; Sandalack, B.A.; Giles–Corti, B.; Doyle-Baker, P.K.; Shiell, A. The relationship between cluster-analysis derived walkability and local recreational and transportation walking among canadian adults. *Health Place* **2012**, *18*, 1079–1087. [CrossRef] [PubMed]

26. Choi, J.; Lee, M.; Lee, J.K.; Kang, D.; Choi, J.Y. Correlates associated with participation in physical activity among adults: A systematic review of reviews and update. *BMC Public Health* **2017**, *17*, 356. [CrossRef] [PubMed]

27. Cerin, E.; Conway, T.L.; Cain, K.L.; Kerr, J.; De Bourdeaudhuij, I.; Owen, N.; Reis, R.S.; Sarmiento, O.L.; Hinckson, E.A.; Salvo, D.; et al. Sharing good news across the world: Developing comparable scores across 12 countries for the neighborhood environment walkability scale (news). *BMC Public Health* **2013**, *13*, 309. [CrossRef] [PubMed]

28. Jack, E.; McCormack, G.R. The associations between objectively-determined and self-reported urban form characteristics and neighborhood-based walking in adults. *Int. J. Behav. Nutr. Phys. Act.* **2014**, *11*, 71. [CrossRef]

29. Christian, H.E.; Bull, F.C.; Middleton, N.J.; Knuiman, M.W.; Divitini, M.L.; Hooper, P.; Amarasinghe, A.; Giles-Corti, B. How important is the land use mix measure in understanding walking behaviour? Results from the reside study. *Int. J. Behav. Nutr. Phys. Act.* **2011**, *8*, 55. [CrossRef] [PubMed]

30. Duncan, D.T.; Meline, J.; Kestens, Y.; Day, K.; Elbel, B.; Trasande, L.; Chaix, B. Walk score, transportation mode choice, and walking among french adults: A gps, accelerometer, and mobility survey study. *Int. J. Environ. Res. Public Health* **2016**, *13*, 611. [CrossRef]

31. Suminski, R.R.; Poston, W.S.; Petosa, R.L.; Stevens, E.; Katzenmoyer, L.M. Features of the neighborhood environment and walking by U.S. Adults. *Am. J. Prev. Med.* **2005**, *28*, 149–155. [CrossRef]

32. Chiu, M.; Shah, B.R.; Maclagan, L.C.; Rezai, M.R.; Austin, P.C.; Tu, J.V. Walk score(r) and the prevalence of utilitarian walking and obesity among ontario adults: A cross-sectional study. *Health Rep.* **2015**, *26*, 3–10.

33. Carr, L.J.; Dunsiger, S.I.; Marcus, B.H. Walk score as a global estimate of neighborhood walkability. *Am. J. Prev. Med.* **2010**, *39*, 460–463. [CrossRef]

34. Carr, L.J.; Dunsiger, S.I.; Marcus, B.H. Validation of walk score for estimating access to walkable amenities. *Br. J. Sports Med.* **2011**, *45*, 1144–1148. [CrossRef]

35. Nykiforuk, C.I.; McGetrick, J.A.; Crick, K.; Johnson, J.A. Check the score: Field validation of street smart walk score in alberta, canada. *Prev. Med. Rep.* **2016**, *4*, 532–539. [CrossRef]

36. Hajna, S.; Ross, N.A.; Joseph, L.; Harper, S.; Dasgupta, K. Neighbourhood walkability, daily steps and utilitarian walking in canadian adults. *BMJ Open* **2015**, *5*, e008964. [CrossRef]

37. Thielman, J.; Manson, H.; Chiu, M.; Copes, R.; Rosella, L.C. Residents of highly walkable neighbourhoods in canadian urban areas do substantially more physical activity: A cross-sectional analysis. *CMAJ Open* **2016**, *4*, E720–E728. [CrossRef]

38. Al-Hazzaa, H.M.; Abahussain, N.A.; Al-Sobayel, H.I.; Qahwaji, D.M.; Musaiger, A.O. Physical activity, sedentary behaviors and dietary habits among saudi adolescents relative to age, gender and region. *Int. J. Behav. Nutr. Phys. Act.* **2011**, *8*, 140. [CrossRef] [PubMed]

39. McCormack, G.R.; Giles-Corti, B.; Bulsara, M. The relationship between destination proximity, destination mix and physical activity behaviors. *Prev. Med.* **2008**, *46*, 33–40. [CrossRef]

40. Cerin, E.; Saelens, B.E.; Sallis, J.F.; Frank, L.D. Neighborhood environment walkability scale: Validity and development of a short form. *Med. Sci. Sports Exerc.* **2006**, *38*, 1682–1691. [CrossRef]

41. Landis, J.R.; Koch, G.G. The measurement of observer agreement for categorical data. *Biometrics* **1977**, *33*, 159–174. [CrossRef] [PubMed]

42. Humpel, N.; Owen, N.; Leslie, E. Environmental factors associated with adults' participation in physical activity: A review. *Am. J. Prev. Med.* **2002**, *22*, 188–199. [CrossRef]

43. Madsen, T.; Schipperijn, J.; Christiansen, L.B.; Nielsen, T.S.; Troelsen, J. Developing suitable buffers to capture transport cycling behavior. *Front. Public Health* **2014**, *2*, 61. [CrossRef] [PubMed]

44. Spielman, S.E.; Yoo, E.H. The spatial dimensions of neighborhood effects. *Soc. Sci. Med.* **2009**, *68*, 1098–1105. [CrossRef] [PubMed]

45. Adams, M.A.; Ryan, S.; Kerr, J.; Sallis, J.F.; Patrick, K.; Frank, L.D.; Norman, G.J. Validation of the neighborhood environment walkability scale (news) items using geographic information systems. *J. Phys. Act. Health* **2009**, *6* (Suppl. 1), S113–S123. [CrossRef]

46. Sallis, J.F.; Saelens, B.E. Assessment of physical activity by self-report: Status, limitations, and future directions. *Res. Q Exerc. Sport* **2000**, *71*, S1–S14. [CrossRef] [PubMed]

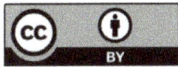

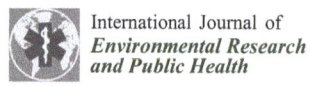

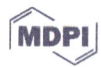

*Article*

# Modal Shift from Cars and Promotion of Walking by Providing Pedometers in Yokohama City, Japan

**Kimihiro Hino [1,*], Ayako Taniguchi [2], Masamichi Hanazato [3] and Daisuke Takagi [4]**

1   Department of Urban Engineering, Graduate School of Engineering, The University of Tokyo, Tokyo 113-8656, Japan
2   Department of Risk Engineering, Graduate School of Systems and Information Engineering, University of Tsukuba, Ibaraki 305-8573, Japan; taniguchi@risk.tsukuba.ac.jp
3   Center for Preventive Medical Sciences, Chiba University, Chiba 263-8522, Japan; hanazato@chiba-u.jp
4   Graduate School of Medicine, School of Public Health, The University of Tokyo, Tokyo 113-0033, Japan; dtakagi-utokyo@umin.ac.jp
*   Correspondence: hino@ua.t.u-tokyo.ac.jp; Tel.: +81-3-5841-6225

Received: 16 April 2019; Accepted: 14 June 2019; Published: 17 June 2019

**Abstract:** Mobility management is a transportation policy aiming to change travel behavior from car use to sustainable transportation modes while increasing people's physical activity. Providing pedometers and visualizing step counts, popular interventions in public health practice, may constitute a mobility management program. However, the ease of modal shifts and changeability of walking habits differ across neighborhood environments. Using questionnaire data from 2023 middle-aged and older participants from Yokohama, Japan, in May 2017, this study examined (1) the relationship between the physical and social environments of Yokohama Walking Point Program participants who volunteered to use free pedometers and their modal shifts from cars to walking and public transport, and (2) whether participants' modal shifts were associated with increases in step counts. Multivariate categorical regression analyses identified the frequency of greetings and conversations with neighbors as well as health motivation as important explanatory variables in both analyses. Participants living in neighborhoods far from railway stations and in neighborhoods with a high bus stop density tended to shift to walking and public transport, a modal shift that was highly associated with increased step counts. These results suggest that mobility management should be promoted in collaboration with public health and city planning professionals.

**Keywords:** mobility management; public transport; step counts; city planning; compact city; neighborhood

---

## 1. Introduction

Although considerable evidence exists demonstrating that physical inactivity increases the risk of major non-communicable diseases and shortens life expectancy, much of the world's population is inactive [1,2]. Recently, researchers have urged city planning policies to increase opportunities for physical activity (PA) by encouraging active transport (e.g., walking and cycling) and public transport use (e.g., railway and local bus) and reducing private car use [3–5]. One such policy concerns the creation of compact cities in which major facilities are concentrated within the city center, around public transport hubs, enabling residents to walk to public transport. This model is in contrast to sprawled cities in which residents are dependent on cars [5,6].

The Japanese government at the national and municipal levels have sought to promote compact city policies in light of the need to reduce environmental load and the reality of an increasing older population. The Japanese city of Toyama's city planning policies are reflective of the trend towards compact cities, with the municipality promoting public transit-oriented development and vitalization through initiatives such as the opening of the first light-rail transit in Japan and the subsidizing of costs for the acquisition of dwellings in the city center and along public transport lines [7,8]. Nonetheless, the realization of a truly compact city requires tens of years to come to fruition; as such, it is necessary to implement policies beyond those that look to change the physical environment, policies that promote a modal shift from cars to walking and public transport (hereafter simply referred to as "modal shift"), in addition to policies that look to reshape the urban structure.

Mobility management (MM) is one example of such non-physical transportation management policies. MM aims to change travel behaviors from car use to sustainable transportation modes (i.e., public transport and active transport) using communicative measures such as the provision of specific information on public transport, travel education, and word-to-mouth recommendation [9,10]. We use the term MM according to these definitions hereafter in this study, while MM is often referred to as travel planning in the United Kingdom [11] and voluntary travel behavior change in Australia [12]. Drawing on research from social and environmental psychology, studies on MM have accumulated since the mid-1990s, with such research contributing to the identification and development of effective methods of promoting modal shifts [13]. In addition, factors that influence the choice of travel mode, such as travel time and family structure, have been investigated [14–16].

MM practices have been reported not only in developed but in developing countries as well. In Metropolitan Manila, Philippines, a rideshare app for university students was developed to promote behavioral change [17,18]. In Japan, typical MM practices include personal conversations, workshops, education initiatives in schools, and travel feedback programs, practices that look to address social problems caused by car overuse [19]. A MM program in Yamato, Kanagawa, in which participants were provided pedometers in addition to leaflets and town guides, succeeded in decreasing their car use and increasing their PA [20].

In public health research and practice, providing pedometers and visualizing step counts is also a popular intervention for promoting PA [21–23]. Compared to other devices used to visualize step counts, a pedometer is cheaper and easier for every population to use. A systematic review of studies which assessed pedometer use among adults suggests that pedometer use is associated with significant increases in PA and improvements in several key health outcomes [24]. However, the ease with which modal shifts and the changeability of walking habits occur differs according to participants' neighborhood environments. Several studies have shown that public transport users spend greater amounts of time walking [25,26], with access to public transport associated with increased PA [27–29] and walking [30,31]. For example, an analysis of 6822 adults from 14 cities in 10 countries found that public transport density is significantly, positively, and linearly correlated with increased PA [32]. In addition, a longitudinal study confirmed that access to bus stops and railway stations is a key determinant of walking as a mode of transportation [33]. Based on existing studies demonstrating a relationship between public transport and PA/walking habits, the ease with which modal shifts and changeability of walking habits occur must be analyzed in light of participants' access to public transport in order for effective intervention to occur.

This study engages in such an analysis within the context of a program in the Japanese city of Yokohama, in which participants volunteered to use free pedometers to promote PA and improve their health. The first part of this study examines the relationship between participant attributes and their surrounding physical environments (i.e., distance to the nearest railway stations and bus stop density) and social environments (i.e., frequency of interaction with neighbors) on one hand, and modal shift on the other. In the second part of this study, we explore if and how modal shifts are associated with increases in step counts while controlling for other factors. This study contributes to the existing literature by identifying how neighborhood environments influence middle-aged and older people's active behaviors in the context of a super-aged society such as Japan, which has the world's highest proportion of older adults among its population [34].

## 2. Materials and Methods

### 2.1. Yokohama Walking Point Program

Located 30–40 km from Tokyo, Yokohama is the second-most populous city in Japan and was developed as an international port city. The city has a population of approximately 3.7 million people, of whom 24% are 65 years or older as of January 2017. The city's railway network has been developed, with many lines running towards central Tokyo. The railway is approximately 308 km long, and there are 157 railway stations in Yokohama. The local bus network has been expanded around the railway stations, enabling approximately 90% of citizens access to the railway stations within 15 minutes. According to the latest Person Trip Survey from 2008, railway and local bus use constituted 33.9% and 5.8% of the main modes of transportation, respectively, with these figures being higher than in other nearby major cities [35]. Nevertheless, approximately 20% of greenhouse gas emissions in Yokohama are caused by the transportation sector, half of which can be attributed to private cars [36]. Thus, shifting from private cars to public transport is one of the policy targets of the city as it looks to reduce its environmental footprint, improve the sustainability of public transport, and promote citizen health [36].

In November 2014, the city launched the Yokohama Walking Point Program (YWPP) to encourage citizens to improve their health and healthy life expectancy, as the average age of the population and the nature of diseases change. It provided free pedometers (Omron HJ-326F, Japan), purchased with the city budget, for volunteer participants aged 40 years and above. In June 2016, participation qualification was expanded to citizens aged 18 years and above. Participants were awarded points based on their step counts by scanning their pedometers via special readers installed at approximately 1000 stores and other facilities in the city. Accumulation of a certain number of points made participants eligible to win prizes. The scanned data were sent to a data server through the Internet, and participants could monitor step counts and rank among all participants using a computer or smartphone [37,38]. Every time the average monthly step counts from all participants exceed a set target, 200,000 yen is donated to the United Nations World Food Programme.

### 2.2. Data Collection

Participants' sex, age, neighborhood-level address, and number of months participating in YWPP were acquired from the YWPP registration information. Distance to the nearest railway station was measured from the center of each neighborhood, and bus stop density was calculated for each neighborhood using data from the National Land Numerical Information download service [39].

The other data were measured in the questionnaire survey that Yokohama city conducted in May 2017 among 6000 participants selected from 231,600 participants. They were randomly and proportionally selected from three stratified groups by data sending rate: participants whose data sending rate was 80% or more, less than 80%, and those who never sent data. Among the selected participants, 3493 replied to the survey, with a response rate of 58.2%. Since the original age eligibility requirement for the program was 40 years and older until June 2016, 141 respondents were aged below 40 and were thus excluded from analysis. Ultimately, a total of 2023 participants who answered all necessary questions were included in the survey analysis. The questionnaire asked primarily about the participants' changes in walking habits and health attitudes as well as their modal shifts after participating in the program for a period of time. Translated questions asked in the survey are presented in Table A1.

### 2.3. Variables

#### 2.3.1. Outcome Variables

In the first analysis, modal shift with four options, ranging from "Yes" to "No", served as the outcome variable. In the second analysis, increases in step counts served as the outcome variable.

Although it originally had four options, ranging from "increased" to "decreased", "decreased" was selected by only 0.5% of participants and thus merged with "not changed".

### 2.3.2. Explanatory Variables

The explanatory variables in both analyses were distance to the nearest railway station, bus stop density, and frequency of greetings and conversation with neighbors. Participants' modal shift, which was the outcome variable in the first analysis, was added as an explanatory variable in the second analysis.

As the number of bus stops (2735) was much higher than the number of neighborhoods (758) in Yokohama, we used bus stop density rather than distance to a bus stop as an explanatory variable. The mean distance to the nearest railway station was 807.6 (±634.6) m and the mean bus stop density per $km^2$ was 7.6 (±9.3). The two variables were disaggregated into four categories by three thresholds: approximately the mean and the mean ± 1/2 SD.

Frequency of greetings and conversation with neighbors was surveyed with five options ranging from "increased" to "decreased". Not only physical but social features of neighborhoods can also affect health by constraining or enhancing health-related behaviors [40]. Also, relationships between neighbors have been shown to have a positive association with engagement in PA [41].

### 2.3.3. Control Variables

The control variables in both analyses were participants' sex, age, occupation, self-rated health, diagnosis of a metabolic syndrome prior to participation, motivation for participation in YWPP, and months participating in YWPP.

Participants' ages were categorized as non-older adults (<65 years), early-stage older adults (65–74 years), and later-stage older adults (>75 years), based on categories provided by the long-term care insurance system in Japan [42]. Self-rated health [43–45], pre-existing metabolic syndromes [46,47], and motivation [48,49] were found to be associated with walking/PA in previous studies. Months participating in YWPP was considered because the effect of pedometers on participants' walking levels might vary over time [50].

Regarding motivation for participation, we identified four categories—health motivation, profit motivation, data confirmation motivation, and interaction motivation—based on the result of a hierarchical cluster analysis of the original 10 hypothesized options from which participants could select multiple answers (Table A2).

Survey options selected by a small percentage of participants were merged into four variables—occupation, self-rated health, frequency of greetings and conversations with neighbors, and change in step counts—as shown in Table 1.

### 2.4. Statistical Analysis

Multivariate categorical regression was used in both analyses. Categorical regression quantifies categorical variables using optimal scaling and assigns numerical values to categories. It simultaneously scales nominal, ordinal, and numerical variables and treats quantified categorical variables in the same way as numerical variables. Scaling all variables at the numerical level results in standard multiple regression analysis of the transformed variables [51]. In our analyses, all variables including outcome variables were transformed into numerical variables.

The output of the analysis comprises regression coefficients, their statistical significance, and Pratt's relative importance measure of predictors, which is large for predictors that are crucial to the regression and useful in interpreting predictor contributions to the regression, for all explanatory and control variables [51].

The significance level was set at $p < 0.05$. All statistical analyses were conducted using IBM SPSS Statistics 23 (IBM Corp., Armonk, NY, USA).

**Table 1.** Characteristics of the study samples and questionnaire results (*n* = 2023).

| Variables | Options | *n* | % |
|---|---|---|---|
| **Control variables** | | | |
| Sex | Male | 869 | 43.0 |
| | Female | 1154 | 57.0 |
| Age (years) | <65 | 781 | 38.6 |
| | 65–74 | 778 | 38.5 |
| | 75+ | 464 | 22.9 |
| Occupation | Full-time | 367 | 18.1 |
| | Part-time/self-employed | 407 | 20.1 |
| | Non-worker/other | 1249 | 61.7 |
| Self-rated health (before participation) | Healthy | 646 | 31.9 |
| | Rather healthy | 1158 | 57.2 |
| | (Rather) unhealthy | 219 | 10.8 |
| Diagnosis of metabolic syndrome (before participation) | Yes | 262 | 13.0 |
| | Preliminary | 238 | 11.8 |
| | No | 1523 | 75.3 |
| Motivation for participation in YWPP (Multiple Answers) | Health | 1607 | 79.4 |
| | Profit | 1282 | 63.4 |
| | Data confirmation | 945 | 46.7 |
| | Interaction | 574 | 28.4 |
| Months participating in YWPP | <12 | 421 | 20.8 |
| | 12–24 | 512 | 25.3 |
| | 24+ | 1090 | 53.9 |
| **Explanatory variables** | | | |
| Frequency of greetings and conversations with neighbors | Increased | 195 | 9.6 |
| | Slightly increased | 621 | 30.7 |
| | Not changed/(slightly) decreased | 1207 | 59.7 |
| Distance to the nearest railway station | <500 m | 583 | 28.8 |
| | 500–800 m | 556 | 27.5 |
| | 800–1100 m | 286 | 14.1 |
| | 1100 m+ | 598 | 29.6 |
| Bus stop density (per km$^2$) | <3 | 330 | 16.3 |
| | 3–7.5 | 969 | 47.9 |
| | 7.5–12 | 534 | 26.4 |
| | 12+ | 190 | 9.4 |
| **Outcome variables** | | | |
| Modal shift | Yes | 548 | 27.1 |
| | Mostly yes | 578 | 28.6 |
| | Mostly no | 432 | 21.4 |
| | No | 465 | 23.0 |
| Change in step counts | Increased | 910 | 45.0 |
| | Slightly increased | 408 | 20.2 |
| | Not changed/decreased | 705 | 34.9 |

## 3. Results

### 3.1. Sample Statistics

Participant characteristics and questionnaire results are presented in Table 1. Regarding outcome variables, more than half of the participants disclosed that they had "shifted from cars to public transport/slightly shifted", and approximately two-thirds of participants reported that their step counts had "increased/slightly increased" after participation in YWPP. Approximately 40% reported that their frequency of greetings and conversations with neighbors "increased/slightly increased".

Regarding the control variables, males constituted 43.0% of the sample. The mean age of the participants was 65.7 (±11.1) years, with 61.4% being more than 65 years old as of the end of May 2017. Only 18.1% of the participants had full-time jobs, reflecting the old age of the sample population. Approximately 90% reported that prior to participation in the program, they had been "healthy/rather healthy", with less than 25% having been diagnosed with a metabolic syndrome. More than half had participated in YWPP for more than 24 months at the time of the survey. As the motivation for participation in YWPP, health, profit, data confirmation, and interaction were selected by 79.4%, 63.4%, 46.7%, and 28.4% of the participants, respectively.

## 3.2. Modal Shift

The left side of Table 2 shows the results of the first analysis, and Table 3 shows the numerical values assigned to the categorical variables. The variables with the most and the second-most importance were, respectively, health motivation and frequency of greetings and conversations with neighbors.

**Table 2.** Results of categorical regression.

| Outcome Variables | Modal Shift | | | | Change in Step Counts | | | |
|---|---|---|---|---|---|---|---|---|
| | B | p | | Importance | B | p | | Importance |
| Sex | 0.048 | 0.031 | * | 0.013 | 0.026 | 0.147 | | 0.002 |
| Age (years) | 0.040 | 0.082 | | 0.046 | 0.067 | 0.000 | *** | 0.020 |
| Occupation | 0.056 | 0.007 | ** | 0.057 | 0.062 | 0.001 | ** | 0.033 |
| Self-rated health [a] | −0.001 | 1.000 | | 0.000 | −0.039 | 0.141 | | 0.007 |
| Diagnosis of metabolic syndrome [a] | 0.043 | 0.009 | ** | 0.019 | 0.016 | 0.294 | | 0.002 |
| Motivation:   Health | 0.203 | 0.000 | *** | 0.383 | 0.158 | 0.000 | *** | 0.172 |
| rofit | 0.029 | 0.136 | | 0.011 | 0.017 | 0.260 | | −0.001 |
| Data confirmation | 0.036 | 0.079 | | 0.007 | 0.027 | 0.123 | | 0.004 |
| Interaction | 0.030 | 0.113 | | 0.020 | 0.059 | 0.003 | ** | 0.030 |
| Months participating in YWPP | 0.057 | 0.001 | *** | 0.036 | 0.018 | 0.223 | | 0.005 |
| Frequency of greetings and conversations with neighbors | 0.199 | 0.000 | *** | 0.375 | 0.103 | 0.000 | *** | 0.097 |
| Distance to the nearest railway station | 0.038 | 0.008 | ** | 0.014 | 0.019 | 0.139 | | 0.002 |
| Bus stop density (per km$^2$) | 0.051 | 0.000 | *** | 0.019 | 0.035 | 0.006 | ** | 0.003 |
| Modal shift | | | | | 0.369 | 0.000 | *** | 0.623 |
| p | 0 | | | | 0 | | | |
| Adjusted R$^2$ | 0.129 | | | | 0.260 | | | |

B: regression coefficient (beta); p: statistical significance of coefficient (* < 0.05, ** < 0.01, *** < 0.001); importance: Pratt's relative importance measure of predictors; [a] before participation.

Regarding physical environment, distance to the nearest railway station as well as bus stop density were also significantly associated with the outcome variable. Participants living in neighborhoods far from railway stations (more than 1100 m) and those with a high bus stop density (more than 12 per km$^2$) tended to shift from cars to public transport. Figure 1 shows the spatial distribution of such neighborhoods—neighborhoods far from railway stations were located in suburban hilly areas and coastal industrial zones, while most neighborhoods with a high bus stop density were located near city centers.

Regarding the other control variables, being male, unemployed, diagnosed with a metabolic syndrome before participation, and longer months participating in YWPP were positively associated with modal shifts, while age and self-rated health were not. The adjusted R$^2$ of the regression was 0.129.

**Table 3.** Numerical values assigned to the categories.

| Variables | Categories | Outcome Variables | |
|---|---|---|---|
| | | Modal Shift | Change in Step Counts |
| Sex | Male | −1.152 | −1.152 |
| | Female | 0.868 | 0.868 |
| Age (years) | <65 | 1.261 | 0.352 |
| | 65–74 | −0.810 | −1.168 |
| | 75+ | −0.764 | 1.366 |
| Occupation | Full-time | 1.684 | 1.310 |
| | Part-time/self-employed | 0.807 | 1.234 |
| | Non-worker/other | −0.758 | −0.787 |
| Self-rated health [a] (before participation) | Healthy | −0.598 | −0.390 |
| | Rather healthy | −0.200 | −0.325 |
| | (Rather) unhealthy | 2.823 | 2.869 |
| Diagnosis of metabolic syndrome (before participation) | Yes | −1.157 | 1.468 |
| | Preliminary | −2.254 | −2.453 |
| | No | 0.551 | 0.131 |
| Motivation | | | |
| Health | Yes | −0.509 | −0.509 |
| | No | 1.965 | 1.965 |
| Profit | Yes | 0.760 | −0.760 |
| | No | −1.315 | 1.315 |
| Data confirmation | Yes | −1.068 | −1.068 |
| | No | 0.936 | 0.936 |
| Interaction | Yes | −1.589 | −1.589 |
| | No | 0.629 | 0.629 |
| Months participating in YWPP | <12 | 1.824 | 0.975 |
| | 12–24 | −1.061 | 1.164 |
| | 24+ | −0.206 | −0.923 |
| Frequency of greetings and conversations with neighbors [a] | Increased | −2.455 | −2.027 |
| | Slightly increased | −0.614 | −0.883 |
| | Not changed/(slightly) decreased | 0.713 | 0.782 |
| Distance to the nearest train station | <500 m | 1.054 | 0.460 |
| | 500–800 m | 0.516 | −0.380 |
| | 800–1100 m | −0.167 | 2.008 |
| | 1100 m+ | −1.428 | −1.056 |
| Bus stop density (per km$^2$) | <3 | 1.613 | -0.986 |
| | 3–7.5 | −0.156 | 0.506 |
| | 7.5–12 | 0.154 | 0.607 |
| | 12+ | −2.436 | −2.573 |
| Modal shift [a] | Yes | −1.394 | −1.146 |
| | Rather yes | −0.191 | −0.498 |
| | Rather no | 0.655 | 0.503 |
| | No | 1.272 | 1.503 |
| Change in step counts [a] | Increased | | −0.887 |
| | Slightly increased | | −0.334 |
| | Not changed/decreased | | 1.338 |

[a] The order of the categories is preserved in the optimally scaled variables.

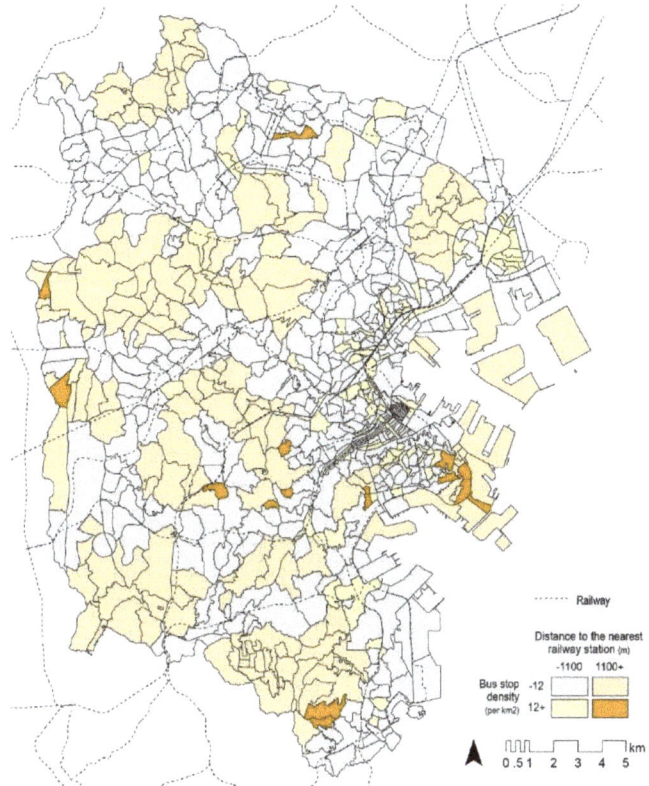

**Figure 1.** Spatial distribution of accessibility to public transport.

*3.3. Change in Step Counts*

The right side of Table 2 shows the results of the second analysis, with Table 3 showing the numerical values assigned to categorical variables. The variable with the most importance by far was modal shift. This was followed by health motivation and by frequency of greetings and conversations with neighbors, both of which were highly associated with the outcome variable in the first analysis.

Regarding physical environment, bus stop density was significantly associated with increased step counts. Those living in neighborhoods more than 1100 m away from the nearest railway station tended to increase their step counts, although the variable was not statistically significant.

Regarding the other control variables, ages between 65 and 74 years, non-workers, and interaction motivation were positively associated with increased step counts, while sex, self-rated health, and months participating in YWPP were not. The adjusted $R^2$ of the regression was 0.260, which was higher than the first analysis.

## 4. Discussion

This study examined aspects of the physical and social environments of middle-aged and older participants, who volunteered to use free pedometers, that are associated with modal shifts and increases in step counts in Yokohama, Japan. Although the adjusted $R^2$ of the regression was not high in the two analyses, eight and seven variables were statistically significant in the respective analyses.

The results of the first analysis showed that participants living in neighborhoods far from railway stations and in neighborhoods with a high bus stop density tended to engage in modal shifts. This shift may have occurred because local buses are used for shorter trips than railways, and participants changed their short trip transport mode from cars to buses. On the other hand, participants living near railway stations seemed unable to change their transport mode while participating in the program. This may be because these participants had used cars less frequently than suburban participants prior to participation because of the general features of the city's transit-oriented development, such as "less convenience for cars and special consideration for pedestrians" [26].

The second half of the study showed that participants' modal shifts were most associated with increases in their step counts. These results suggest that participation in YWPP promoted modal shifts and walking instead of driving. As seen with modal shifts, living in neighborhoods with a high bus stop density tended to increase participants' step counts. Although not statistically significant, participants living in neighborhoods far from railway stations tended to increase their step counts. Particularly in light of the results of a previous study on a Japanese rural city that demonstrated that distance to bus stops had significant relationship with PA, but distance to railway stations did not [52], future studies should explore the role of public transport not only by distinguishing railway and bus modalities, but urban and rural environmental differences as well.

Participants' frequency of greetings and conversations with others, as a proxy for social environment, was positively associated with modal shifts and increases in step counts. Considering the causal relationship, identified by a quasi-longitudinal study [53], in which changes in socializing with neighbors had a positive impact on walking activities, the provision of pedometers in our study might encourage opportunities for communication with other participants and promote participants to go out and use public transport together.

With regard to control variables, motivation to participate in YWPP must be highlighted. Health motivation had a positive association with both modal shift and increased step counts, while self-rated health before participation was not statistically significant. Interaction motivation was also positively associated with increased step counts, a finding potentially driven by the fact that expanded social connections may have contributed to increased frequencies of going out, as discussed above. On the other hand, the other categories of motivations—profit motivation and data confirmation motivation—were not found to be statistically significant in either analysis. These aspects of YWPP appear to not be useful in promoting modal shifts and increased walking.

While participants with preliminary metabolic syndromes tended to report relatively high levels of modal shifts, those with metabolic syndrome did not do so. This result is consistent with previous studies demonstrating that the conditions of overweight and obesity are causally associated with future inactivity [54,55]. These findings suggest the importance of intervention at an early stage because PA promotion for obese and overweight people is more difficult. Considering the fact that health motivation was found to be positively associated with both modal shifts and increased step counts, providing pedometers and PA education during health examinations may be effective at preventing and treating metabolic syndrome.

In Japan, many municipalities list health promotion as a benefit of compact cities as well as the reduction of environmental load [6]. In depopulated areas, however, bus routes may decrease in frequency or even withdraw from these areas entirely, a reality that is undesirable from the viewpoint of health promotion. As such, bus routes and availability should be sustained. During the realization of compact cities, non-physical policies such as MM programs should be promoted in the short-term, informed by collaboration between public health and city planning professionals. Pedometer intervention may prove to be a critical component of such policies, one that contributes to a healthy active urban population.

While making an important contribution to existing research on neighborhood environments and people's active behaviors, this study has some limitations. Retrospective questions on participants' public transport use, step counts, self-reported health, and communication frequency with neighbors may be subject to recall bias. Changes in step counts reported in our questionnaire might also be subject to self-reporting bias, as we lacked measures of step counts before the pedometer intervention. In addition, study participants may not be representative of the general population of Yokohama city in that they were motivated to have pedometers, suggesting a higher baseline interest in PA than others. We cannot know precisely the effect of pedometers in reality as in a control experiment due to the absence of comparison with non-participants. Lastly, only the physical environment of neighborhoods in which participants lived was considered in this study. Future studies should examine more detailed factors for modal shifts and the promotion of walking through pedometer use by considering physical and social environments not only around participant homes, but workplaces and favorite places as well. This may be done using travel diary data or GPS data.

## 5. Conclusions

This study examined the relationship between the physical and social environments of middle-aged and older YWPP participants who volunteered to use free pedometers, and their modal shifts from cars to walking and public transport. This study further considered if participants' modal shifts were associated with increases in their step counts using questionnaire data. The results of multivariate categorical regression analysis find that the frequency of greetings and conversations with neighbors as well as health motivation are highly associated with modal shift. Regarding physical environment characteristics, participants living in neighborhoods far from railway stations and in neighborhoods with a high bus stop density tended to shift to walking and public transport. In addition, modal shift was by far the most associated with increased step counts. This study's results suggest that pedometer intervention could be an effective component of MM programs that promote healthier, active cities.

**Author Contributions:** Formal analysis, K.H.; Funding acquisition, K.H. and A.T.; Writing—original draft, K.H.; Writing—review and editing, A.T., M.H., and D.T.

**Funding:** This research was supported by JSPS KAKENHI, grant numbers 18H01602 and 26249073.

**Acknowledgments:** We thank the staff of Yokohama city for their generous support of this research. Due to a confidentiality agreement with survey respondents, raw data of the questionnaire cannot be shared.

**Conflicts of Interest:** The authors declare no conflict of interest.

## Appendix A

Table A1. Questions asked in the survey.

| Variables | Questions Asked in the Survey |
| --- | --- |
| Self-rated health (before participation) | How did you feel about your health? (before participation) |
| Diagnosis of metabolic syndrome (before participation) | Have you been diagnosed with metabolic syndrome in a periodic health examination or a medical examination? (before participation) |
| Frequency of greetings and conversations with neighbors | Did the frequency of greetings and holding conversations with neighbors increase compared to the frequency pre-participation in YWPP? |
| Modal shift | Did the frequency of walking or using public transport increase while decreasing the frequency of car or motor bike use when going out (e.g., commuting and going shopping) after participating in YWPP? |
| Change in step counts | Did your daily step count change after participating in YWPP? |

**Table A2.** Motivation for participation in YWPP (multiple answer).

| Categories | Options | n | % |
|---|---|---|---|
| Health motivation | Can promote health while enjoying | 1406 | 69.5 |
| | Good chance to begin walking | 666 | 32.9 |
| | Can feel healthy | 261 | 12.9 |
| Profit motivation | Can get a pedometer | 926 | 45.8 |
| | Can win prizes | 715 | 35.3 |
| | Can donate | 255 | 12.6 |
| Data confirmation motivation | Can confirm data of step counts and rank | 945 | 46.7 |
| Interaction motivation | Can walk with families and friends | 502 | 24.8 |
| | Can interact with other participants | 125 | 6.2 |
| (None) | Can participate with office colleagues | 41 | 2.0 |

Measure: Phi 4-point correlation, cluster method: centroid clustering. Nine options were categorized into four using hierarchical cluster analysis. The last option (Can participate with office colleagues) was not included in any category because it was not clustered with any of the other nine options and its selection rate was the lowest. When a participant selected any options in category A, the binary variable of the category A was 1.

## References

1. Lee, I.-M.; Shiroma, E.J.; Lobelo, F.; Puska, P.; Blair, S.N.; Katzmarzyk, P.T.; Lancet Physical Activity Series Working Group. Effect of physical inactivity on major non-communicable diseases worldwide: An analysis of burden of disease and life expectancy. *Lancet* **2012**, *380*, 219–229. [CrossRef]
2. World Health Organization. *Global Action Plan on Physical Activity 2018–2030: More Active People for a Healthier World*; World Health Organization: Geneva, Switzerland, 2018.
3. Giles-Corti, B.; Vernez-Moúdon, A.; Reis, R.; Turrell, G.; Dannenberg, A.L.; Badland, H.; Foster, S.; Lowe, M.; Sallis, J.F.; Stevenson, M.; et al. City planning and population health: A global challenge. *Lancet* **2016**, *388*, 2912–2924. [CrossRef]
4. Sallis, J.F.; Bull, F.; Burdett, R.; Frank, L.D.; Griffiths, P.; Giles-Corti, B.; Stevenson, M. Use of science to guide city planning policy and practice: How to achieve healthy and sustainable future cities. *Lancet* **2016**, *388*, 2936–2947. [CrossRef]
5. Stevenson, M.; Thompson, J.; de Sá, T.H.; Ewing, R.; Mohan, D.; McClure, R.; Roberts, I.; Tiwari, G.; Giles-Corti, B.; Sun, X.; et al. Land use, transport, and population health: Estimating the health benefits of compact cities. *Lancet* **2016**, *388*, 2925–2935. [CrossRef]
6. Mministry of Land Infrastructure Transport and Tourism Promotion of Urban Renovation and Compact Cities. Available online: https://www.mlit.go.jp/common/000996976.pdf (accessed on 16 March 2019).
7. Lee, J.; Kurisu, K.; An, K.; Hanaki, K. Development of the compact city index and its application to Japanese cities. *Urban Stud.* **2015**, *52*, 1054–1070. [CrossRef]
8. Takami, K.; Hatoyama, K. Sustainable regeneration of a car-dependent city: The case of Toyama toward a compact city. In *Sustainable City Regions*; Kidokoro, T., Harata, N., Subanu, L.P., Jessen, J., Motte, A., Seltzer, E.P., Eds.; cSUR-UT Series: Library for Sustainable Urban Regeneration; Springer: Tokyo, Japan, 2008; Volume 7, pp. 183–200, ISBN 978-4-431-78146-2.
9. Fujii, S.; Taniguchi, A. Determinants of the effectiveness of travel feedback programs-a review of communicative mobility management measures for changing travel behaviour in Japan. *Transp. Policy* **2006**, *13*, 339–348. [CrossRef]
10. Taniguchi, A.; Fujii, S. Promoting public transport using marketing techniques in mobility management and verifying their quantitative effects. *Transportation* **2007**, *34*, 37–49. [CrossRef]
11. Enoch, M. *Sustainable Transport, Mobility Management and Travel Plans*; Routledge: Abingdon, UK, 2016; ISBN 9781315611563.
12. Taylor, M.A.P. Voluntary travel behavior change programs in Australia: The carrot rather than the stick in travel demand management. *Int. J. Sustain. Transp.* **2007**, *1*, 173–192. [CrossRef]

13. Bamberg, S.; Fujii, S.; Friman, M.; Gärling, T. Behaviour theory and soft transport policy measures. *Transp. Policy* **2011**, *18*, 228–235. [CrossRef]

14. Nurdden, A.; Rahmat, R.A.O.K.; Ismail, A. Effect of Transportation Policies on Modal Shift from Private Car to Public Transport in Malaysia. *J. Appl. Sci.* **2007**, *7*, 1013–1018.

15. Anwar, A.M.; Yang, J. Examining the Effects of Transport Policy on Modal Shift from Private Car to Public Bus. *Procedia Eng.* **2017**, *180*, 1413–1422. [CrossRef]

16. Tuan, V.A. Mode Choice Behavior and Modal Shift to Public Transport in Developing Countries—The Case of Hanoi City. *J. East. Asia Soc. Transp. Stud.* **2015**, *11*, 473–487.

17. Sunio, V.; Schmöcker, J.; Estuar, R.; Dela, B.L. Development and Usability Evaluation of Blaze Information System for Promoting Sustainable Travel Behaviour in Metro Manila. *J. East. Asia Soc. Transp. Stud.* **2017**, *12*, 2428–2443.

18. Sunio, V.; Schmöcker, J.D. Can we promote sustainable travel behavior through mobile apps? Evaluation and review of evidence. *Int. J. Sustain. Transp.* **2017**, *11*, 553–566. [CrossRef]

19. Taniguchi, A.; Suzuki, H.; Fujii, S. Mobility Management in Japan: Its Development and Meta-Analysis of Travel Feedback Programs. *Transp. Res. Rec.* **2007**, *2021*, 100–109. [CrossRef]

20. Sasaki, H.; Fujimoto, S.; Taniguchi, A.; Nakahara, S. Mobility Management for Health Promotion in Cooperation with Local Government Urban Transport Planning and Public Health Departments. *J. Transp. Health* **2017**, *5*, S90. [CrossRef]

21. Ogilvie, D.; Foster, C.E.; Rothnie, H.; Cavill, N.; Hamilton, V.; Fitzsimons, C.F.; Mutrie, N. Interventions to promote walking: Systematic review. *BMJ* **2007**, *334*, 1204. [CrossRef] [PubMed]

22. Wallmann, B.; Spittaels, H.; De Bourdeaudhuij, I.; Froboese, I. The perception of the neighborhood environment changes after participation in a pedometer based community intervention. *Int. J. Behav. Nutr. Phys. Act.* **2012**, *9*, 33. [CrossRef]

23. Harris, T.J.; Owen, C.G.; Victor, C.R.; Adams, R.; Cook, D.G. What factors are associated with physical activity in older people, assessed objectively by accelerometry? *Br. J. Sports Med.* **2009**, *43*, 442–450. [CrossRef]

24. Bravata, D.M.; Smith-Spangler, C.; Sundaram, V.; Gienger, A.L.; Lin, N.; Lewis, R.; Stave, C.D.; Olkin, I.; Sirard, J.R. Using pedometers to increase physical activity and improve health: A systematic review. *JAMA* **2007**, *298*, 2296–2304. [CrossRef]

25. Besser, L.M.; Dannenberg, A.L. Walking to Public Transit. *Am. J. Prev. Med.* **2005**, *29*, 273–280. [CrossRef] [PubMed]

26. Brown, B.B.; Yamada, I.; Smith, K.R.; Zick, C.D.; Kowaleski-Jones, L.; Fan, J.X. Mixed land use and walkability: Variations in land use measures and relationships with BMI, overweight, and obesity. *Health Place* **2009**, *15*, 1130–1141. [CrossRef] [PubMed]

27. McCormack, G.R.; Giles-Corti, B.; Bulsara, M. The relationship between destination proximity, destination mix and physical activity behaviors. *Prev. Med.* **2008**, *46*, 33–40. [CrossRef] [PubMed]

28. De Bourdeaudhuij, I.; Sallis, J.F.; Saelens, B.E. Environmental correlates of physical activity in a sample of Belgian adults. *Am. J. Health Promot.* **2003**, *18*, 83–92. [CrossRef] [PubMed]

29. Sallis, J.F.; Spoon, C.; Cavill, N.; Engelberg, J.K.; Gebel, K.; Parker, M.; Thornton, C.M.; Lou, D.; Wilson, A.L.; Cutter, C.L.; et al. Co-benefits of designing communities for active living: An exploration of literature. *Int. J. Behav. Nutr. Phys. Act.* **2015**, *12*, 30. [CrossRef] [PubMed]

30. Pikora, T.J.; Giles-Corti, B.; Knuiman, M.W.; Bull, F.C.; Jamrozik, K.; Donovan, R.J. Neighborhood environmental factors correlated with walking near home: Using SPACES. *Med. Sci. Sports Exerc.* **2006**, *38*, 708–714. [CrossRef] [PubMed]

31. Van Dyck, D.; Deforche, B.; Cardon, G.; De Bourdeaudhuij, I. Neighbourhood walkability and its particular importance for adults with a preference for passive transport. *Health Place* **2009**, *15*, 496–504. [CrossRef] [PubMed]

32. Sallis, J.F.; Cerin, E.; Conway, T.L.; Adams, M.A.; Frank, L.D.; Pratt, M.; Salvo, D.; Schipperijn, J.; Smith, G.; Cain, K.L.; et al. Physical activity in relation to urban environments in 14 cities worldwide: A cross-sectional study. *Lancet* **2016**, *387*, 2207–2217. [CrossRef]

33. Knuiman, M.W.; Divitini, M.L.; Foster, S.A.; Christian, H.E.; Giles-Corti, B.; Bull, F.C.; Badland, H.M. A Longitudinal Analysis of the Influence of the Neighborhood Built Environment on Walking for Transportation: The RESIDE Study. *Am. J. Epidemiol.* **2014**, *180*, 453–461. [CrossRef]

34. Koohsari, M.; Nakaya, T.; Oka, K. Activity-Friendly Built Environments in a Super-Aged Society, Japan: Current Challenges and toward a Research Agenda. *Int. J. Environ. Res. Public Health* **2018**, *15*, 2054. [CrossRef]

35. Committee on Transportation Policy in Yokohama City. *A Report on Transportation Policy in Yokohama City*; Committee on Transportation Policy in Yokohama City: Yokohama, Japan, 2010.

36. Yokohama City. *Yokohama City Transportation Plan*; Yokohama City: Yokohama, Japan, 2018.

37. Hino, K.; Lee, J.S.; Asami, Y. Associations between seasonal meteorological conditions and the daily step count of adults in Yokohama, Japan: Results of year-round pedometer measurements in a large population. *Prev. Med. Rep.* **2017**, *8*, 15–17. [CrossRef]

38. Hino, K.; Asami, Y.; Lee, J.S. Step Counts of Middle-Aged and Elderly Adults for 10 Months Before and After the Release of Pokémon GO in Yokohama, Japan. *J. Med. Internet Res.* **2019**, *21*, e10724. [CrossRef] [PubMed]

39. Ministry of Land Infrastructure Transport and Tourism National Land Numerical Information Download Service. Available online: http://nlftp.mlit.go.jp/ksj/index.html (accessed on 16 March 2019).

40. Kawachi, I.; Berkman, L.F. *Neighborhoods and Health*; Oxford University Press: New York, NY, USA, 2003; pp. 1–352.

41. Seino, S.; Kitamura, A.; Nishi, M.; Tomine, Y.; Tanaka, I.; Taniguchi, Y.; Yokoyama, Y.; Amano, H.; Narita, M.; Ikeuchi, T.; et al. Individual- and community-level neighbor relationships and physical activity among older Japanese adults living in a metropolitan area: A cross-sectional multilevel analysis. *Int. J. Behav. Nutr. Phys. Act.* **2018**, *15*, 1–11. [CrossRef]

42. Ministry of Health. Labour and Welfare Long-term Care Insurance in Japan. Available online: https://www.mhlw.go.jp/english/topics/elderly/care/index.html (accessed on 26 May 2019).

43. Inoue, S.; Ohya, Y.; Odagiri, Y.; Takamiya, T.; Ishii, K.; Kitabayashi, M.; Suijo, K.; Sallis, J.F.; Shimomitsu, T. Association between Perceived Neighborhood Environment and Walking among Adults in 4 Cities in Japan. *J. Epidemiol.* **2010**, *20*, 277–286. [CrossRef] [PubMed]

44. Inoue, S.; Ohya, Y.; Odagiri, Y.; Takamiya, T.; Kamada, M.; Okada, S.; Oka, K.; Kitabatake, Y.; Nakaya, T.; Sallis, J.F.; et al. Perceived Neighborhood Environment and Walking for Specific Purposes Among Elderly Japanese. *J. Epidemiol.* **2011**, *21*, 481–490. [CrossRef] [PubMed]

45. Turrell, G.; Haynes, M.; Wilson, L.A.; Giles-Corti, B. Can the built environment reduce health inequalities? A study of neighbourhood socioeconomic disadvantage and walking for transport. *Health Place* **2013**, *19*, 89–98. [CrossRef] [PubMed]

46. Naeini, F.; Najafian, J.; Nouri, F.; Mohammadifard, N. Relation between usual daily walking time and metabolic syndrome. *Niger. Med. J.* **2014**, *55*, 29. [CrossRef]

47. Jefferis, B.J.; Parsons, T.J.; Sartini, C.; Ash, S.; Lennon, L.T.; Wannamethee, S.G.; Lee, I.M.; Whincup, P.H. Does duration of physical activity bouts matter for adiposity and metabolic syndrome? A cross-sectional study of older British men. *Int. J. Behav. Nutr. Phys. Act.* **2016**, *13*, 36. [CrossRef]

48. Stephan, Y.; Boiché, J.; Le Scanff, C. Motivation and physical activity behaviors among older women: A self-determination perspective. *Psychol. Women Q.* **2010**, *34*, 339–348. [CrossRef]

49. Brunet, J.; Sabiston, C.M. Exploring motivation for physical activity across the adult lifespan. *Psychol. Sport Exerc.* **2011**, *12*, 99–105. [CrossRef]

50. Robertson, L.B.; Ward Thompson, C.; Aspinall, P.; Millington, C.; McAdam, C.; Mutrie, N. The influence of the local neighbourhood environment on walking levels during the walking for wellbeing in the west pedometer-based community intervention. *J. Environ. Public Health* **2012**, *2012*, 974786. [CrossRef]

51. IBM Corporation. IBM SPSS Statistics V23.0 Documentation. Available online: https://www.ibm.com/support/knowledgecenter/en/SSLVMB_23.0.0/spss/product_landing.html (accessed on 16 March 2019).

52. Kamada, M.; Kitayuguchi, J.; Inoue, S.; Kamioka, H.; Mutoh, Y.; Shiwaku, K. Environmental correlates of physical activity in driving and non-driving rural Japanese women. *Prev. Med.* **2009**, *49*, 490–496. [CrossRef] [PubMed]

53. Handy, S.; Cao, X.; Mokhtarian, P.L. Self-selection in the relationship between the built environment and walking: Empirical evidence from Northern California. *J. Am. Plan. Assoc.* **2006**, *72*, 55–74. [CrossRef]

54. Ekelund, U.; Brage, S.; Besson, H.; Sharp, S.; Wareham, N.J. Time spent being sedentary and weight gain in healthy adults: Reverse or bidirectional causality? *Am. J. Clin. Nutr.* **2008**, *88*, 612–617. [CrossRef] [PubMed]
55. Metcalf, B.S.; Hosking, J.; Jeffery, A.N.; Voss, L.D.; Henley, W.; Wilkin, T.J. Fatness leads to inactivity, but inactivity does not lead to fatness: A longitudinal study in children (EarlyBird 45). *Arch. Dis. Child.* **2011**, *96*, 942–947. [CrossRef] [PubMed]

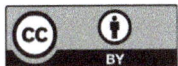

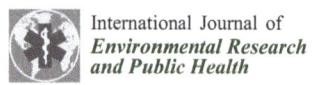
International Journal of
*Environmental Research
and Public Health*

*Review*

# Walkability, Overweight, and Obesity in Adults: A Systematic Review of Observational Studies

João Paulo dos Anjos Souza Barbosa [1,2,*], Paulo Henrique Guerra [2,3],
Crislaine de Oliveira Santos [2,4], Ana Paula de Oliveira Barbosa Nunes [2], Gavin Turrell [5]
and Alex Antonio Florindo [1,2,4]

[1] Nutrition Department, Graduate Program in Public Health Nutrition, School of Public Health, University of São Paulo, Sao Paulo City 01246-904, Brazil
[2] Physical Activity Epidemiology Group, University of Sao Paulo, Sao Paulo City 03828-000, Brazil
[3] Federal University of Fronteira Sul, Chapecó Campus, Chapecó 89815-899, Brazil
[4] School of Arts, Sciences and Humanities, Graduate Program in Physical Activity Sciences, University of Sao Paulo, Sao Paulo City 03828-000, Brazil
[5] Centre for Urban Research, School of Global, Urban and Social Studies, RMIT University, Melbourne, VIC 3000, Australia
* Correspondence: jpdosanjos@usp.br

Received: 23 March 2019; Accepted: 13 July 2019; Published: 28 August 2019

**Abstract:** We conducted a systematic review to describe and summarize possible associations between the walkability index, overweight, and obesity. Systematic searches using seven electronic databases and reference lists were conducted to identify papers published until December 2017. Observational studies, describing associations using regression-based statistical methods, published in English and Portuguese, reporting markers of overweight and obesity, and involving adults (≥18 years) were included. Of the 2469 references initially retrieved, ten were used for the descriptive synthesis. Seven studies showed significant inverse associations between walkability and overweight and obesity, however, all were cross-sectional studies. High risk of bias scores were observed in "selection bias" and "withdrawals and dropouts". All studies were published in high-income countries with sample sizes ranging among 75 to 649,513 participants. Weight and height as measures for determining BMI tended to be self-reported. Indicators of walkability, such as land-use mix, street connectivity and residential density were used as components of the indices. Based on this review, more studies should be conducted in low, middle, and middle-high income countries, using longitudinal designs that control neighborhood self-selection; other indicators of the neighborhood environment, such as food access, physical activity facilities, sidewalks, and safety and crime prevention should be considered.

**Keywords:** walkability; environment; overweight; obesity; review

## 1. Introduction

Overweight and obesity have risen dramatically over the last 40 years and they now constitute serious public health threats that are contributing to increasing rates of non-communicable disease such as type 2 diabetes and cardiovascular disease [1–3]. A recent publication gathering data from 239 prospective studies involving over 10 million individuals in four continents showed that the risk of mortality increases linearly with overweight (body mass index—BMI ≥ 25 kg/m$^2$) and mainly obesity (BMI ≥ 30 kg/m$^2$), regardless of age or sex [4]. A study of trends observed across 19 million participants shows a significant increase in BMI occurring over the last four decades, particularly in low- and middle-income countries. Between 1975 and 2014, the prevalence of age-standardized obesity increased 3.2% in 1975 to 10.8% in 2014 in men, and from 6.4 to 14.9% in women [5].

The major challenge faced relates to the fact that overweight and obesity are multi-factorial problems related mainly to behavioral variables, such as physical activity and diet [6], and these variables are related to health policies and living environments [7]. The built environment is defined as the physical form of neighborhoods, including patterns of land use, built and natural structures, and transportation systems [8]. The presence of an "obesogenic environment" hampers the adoption of healthy behaviors, such as maintaining a healthy diet, engaging in physical activity and limiting sedentary behavior [9–13]. Hence, obesogenic environments have emerged as the sum of influences that the surroundings, opportunities, or conditions of life have on promoting obesity in individuals or populations [9].

Walkability constitutes part of the built environment concept that can be operationalized when taking into account the setting and population under study and that appeared in the health field in the mid-2000s [14]. However, different built environment features have been used to calculate walkability scores, depending on the places in which studies have been conducted. In addition, some studies have shown that such results can vary according to the socioeconomic level of a given location and to neighborhood self-selection patterns [15–18]. Further, in upper middle income countries, other factors such as high population density levels and rates of violence, were related to rates of overweight and obesity [19]. Three previous systematic reviews stressed the importance of walkability in relation to obesity although they had a broader scope for both exposure and outcomes. The reviews examined more general issues, one of them synthesized current evidence on longitudinal relationships between a built environment and cardio-metabolic health outcomes among adults [20], the second was focused on obesogenic environments in high income countries [21], and the last review investigated which GIS-based measures of walkability (density, land-use mix, connectivity, and walkability indices) in urban and suburban neighborhoods were used and which of them were associated with active transportation and weight-related measures in adults [22].

Given these findings, a broad and up-to-date review of observational studies specifically on walkability, overweight, and obesity is crucial to better understand these relationships in different countries, how built environment components forming walkability are devised and assessed, how statistical models have been specified, and the main results that are found. Therefore, our main objective is to describe and summarize the evidence on associations between walkability, overweight, and obesity in adults. This review will also provide the basis for built environment interventions to help address the overweight and obesity crisis.

## 2. Methods

The protocol of this review was registered on PROSPERO database (CRD42017071830). Its report is based on PRISMA checklist items [23].

The following inclusion criteria were adopted: (1) Observational studies (e.g., cross-sectional, cohort, time-series or case-control); (2) describing associations using regression-based statistical methods; (3) published in English and Portuguese; (4) reporting on overweight and obesity markers (5) that used walkability indices; and (6) using samples of adults (≥18 years). Articles not addressing the concept of walkability or that used separate indicators, that did not use markers of overweight or obesity, studies with children or adolescents, and qualitative and protocol studies were excluded.

To retrieve potential references, seven electronic databases were used: Pubmed, Scielo, Lilacs, Web of Science, Scopus, Physical Education Index, and SportDiscus. Systematic searches were conducted in accordance with the strategy (Supplementary Materials S1: Search string) applied by Pubmed: (((((((((((Neighborhood buffer[Text Word]) OR Neighborhood context[Text Word]) OR Walking locations[Text Word]) OR Space syntax[Text Word]) OR Street layout[Text Word]) OR Street design[Text Word]) OR Urban design[Text Word]) OR Urban form[Text Word]) OR Urban planning[Text Word]) OR Walkability[Text Word]) OR Walkable[Text Word])) AND ((((((Obesity[TextWord]) OR Overweight[Text Word]) OR Body Size[Text Word]) OR Body Weight[Text Word]) OR Body Mass Index[Text Word]) OR Adiposity[Text Word]). Using Lilacs and Scielo, searches were made in Portuguese using other terms such *"caminhabilidade"* and *"obesidade"*, *"sobrepeso"*, *"índice de massa corporal"*. Searches covered references available to December 2017. To avoid potential losses, manual searches through reference lists of the included studies were also performed.

Three researchers selected studies independently. Based on the systematic search results, titles and abstracts were screened, and then eligibility through a full text assessment was determined by all three researchers. Doubts and disagreements were resolved through a consensus meeting with a senior reviewer.

Data extraction involved the use of relevant information: Author (year), country/city/province/state (year of data collection), sampling, (n) sample, percentage of females, age (mean or range in years), and study type. Assessment of walkability variables: Geographic scale (e.g., census sectors, home addresses, post codes or geocoding buffers); geocoding of facilities; how walkability indicators were created and calculated. Assessments of overweight and obesity: How the markers were used (as categorical or dichotomous continuous variables); and the regression model used for analyses. Variables related to walkability, overweight, and obesity were extracted from included studies as significant or not significant associations at the 95% confidence interval or *"p"* values to better describe the odds ratio, beta coefficient, prevalence ratio, relative risks or other values with variables adjusted.

Risk of bias was evaluated with an adapted 12-item version, of the Effective Public Health Practice Project (EPHPP), proposed by Thomas et al. [24]. Other details of the assessment tool are given in Supplementary Materials S2. Original articles were assessed across seven methodological domains: (a) Selection bias (characteristics of the sample); (b) study design (information on the representativeness of the study, sampling methods); (c) confounders (control of relevant confounding factors of the analysis); (d) blinding (of assessors, outcomes and participants); (e) information on tools used to assess walkability and overweight/obesity (reports on previous validity and information, allowing for the reproducibility of the assessment of walkability and overweight/obesity); (f) withdrawals and dropouts (reported numbers and/or ratios and percentages of participants that completed the study); and (g) analysis (use of appropriate methods for analyses). The studies included were then classified by two previously trained researchers as presenting low, moderate or high levels of bias.

## 3. Results

Systematic searches retrieved 2469 potential articles. After the identification and removal of duplicate references (n = 116), 2353 references were screened by their titles and abstracts. Of these references, 69 were assessed from the full text. In view of the 59 rejected articles (for not addressing the main focuses of this review (n = 55) and for not reflecting qualitative and protocol studies (n = 4), 10 articles were used for the descriptive synthesis [15,25–33] (Figure 1).

Sample sizes ranged from 75 [29] to 649,513 participants [30] (Table 1). Regarding available data on as a percentage of female participants (n = 7), females predominated in four studies [15,27,28,31], and only three studies involved a lower percentage of females than males [25,29,32]. The youngest participants were 18 years old and the oldest was 90 years of age [25,32]. All studies were conducted in high-income countries, particularly in the United States (n = 6) [15,27,29,30,32,33], Canada [25,26,28], and Australia [31] (Table 1).

Six studies employed a cross-sectional design (58.3%) (Table 1) [15,29–33], two employed a longitudinal design [25,27] one applied both cross-sectional and longitudinal methods (n = 1) [26] and one used time-series analysis methods [28].

Of the three studies employing a longitudinal design, none showed significant results [25–27]. Most of the studies that found an inverse association between walkability and overweight and obesity were cross-sectional (n = 6) [15,29–33]. The study that used time-series analysis presented significant results for the walkability index and a lower prevalence of obesity [28].

Regarding assessments used to the measure walkability (Table 2), most studies investigated main spatial information through neighborhood geocoding by geospatial sector of interest (e.g., census tracts, home addresses or post codes) (n = 7) [25–28,30,32,33]. Of these studies, two used home addresses [27,32]. One measured walkability attributes (e.g., population density, street connectivity, food, and physical activity resources) within three Euclidean kilometers using time-varying geographic information system (GIS) data [34] linked to participants' geocoded home addresses [27]. Others used Mapping Analytics Inc., home addresses, walkability indicator population density levels, types of residences, median residence periods, and travel patterns [32].

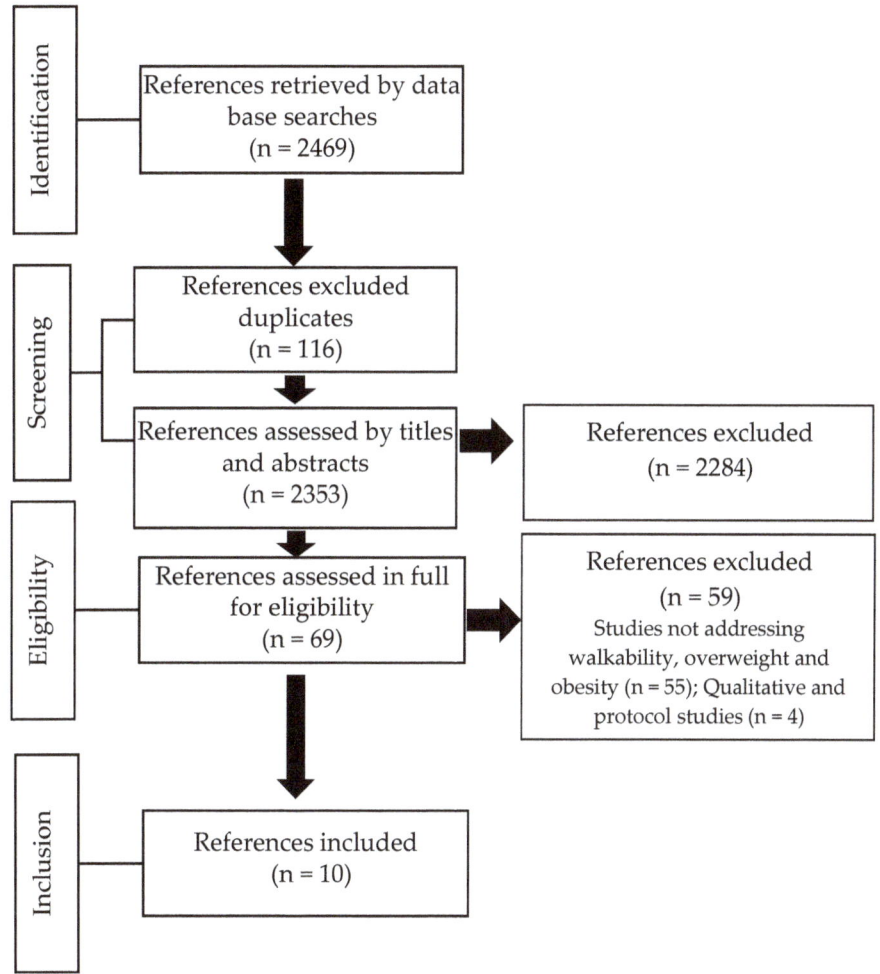

**Figure 1.** Systematic review flowchart.

Different buffer areas around residents' homes were employed in two studies, e.g., a 1-km network buffer measured on the street network of each individual's geocoded residence [15,29], and one study employed network buffers of 800 and 1600 m [31].

Variables used to measure walkability included residential and population density (n = 9; 91.6%), street connectivity (n = 8; 83.3%), and land-use mix (n = 5; 58.3%). Five studies defined walkability as the sum of the scores of main indicators with the index divided into quintiles [28] or quartiles [15] or expressed as a continuous score [30,32].

Scales and standard stadiometers (n = 3) [27,30,32] or self-reported measures (n = 7) [15,25,26,28,29,31,33] were used to measure weights and heights and to derive BMI scores to classify individuals as overweight (25–29.9 kg/m$^2$) and/or obese (≥30 kg/m$^2$). One study evaluated waist circumferences calculated from anthropometry measurements [27].

While various statistical analyses were employed, most studies used logistic regression analyses (n = 5) [15,27,30,31,33], while multi-level analyses were adopted in one study [25], one study used Poisson regression analysis [28] and another three studies used linear regression [26,29,32].

Eight studies adjusted and controlled variables employing different analysis models [25–32]. The main variables used for adjustment included sex, age, neighborhood socioeconomic status, ethnicity, physical activity, sedentary behavior, fruit and vegetable consumption, general health status, residential time, and the total number of household vehicles. Regarding the analyses by risk of bias, all included studies [15,25–33] were evaluated as low risk of bias in the domains "control of confounders", "assessment tools", and "statistical analysis" items. Moderate scores were observed in terms of "techniques used for sampling" (n = 7) [25,26,28–30,32,33], "report the blindness of the outcome assessor" (n = 10) [15,25–33], and "withdrawals and dropouts" (n = 4) [25,26,28,29]. High risk of bias scores were showed in "selection bias" (n = 1) [32] and "withdrawals and dropouts" (n = 5) [15,30–33] (Figure 2).

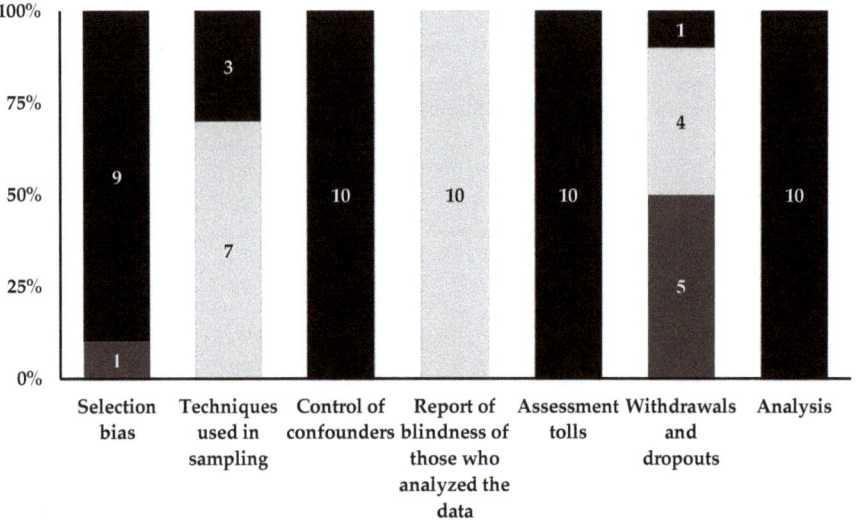

**Figure 2.** Risk of bias assessment of included articles (Black: low; Light grey: moderate; Dark grey: high). The numbers within the bars indicate the number of articles that were classified in the risk of bias classifications.

Some of the previously reported results are noteworthy (Table 3), such as an increased prevalence of obesity observed in less walkable neighborhoods for quintiles of an 11-year period for adults in Canada [28]. One study focused on 2088 adults in Atlanta, USA shows that being poorer, older, Black, and from a larger household is related to greater odds of being obese [15]. Higher walkability scores are associated with lower rates of obesity (OR = 0.67; 95% CI 0.49–0.89) [15]. Lathey et al. (2009) found inverse associations for moderate (OR = 0.62; $p < 0.05$) and high (OR = 0.50; $p < 0.001$) walkability relative to low walkability indices for obese adult residents in Arizona, USA (June 2003 to June 2005) [30].

When stratifying by sex, walkability indicators present relations with obesity for both sexes and particularly for variables measuring destination diversity [33] like the land use diversity of a given neighborhood.

When measuring "street design" in association with obesity, individuals living in highly compared with less walkable areas were less likely to be obese (1600 m OR: 0.84, 95% CI: 0.7 to 1; 800 m OR: 0.75, 95% CI: 0.62 to 0.9) [31].

Regarding other variables concerning walkability, only one study showed an inverse association between the proportion of inhabitants who walk to work and housing age (length of residence) to both men and women according to indicators of overweight and obesity. According to this study, the estimate of beta values was found to range from −6829 ($p < 0.001$) to −0.015 according to the BMI [33].

Three studies did not find associations between walkability, overweight, and obesity [25–27]. Two were longitudinal studies [25,27] while the other presented the results of cross-sectional and longitudinal analyses [26]. Despite not having found significant associations, it is important to note that these studies evaluated the changes in variables related to walkability as well as those of overweight and obesity. In addition, they referred to and discussed residential and neighborhood self-selection.

**Table 1.** Descriptive characteristics of the reviewed studies (n = 10).

| Reference | Country/City or Province or State (Year of Data Collection) | Sampling | Sample Size (n) | %F | Age (Mean or Range in Years) | Study Type |
|---|---|---|---|---|---|---|
| Berry et al., (2010b) [26] | Canada/Alberta (2002/2008) | nd | 1736 ** | nd | <50/≥50 | CS and L |
| Berry et al., (2010a) [25] | Canada/Alberta (2002/2008) | nd | 500 | 47.8 | 18–90 | L |
| Braun et al., (2016) [27] | USA (2000/2006) | R | 1079 | 54.8 | 44.7 | L |
| Creatore et al., (2016) [28] | Canada/Ontario (2001/2012) | nd | 5500 | 51.3 | 30–64 (1) | TS |
| Frank et al., (2006) [29] | USA/Washington (1999) | R | 75 | 44.5 | 20–65 | CS |
| Frank et al., (2007) [15] | USA/Atlanta (2001–2002) | R | 2088 | 50.6 | 40.9 | CS |
| Hoehner et al., (2011) [32] | USA/Texas (1987–2005) | nd | 16,543 | 30.3 | 18–90 (2) | CS |
| Lathey et al., (2009) [30] | USA/Arizona (2003–2005) | C | 649,513 | nd | 35.5 | CS |
| Muller-Riemenschneider et al., (2013) [31] | Australia/Perth (2003–2006) | R | 5970 | 58.0 | 25–≥65 (3) | CS |
| Smith et al., (2008) [33] | USA/Utah (2007–2008) | C | 453,927 | nd | 25–64 | CS |

Legends: ** longitudinal data for 572 participants and cross-sectional data for 1,164 participants; (1): Higher prevalence of people among 30–49 years old (66.7%); (2): Higher prevalence of people among 40–49 years old (39.1%); (3): Higher prevalence of people among 45–64 years old (40.7%); C: convenience; nd: not described; R: randomised; USA: United States of America; CS: Cross-sectional study; L: Longitudinal study; TS: Time-series study; %F: Percentage of females.

**Table 2.** Methodological characteristics of the descriptive studies.

| Reference | Assessment of Walkability/Study Scale/Geocoding of Facilities | Walkability Indicators Evaluated | Walkability Index Calculated | Assessment of Overweight and Obesity/Markers of Overweight and Obesity | Regression Model Used for Analyses of Associations |
|---|---|---|---|---|---|
| Berry et al., (2010b) [26] | Geocoding of neighborhoods from census data | Residential density (density of dwellings per area in residential use), land-use mix (floor areas of the following five uses: residential, retail, office, education/institutional (including religious establishments) and entertainment) and street connectivity (density of true intersections in each neighborhood). | The walkability index was calculated based on Frank et al.'s formula not including the z-score for the retail floor area, and z-scores for walkability were then classified with quantiles (five classes of equal intervals divided into very high, high, moderate, low and very low walkability neighborhood groups). | Self-reported weight and height/BMI | Linear regression/standardized and unstandardized coefficient - β |
| Berry et al., (2010a) [25] | Geocoding of neighborhoods from census data | Residential density (density of dwellings per area in residential use), land use mix (floor areas of the following five uses: residential, retail, office, education/institutional (including religious establishments) and entertainment) and street connectivity (density of true intersections in each neighborhood). | The walkability index was calculated based on Frank et al.'s formula not including the z-score for the retail floor area, and z-scores for walkability were then classified using quantiles (five classes of equal intervals divided into very high, high, moderate, low and very low walkability neighborhood groups). | Self-reported weight and height/BMI | Ordinal regression model/standardized and unstandardized coefficient - β |

Table 2. Cont.

| Reference | Assessment of Walkability/Study Scale/Geocoding of Facilities | Walkability Indicators Evaluated | Walkability Index Calculated | Assessment of Overweight and Obesity/Markers of Overweight and Obesity | Regression Model Used for Analyses of Associations |
|---|---|---|---|---|---|
| Braun et al., (2016) [27] | Geocoding from home addresses | Population density, street connectivity and food and physical activity resources within three Euclidean kilometers of each respondent's residential location. | The walkability index was determined from measures of population density, street connectivity, and food and physical activity resources measured from participants' pre- and post-move residential locations. | Anthropometric measurements determined from exams/BMI and WC | Fixed effect regression models (logistic and linear)/odds ratio and standardized and unstandardized coefficient - β |
| Creatore et al., (2016) [28] | Geocoding of neighborhoods from the Canadian census | Population density (number of persons per square kilometer), residential density (number of occupied residential dwellings per square kilometer), walkable destinations (number of retail stores, services [e.g., libraries, banks, community centers], and schools a ten minute walk away) and street connectivity (number of intersections with at least 3 converging roads or pathways) | Neighborhood walkability derived from a validated index with standardized scores of 0 to 100 and with higher scores denoting more walkability. Neighborhoods were ranked and classified into quintiles from lowest (quintile 1) to highest (quintile 5) walkability. | Self-reported weight and height/BMI | Poisson Regression |
| Frank et al., (2006) [29] | Geocoding, 1 km network buffer | Net residential density (residential units divided by acres in residential use), street connectivity (intersections per square kilometre), land use mix (A/ln (N)) by entropy), and the retail floor area ratio (FAR) (the retail building floor area divided by the retail land area) | Sum of $z$-scores of land-use mix and net residential and intersection density | Self-reported weight and height/BMI | Linear regression/standardized and unstandardized coefficient - β |
| Frank et al., (2007) [15] | Geocoding, 1 km network buffer | Net residential density (residential units divided by acres in residential use), street connectivity (intersections per square kilometer), land use mix (A/ln (N)) by entropy), the retail floor area ratio (FAR) (the retail building floor area divided by the retail land area) | Sum of $z$-score land-use mix, net residential density and intersection density and divided into quartiles (lowest quartile, second quartile, third quartile and highest quartile) | Self-reported weight and height/BMI | Logistic regression/odds ratio and linear regression/standardized coefficient - β |
| Hochner et al., (2011) [?2] | Geocoding of neighborhoods by home address and residential block group | Traditional core (higher values corresponding to block groups with older homes and residents with shorter commute units), high density (higher values corresponding to block groups of higher populations and housing unit densities) and non-auto commuting (higher values corresponding to block-groups with a higher proportion of commute trips made by walking, bicycling, or public transport) | Block-group level measures of population density, housing type, median home age, and commuting patterns representing neighborhood walkability divided into different factors such as traditional core, high density and non-auto commuting. These factors were interpreted and analyzed separately | Weight and height/BMI | Fit regression model/standardized and unstandardized coefficient (β) |
| Lathey et al., (2009) [30] | Geocoding by census block group | Population density, land use, connectivity, locations for social interaction | The walkability index was calculated and divided into three groups: low (reference), average and high prevalence. | Weight and height/BMI | Multinomial logistic regression/odds ratio |

**Table 2.** *Cont.*

| Reference | Assessment of Walkability/Study Scale/Geocoding of Facilities | Walkability Indicators Evaluated | Walkability Index Calculated | Assessment of Overweight and Obesity/Markers of Overweight and Obesity | Regression Model Used for Analyses of Associations |
|---|---|---|---|---|---|
| Muller-Riemenschneider (2013) [31] | Geocoding, 800 and 1600 m network buffers | Residential density (the ratio of residential dwellings to residential area in hectares), street connectivity (the ratio of three or more intersections to area in km2), land use mix (calculated with an entropy formula adapted from that developed by Frank et al. 2005 that considers the proportion of area covered by each land use type from the summed area for all land use types of interest divided by the number of land use classes) | The walkability index was calculated by summing the z-scores of each component | Self-reported weight and height/BMI | Logistic regression/odds ratio |
| Smith et al., (2008) [33] | Geocoding of neighborhoods by census block group - 2000 census for Salt Lake County, Utah | Population density, street connectivity, proportion of residents walking to work, the age of housing | Four D (density: population per square mile, design: intersections over 0.25 miles, diversity: proportion walking to work, and diversity: housing age) representing neighborhood walkability. These factors were interpreted and analyzed separately | Self-reported weight and height/BMI | Logistic regression/odds ratio and Linear regression/standardized coefficient - β |

Legends: BMI: body mass index; WC: waist circumference.

**Table 3.** Synthesis of results.

| Reference | Walkability Variables | Variable of Walkability (Score or Categorical) | Overweight and/or obese | Variable for Overweight and Obesity (Continuous/Categorical) | β-Values | Other-Values | OR-Values | 95% CI | $p$-Value | Variables Adjusted | An Association (+) or No Association (ns) Found |
|---|---|---|---|---|---|---|---|---|---|---|---|
| | | | | | | Walkability-Index | | | | | |
| 12pt Berry et al., (2011a) [25] | Lowest Walkability index / Low Walkability index / Moderate Walkability index / High Walkability index / Highest Walkability index (Reference) | Categorical | BMI | Continuous | 0.479 / 0.251 / 0.149 / 0.3 / - | | | | 0.096 / 0.339 / 0.562 / 0.232 / - | Age, sex, marital status, education, physical activity, fruit and vegetable consumption, neighborhood socioeconomic status | ns |
| Creatore et al., (2016) [28] | Walkability index (Population density, residential density, walkable destinations (land use) and street connectivity) in quintiles absolute change adjusted values (prevalence) | Categorical | BMI | Categorical | | Less walkable neighborhood (quintile 1) vs. most walkable neighborhood (quintile 5) = 43.3% vs. 53.5% Absolute difference = 10.2% (95% CI, 13.5% to 6.8%) $p < 0.001$ — Adjusted prevalence: Quintile 1 (%) = 5.4; Quintile 2 (%) = 6.7; Quintile 3 (%) = 9.2; Quintile 4 (%) = 2.8; Quintile 5 (%) = 2.1 | | 2.1%–8.8% / 2.3%–11.1% / 6.2%–12.1% / −1.4%–7.0% / −1.4%–5.5% | 0.002 / 0.003 / <0.001 / 0.20 / 0.20 | Age, sex, income and ethnicity | + |

**Table 3.** *Cont.*

| Reference | Walkability Variables | Variable of Walkability (Score or Categorical) | Overweight and/or obese | Variable for Overweight and Obesity (Continuous/Categorical) | β-Values | Other-Values | OR-Values | 95% CI | p-Value | Variables Adjusted | An Association (+) or No Association (ns) Found |
|---|---|---|---|---|---|---|---|---|---|---|---|
| | | | | | **Walkability-Index** | | | | | | |
| Lathey et al., (2009) [33] | Walkability index (population density, land use, connectivity, locations for social activity) low (reference), medium and high | Categorical | BMI | Categorical | | | Low (reference) / Average = 0.62 / High = 0.50 | | <0.05 / <0.001 | Demographic and socioeconomic characteristics of a neighborhood | + |
| Muller Riemenschneider et al., (2013) [31] | Less walkable vs. highly walkable neighborhoods (1600 m buffers) Less walkable vs. highly walkable neighborhoods (800 m buffers) | Categorical | BMI (≥30 Kg/m2) | Categorical | | | Overall = 0.86 / Male = 0.82 / Female = 0.88 / Overall = 0.78 / Male = 0.76 / Female = 0.80 | 0.70–1.05 / 0.59–1.14 / 068–1.14 / 0.64–0.96 / 0.55–1.04 / 0.61–1.04 | 0.139 / 0.229 / 0.336 / 0.018 / 0.089 / 0.093 | Age, sex, education level, household income, marital status, physical activity and sedentary behaviour | + |
| Braun et al., (2016) [27] | Walkability index (population density, street connectivity, variables related to food and physical activity) | Score | BMI / WC | Continuous | Fixed effects: Traditional core = −0.194; −0.022, −0.232 | Random-effects: −0.018, −0.26 | | | Fixed effects: 0.778, 0.391 / Random effects: 0.793, 0.283 | Fixed effects adjusted for time (days between exams) and time-varying sociodemographic and health covariates (income, household size, marital status, employment status, smoking status, and health problems that interfere with physical activity) Random effects adjusted for time (days between exams), sociodemographic and health covariates (baseline age, sex, race/ethnicity, educational attainment, income, household size, marital status, employment status, smoking status, and health problems that interfere with physical activity), and reasons for moving to the current neighborhood | ns |
| Hoehner et al., (2011) [32] | Walkability factors of (traditional core, high density and non-auto commuting) | Score | BMI (women) / BMI (men) | Continuous | High-density = −0.171 Non-auto commuting = −0.028 Traditional-core = −0.210 High-density = −0.158 Non-auto commuting = −0.100 | | | | <0.01 / NS / NS / <0.05 / <0.001 / <0.05 | Age, urbanization (moved neighborhood group level percentage of non-Hispanic Blacks and Hispanics, percentage falling below the 200% poverty level, participation in outdoor physical activities (walking, jogging, or bicycling) and cardiorespiratory fitness. | + |

**Table 3.** Cont.

| Reference | Walkability Variables | Variable of Walkability (Score or Categorical) | Overweight and/or obese | Variable for Overweight and Obesity (Continuous/Categorical) | β-Values | Other-Values | OR-Values | 95% CI | p-Value | Variables Adjusted | An Association (+) or No Association (ns) Found |
|---|---|---|---|---|---|---|---|---|---|---|---|
| | | | | **Walkability-Index** | | | | | | | |
| Berry et al., (2010b) [26] | Residential density, land use mix and connectivity | Score and categorical | BMI-(longitudinal) | Continuous | −0.068 | | | | 0.116 | Age, sex, marital status, education, physical activity, fruit and vegetable consumption, proximity to workplace, proximity to outdoor recreation amenities, quality of schools, quality of walking infrastructure, neighborhood socioeconomic status | ns |
| | | | BMI (cross-sectional) | | −0.051 | | | | 0.091 | | |
| Frank et al., (2006) [29] | Walkability index (residential density, street connectivity/land use, proportion of built area) | Score and categorical | BMI | Continuous | Unstandardized -coefficient −0.149 / Standardized -coefficient −0.113 | | | | <0.001 | Sex, age, education, ethnicity, children under the age of 18 and household income | + |
| Frank et al., (2007) [15] | Walkability index (residential density, street connectivity/land use, proportion of built area) in quartiles | Score and categorical | BMI | Categorical | — | Lowest quartile (reference) Second quartile = 0.98 Third quartile = 0.83 Highest quartile = 0.67 | 0.70–1.38 0.59–1.16 0.49–0.89 | NS NS <0.05 | No variables adjusted | + |
| | | | | **Other variables** | | | | | | | |
| Smith et al., (2008) [33] | Density: population density Design: street connectivity Diversity: proportion of residents walking to work Diversity: age of housing | Score and categorical | BMI (women) | Categorical-and-continuous | 0.000 0.000 −6.829 −0.015 | | | | 0.663 0.981 <0.001 <0.001 | No variables adjusted | + |
| | Density: population density Design: street connectivity Diversity: proportion of residents walking to work Diversity: age of housing | | BMI (men) | | −0.001 −0.002 −5.376 −0.019 | | | | 0.336 0.092 <0.001 <0.001 | | |

Legends: 95% CI: 95% confidence interval; BMI: body mass index; WC: waist circumference; OR: odds ratio; ns: no association found; bold values: significant p-Values.

## 4. Discussion

The aim of this study was to describe and summarize the evidence on associations between walkability and overweight and obesity. Seven out of ten included studies show significant inverse associations between walkability and overweight and obesity. Most studies show that less walkable neighborhoods are related to body weight outcomes in adult populations. Indicators measuring walkability index mainly include residential and population density, street connectivity and land-use mix. Some studies employed different buffer sizes around residents' homes of 800 to 1600 m measured along street networks and network buffers. No studies involving longitudinal design had significant results.

Largest associations were found by cross-sectional studies, which generally support the incapacity to establish causality. In addition, all studies were conducted in high-income countries, which differ from low- and middle-income countries in their application of policies, higher levels of urbanization, broader employment opportunities, and greater availability and quality of public services (e.g., public transportation) [35,36].

The main indicators used to calculate the walkability index are commonly used in studies involving health areas and active transportation [37]. Other indicators include different aspects of urban design (e.g., block group-level measures), residence types and displacement patterns (e.g., traditional core, high density and non-auto commuting) [32]. Most walkability indices have been created by z scores of the different indicators and divided by the number of indicators as residential density, land-use mix and street connectivity. Some walkability indices were categorized in quintiles or quartiles or expressed as continuous scores and for this review we used the studies when the walkability index was calculated. Interestingly, from our synthesis, only one study used specific indicators of food environments and physical activity as indicators of the walkability index [27]. While these indicators may be related to land-use-mix variables, the use of such indicators helps strengthen the index given their known association with overweight and obesity [38–41].

Another important issue to discuss concerns the sizes of neighborhood buffers used. Buffers of 800 to 1600 m around residences were used in certain works [15,29,31]. Muller–Riemenschneider et al. investigated 800 and 1600 m buffers based "street design" in association with obesity levels and found individuals living in high compared with less walkable areas were less likely to be obese (1600 m OR: 0.84, 95% CI: 0.7 to 1; 800 m OR: 0.75, 95% CI: 0.62 to 0.9) [31]. Frank et al. used 1 km network buffers [15,29] around households based on street segments and found inverse associations between the walkability index and obesity. Using 1 km network buffers, one study of adults (n = 10,878) living in Atlanta, Georgia, USA from 2000 to 2002 shows that each quartile increase in land-use mix is associated with a 12.2% reduction in the likelihood of obesity across sex and race [42]. However, walkability was not used because the authors used main indicators separately and these were interpreted as measures of walkability.

Thus, studies examining the relationship between the walkability index and overweight and obesity appear to exhibit no consensus regarding buffer sizes. While some use distances that individuals can travel by walking for 10 or 15 minutes, which usually vary from 500 to 1600 m [43], other studies use buffers of 400 m to 8 km [8], denoting the difficulty of establishing a common parameter. The studies included in this review use GIS tools to study household participants and census tracts [25–28,30,32,33]. This poses a challenge to walkability research because some features such as the quality and aesthetics of spaces and facilities cannot be measured with secondary or remote data [33].

Based on assessments of bias risk, the results of the synthesis expose important methodological issues related to such studies, such as in the item "withdrawals and dropouts" for two studies [27,31]. This property can be considered a limitation mainly of longitudinal studies [27], as it is necessary to have a percentage of individuals remaining in the study at the final data collection period, and some longitudinal studies have been able to reassess at least 70% of the individuals with intervals between two or three years [17,44]. This issue should be considered in future studies.

The assessment of certain predictors such as socioeconomic levels, demographic characteristics such as sex and other behavioral characteristics were used in the majority of studies examined in this review. Regarding socioeconomic levels, living in areas of higher socioeconomic levels may play a protective role against obesity [45], and this is interesting because socioeconomic status was used as an adjustment variable in different models and stratified the samples of some studies considered in this review [25,26,28]. Regarding sex, this predictor related to walkability is associated with overweight and obesity in both men and women and particularly among variables of destination diversity [33] (e.g., the land use diversity of a given neighborhood).

Additionally, neighborhood-based changes in walkability can shape other behavioral characteristics, such as leisure, commuting, and physical activity measures [29,46]. Decisions regarding land-use and transport planning can influence, for instance, the safety of walking and cycling as modes of transportation and the convenience of recreational physical activity [35]. This is important given that urban planning that develops neighborhoods with better indicators for walkable neighborhoods promote walking as a mode of transport [35]. Thus, creating smart cities that facilitate physical activity as part of everyday activity can promote health and prevent overweight and obesity in the global population [35]. We found four studies [26,27,31,32] that put physical activity as adjustment variable in different models. It is important to note that the mediating effect of physical activity in such relationship involving walkability and obesity may not be found and some results still remain inconclusive, and this is confirmed in one recent systematic review [20].

Fruit and vegetable consumption is an important predictor with some studies revealing a relationship between diet and certain urban food environment land-use characteristics [34,47–49]. The availability [47] and variety [34,48] of healthy food is associated with diet, and supermarket density is related to higher levels of fruit and vegetable consumption [48] and to a reduced prevalence of obesity [50]. However, according to studies focused on the walkability index covered in this review, fruit and vegetable consumption significantly predicts BMI scores in a cross-sectional analysis model but not in a longitudinal analysis model [26]. One study using only longitudinal data and not using fruit and vegetable consumption as a predictor found that increased levels of obesity observed in lower-income neighborhoods are associated with issues of food accessibility [25]. Therefore, land use policies that protect and support access to healthful foods in urban areas are critical to mitigating differences in terms of access to local food.

*Strengths and Limitations*

The strength of the present study was a broad review of observational studies specifically on walkability, overweight, and obesity, identifying which qualities contributed to walkability and how they measured or quantified these qualities and the association with overweight and obesity.

Most of the positive evidence has been obtained from cross-sectional studies that support the notion that certain neighborhood characteristics are related to low overweight and obesity prevalence [36]. Therefore, caution should be exercised when extrapolating these results due to neighborhood self-selection bias, as people who are not obese and who live a healthier lifestyle that prevents obesity may choose to live in neighborhoods with better living conditions [17,18]. To obtain stronger causal inferences, further longitudinal and quasi-experimental studies should be conducted in addition to natural experimental studies to further our understanding of how walkability at different urban scales affects risk of obesity [36]. Another limitation refers to the type of sampling of the included studies, four did not mention the type of sampling and two were convenience samples, the rest being studies with randomized samples. And because of this, it is possible that unmeasured confounders contributed to some findings.

Weight and height as measures for determining BMI scores were self-reported in the majority of the selected studies, collected through home-based and telephone surveys, and correctly cited reliable and previously validated information [25,28,29,33,51].

A broader variety of methodologies, including variables such as shade from street trees, the widths of sidewalks, safety and crime prevention, and others should also be employed and assessed in terms of walkability. Environmental determinants of obesity, including a healthy diet and certain food environments, such as supermarkets and restaurant chains, among others, are not addressed in the studies reviewed [38–41]. Few studies have explored walkability outside of the neighborhood setting (e.g., in areas surrounding workplaces).

## 5. Conclusions

Most studies have found that less walkable neighborhoods are related to overweight and/or obesity in adult populations. Positive evidence has been obtained from cross-sectional studies and time-series studies, rather than longitudinal studies, and studies have been conducted in high-income countries. In addition, most studies have used a walkability index. Based on these results, the following recommendations can be made: 1) More studies should be conducted in low-income, middle-income, and middle-high-income countries; 2) more longitudinal studies (cohort and natural experiment) that control neighborhood self-selection need to be conducted; 3) other variables of the walkability index, such as food access, physical activity facilities, sidewalk access, and safety and crime prevention measured should be considered; and 4) better operationalizations of GIS evaluation variables (buffers sizes and census tracts) must be developed. Based on cross-sectional and time series studies, potential implications for clinical practice and policy-making can be reported, city planning and policy-related strategies aimed at improving the connectivity of the street network, mix of land uses and density of housing would enable the necessary supportive environments for health-related behaviors and prevention of chronic diseases. Understanding the factors that contribute to walkability can enable urban planners, designers and healthcare professionals to replicate better walkability conditions, providing more opportunities for active routes to help reduce overweight and obesity.

**Supplementary Materials:** The following are available online at http://www.mdpi.com/1660-4601/16/17/3135/s1, Supplementary Materials S1: Search string; Supplementary Materials S2: Explanation of 12-point EHPP tool used for risk of bias analysis.

**Author Contributions:** All of the authors made significant contributions to the development of this study. J.P.d.A.S.B. (proponent of the original idea): Helped develop the research methods and assessments, collected data from original studies, and helped write the manuscript. P.H.G.: Assisted with research method development and with writing the manuscript. C.d.O.S.: Assisted with the assessment, collected data from original studies, and reviewed the final draft. A.P.d.O.B.N.: Assisted with the assessment, collected data from original studies, and reviewed the final draft. G.T.: Assessment, helped write the manuscript, and reviewed the final draft. A.A.F. (senior researcher and proponent of the original idea): Assisted with research method development and assessment and helped to write the manuscript.

**Funding:** Postdoctoral scholarship from the Postdoctoral National Program (PNPD/CAPES—Brazil).

**Acknowledgments:** The author JPASB holds a postdoctoral scholarship from the Postdoctoral National Program (PNPD/CAPES—Brazil). AAF receiving a research fellowship from the Brazilian National Council for Scientific and Technological Development (CNPq) (grant 306635/2016-0).

**Conflicts of Interest:** The authors declare no conflicts of interest.

## References

1.  ABESO. Mapa da Obesidade. Available online: http://www.abeso.org.br/atitude-saudavel/mapa-obesidade (accessed on 22 February 2018).
2.  Berrington de Gonzalez, A.; Hartge, P.; Cerhan, J.R.; Flint, A.J.; Hannan, L.; MacInnis, R.J.; Moore, S.C.; Tobias, G.S.; Anton-Culver, H.; Freeman, L.B.; et al. Body-Mass Index and Mortality among 1.46 Million White Adults. *N. Engl. J. Med.* **2010**, *363*, 2211–2219. [CrossRef]
3.  Sattar, N. Gender aspects in type 2 diabetes mellitus and cardiometabolic risk. *Best Pract. Res. Clin. Endocrinol. Metab.* **2013**, *27*, 501–507. [CrossRef] [PubMed]

4.  Di Angelantonio, E.; Bhupathiraju, S.N.; Wormser, D.; Gao, P.; Kaptoge, S.; de Gonzalez, A.B.; Cairns, B.J.; Huxley, R.; Jackson, C.L.; Joshy, G.; et al. Body-mass index and all-cause mortality: Individual-participant-data meta-analysis of 239 prospective studies in four continents. *Lancet* **2016**, *388*, 776–786. [CrossRef]

5.  NCD Risk Factor Collaboration. Trends in adult body-mass index in 200 countries from 1975 to 2014: A pooled analysis of 1698 population-based measurement studies with 19·2 million participants. *Lancet* **2016**, *387*, 1377–1396. [CrossRef]

6.  Bouchard, C. *Physical Activity and Obesity*; Manole: Barueri, Brazil, 2003.

7.  Sallis James, F.; Floyd Myron, F.; Rodríguez Daniel, A.; Saelens Brian, E. Role of Built Environments in Physical Activity, Obesity, and Cardiovascular Disease. *Circulation* **2012**, *125*, 729–737. [CrossRef]

8.  Brownson, R.C.; Hoehner, C.M.; Day, K.; Forsyth, A.; Sallis, J.F. Measuring the Built Environment for Physical Activity: State of the Science. *Am. J. Prev. Med.* **2009**, *36*, S99–S123.e12. [CrossRef] [PubMed]

9.  Swinburn, B.; Egger, G.; Raza, F. Dissecting Obesogenic Environments: The Development and Application of a Framework for Identifying and Prioritizing Environmental Interventions for Obesity. *Prev. Med.* **1999**, *29*, 563–570. [CrossRef]

10. Armitage, C.J.; Conner, M. Social cognition models and health behaviour: A structured review. *Psychol. Health* **2000**, *15*, 173–189. [CrossRef]

11. Lemmens, V.E.P.P.; Oenema, A.; Klepp, K.I.; Henriksen, H.B.; Brug, J. A systematic review of the evidence regarding efficacy of obesity prevention interventions among adults. *Obes. Rev.* **2008**, *9*, 446–455. [CrossRef]

12. Shaw, K.A.; O'Rourke, P.; Del Mar, C.; Kenardy, J. Psychological interventions for overweight or obesity. *Cochrane Database Syst. Rev.* **2005**. [CrossRef]

13. Booth, K.M.; Pinkston, M.M.; Poston, W.S.C. Obesity and the Built Environment. *J. Acad. Nutr. Diet.* **2005**, *105*, 110–117. [CrossRef] [PubMed]

14. Frank, L.D.; Schmid, T.L.; Sallis, J.F.; Chapman, J.; Saelens, B.E. Linking objectively measured physical activity with objectively measured urban form: Findings from SMARTRAQ. *Am. J. Prev. Med.* **2005**, *28*, 117–125. [CrossRef] [PubMed]

15. Frank, L.D.; Saelens, B.E.; Powell, K.E.; Chapman, J.E. Stepping towards causation: Do built environments or neighborhood and travel preferences explain physical activity, driving, and obesity? *Soc. Sci. Med.* **2007**, *65*, 1898–1914. [CrossRef] [PubMed]

16. Smith, K.R.; Zick, C.D.; Kowaleski-Jones, L.; Brown, B.B.; Fan, J.X.; Yamada, I. Effects of Neighborhood Walkability on Healthy Weight: Assessing Selection and Causal Influences. *Soc. Sci. Res.* **2011**, *40*, 1445–1455. [CrossRef]

17. Giles-Corti, B.; Bull, F.; Knuiman, M.; McCormack, G.; Van Niel, K.; Timperio, A.; Christian, H.; Foster, S.; Divitini, M.; Middleton, N.; et al. The influence of urban design on neighbourhood walking following residential relocation: Longitudinal results from the RESIDE study. *Soc. Sci. Med.* **2013**, *77*, 20–30. [CrossRef] [PubMed]

18. McCormack, G.R.; Shiell, A. In search of causality: A systematic review of the relationship between the built environment and physical activity among adults. *Int. J. Behav. Nutr. Phys. Act.* **2011**, *8*, 125. [CrossRef] [PubMed]

19. Mendes, L.L.; Nogueira, H.; Padez, C.; Ferrao, M.; Velasquez-Melendez, G. Individual and environmental factors associated for overweight in urban population of Brazil. *BMC Public Health* **2013**, *13*, 988. [CrossRef]

20. Chandrabose, M.; Rachele, J.N.; Gunn, L.; Kavanagh, A.; Owen, N.; Turrell, G.; Giles-Corti, B.; Sugiyama, T. Built environment and cardio-metabolic health: Systematic review and meta-analysis of longitudinal studies. *Obes. Rev.* **2019**, *20*, 41–54. [CrossRef]

21. Mackenbach, J.D.; Rutter, H.; Compernolle, S.; Glonti, K.; Oppert, J.-M.; Charreire, H.; De Bourdeaudhuij, I.; Brug, J.; Nijpels, G.; Lakerveld, J. Obesogenic environments: A systematic review of the association between the physical environment and adult weight status, the SPOTLIGHT project. *BMC Public Health* **2014**, *14*, 233. [CrossRef]

22. Grasser, G.; Van Dyck, D.; Titze, S.; Stronegger, W. Objectively measured walkability and active transport and weight-related outcomes in adults: A systematic review. *Int. J. Public Health* **2013**, *58*, 615–625. [CrossRef]

23. Liberati, A.; Altman, D.G.; Tetzlaff, J.; Mulrow, C.; Gøtzsche, P.C.; Ioannidis, J.P.A.; Clarke, M.; Devereaux, P.J.; Kleijnen, J.; Moher, D. The PRISMA statement for reporting systematic reviews and meta-analyses of studies that evaluate healthcare interventions: Explanation and elaboration. *BMJ* **2009**, *339*. [CrossRef]

24. Thomas, B.H.; Ciliska, D.; Dobbins, M.; Micucci, S. A Process for Systematically Reviewing the Literature: Providing the Research Evidence for Public Health Nursing Interventions. *Worldviews Evid. Based Nurs.* **2004**, *1*, 176–184. [CrossRef]

25. Berry, T.R.; Spence, J.C.; Blanchard, C.; Cutumisu, N.; Edwards, J.; Nykiforuk, C. Changes in BMI over 6 years: The role of demographic and neighborhood characteristics. *Int. J. Obes. (Lond.)* **2010**, *34*, 1275–1283. [CrossRef] [PubMed]

26. Berry, T.R.; Spence, J.C.; Blanchard, C.M.; Cutumisu, N.; Edwards, J.; Selfridge, G. A longitudinal and cross-sectional examination of the relationship between reasons for choosing a neighbourhood, physical activity and body mass index. *Int. J. Behav. Nutr. Phys. Act.* **2010**, *7*, 57. [CrossRef] [PubMed]

27. Braun, L.M.; Rodriguez, D.A.; Song, Y.; Meyer, K.A.; Lewis, C.E.; Reis, J.P.; Gordon-Larsen, P. Changes in walking, body mass index, and cardiometabolic risk factors following residential relocation: Longitudinal results from the CARDIA study. *J. Transp. Health* **2016**, *3*, 426–439. [CrossRef]

28. Creatore, M.I.P.; Glazier, R.H.M.D.; Moineddin, R.P.; Fazli, G.S.M.P.H.; Johns, A.M.; Gozdyra, P.M.A.; Matheson, F.I.P.; Kaufman-Shriqui, V.P.; Rosella, L.C.P.; Manuel, D.G.; et al. Association of Neighborhood Walkability With Change in Overweight, Obesity, and Diabetes. *JAMA* **2016**, *315*, 2211–2220. [CrossRef]

29. Frank, L.D.; Sallis, J.F.; Conway, T.L.; Chapman, J.E.; Saelens, B.E.; Bachman, W. Many pathways from land use to health—Associations between neighborhood walkability and active transportation, body mass index, and air quality. *J. Am. Plan. Assoc.* **2006**, *72*, 75–87. [CrossRef]

30. Lathey, V.; Guhathakurta, S.; Aggarwal, R.M. The Impact of Subregional Variations in Urban Sprawl on the Prevalence of Obesity and Related Morbidity. *J. Plan. Educ. Res.* **2009**, *29*, 127–141. [CrossRef]

31. Müller-Riemenschneider, F.; Pereira, G.; Villanueva, K.; Christian, H.; Knuiman, M.; Giles-Corti, B.; Bull, F.C. Neighborhood walkability and cardiometabolic risk factors in australian adults: An observational study. *BMC Public Health* **2013**, *13*, 755. [CrossRef]

32. Hoehner, C.M.; Handy, S.L.; Yan, Y.; Blair, S.N.; Berrigan, D. Association between neighborhood walkability, cardiorespiratory fitness and body-mass index. *Soc. Sci. Med.* **2011**, *73*, 1707–1716. [CrossRef]

33. Smith, K.R.; Brown, B.B.; Yamada, I.; Kowaleski-Jones, L.; Zick, C.D.; Fan, J.X. Walkability and Body Mass Index Density, Design, and New Diversity Measures. *Am. J. Prev. Med.* **2008**, *35*, 237–244. [CrossRef]

34. Thornton, L.E.; Pearce, J.R.; Kavanagh, A.M. Using Geographic Information Systems (GIS) to assess the role of the built environment in influencing obesity: A glossary. *Int. J. Behav. Nutr. Phys. Act.* **2011**, *8*, 71. [CrossRef]

35. Giles-Corti, B.; Vernez-Moudon, A.; Reis, R.; Turrell, G.; Dannenberg, A.L.; Badland, H.; Foster, S.; Lowe, M.; Sallis, J.F.; Stevenson, M.; et al. City planning and population health: A global challenge. *Lancet* **2016**, *388*, 2912–2924. [CrossRef]

36. Garfinkel-Castro, A.; Kim, K.; Hamidi, S.; Ewing, R. Obesity and the built environment at different urban scales: Examining the literature. *Nutr. Rev.* **2017**, *75*, 51–61. [CrossRef]

37. Frank, L.D.; Sallis, J.F.; Saelens, B.E.; Leary, L.; Cain, K.; Conway, T.L.; Hess, P.M. The development of a walkability index: Application to the Neighborhood Quality of Life Study. *Br. J. Sports Med.* **2010**, *44*, 924–933. [CrossRef]

38. Black, J.L.; Macinko, J. The Changing Distribution and Determinants of Obesity in the Neighborhoods of New York City, 2003–2007. *Am. J. Epidemiol.* **2010**, *171*, 765–775. [CrossRef]

39. Chen, S.; Florax, R.J.G.M.; Snyder, S.; Miller, C.C. Obesity and Access to Chain Grocers. *Econ. Geogr.* **2010**, *86*, 431–452. [CrossRef]

40. Drewnowski, A.; Aggarwal, A.; Hurvitz, P.M.; Monsivais, P.; Moudon, A.V. Obesity and Supermarket Access: Proximity or Price? *Am. J. Public Health* **2012**, *102*, e74–e80. [CrossRef]

41. Pereira, M.A.; Kartashov, A.I.; Ebbeling, C.B.; Van Horn, L.; Slattery, M.L.; Jacobs, D.R.; Ludwig, D.S. Fast-food habits, weight gain, and insulin resistance (the CARDIA study): 15-year prospective analysis. *Lancet* **2005**, *365*, 36–42. [CrossRef]

42. Frank, L.D.; Andresen, M.A.; Schmid, T.L. Obesity relationships with community design, physical activity, and time spent in cars. *Am. J. Prev. Med.* **2004**, *27*, 87–96. [CrossRef]

43. McCormack, G.R.; Giles-Corti, B.; Bulsara, M. The relationship between destination proximity, destination mix and physical activity behaviors. *Prev. Med.* **2008**, *46*, 33–40. [CrossRef]

44. Goodman, A.; Sahlqvist, S.; Ogilvie, D.; Consortium, I. New walking and cycling routes and increased physical activity: One-and 2-year findings from the UK iConnect Study. *Am. J. Public Health* **2014**, *104*, e38–e46. [CrossRef]

45. Grafova, I.B.; Freedman, V.A.; Kumar, R.; Rogowski, J. Neighborhoods and Obesity in Later Life. *Am. J. Public Health* **2008**, *98*, 2065–2071. [CrossRef]

46. Adlakha, D.; Hipp, J.A.; Brownson, R.C. Neighborhood-based differences in walkability, physical activity, and weight status in India. *J. Transp. Health* **2016**, *3*, 485–499. [CrossRef]

47. Caspi, C.E.; Sorensen, G.; Subramanian, S.V.; Kawachi, I. The local food environment and diet: A systematic review. *Health Place* **2012**, *18*, 1172–1187. [CrossRef]

48. Thornton, L.E.; Pearce, J.R.; Macdonald, L.; Lamb, K.E.; Ellaway, A. Does the choice of neighbourhood supermarket access measure influence associations with individual-level fruit and vegetable consumption? A case study from Glasgow. *Int. J. Health Geogr.* **2012**, *11*, 29. [CrossRef]

49. Nogueira, R.L.; Fontanelli, D.M.; Aguiar, S.B.; Failla, A.M.; Florindo, A.A.; Barrozo, V.L.; Goldbaum, M.; Cesar, L.C.; Alves, C.M.; Fisberg, M.R. Access to Street Markets and Consumption of Fruits and Vegetables by Adolescents Living in São Paulo, Brazil. *Int. J. Environ. Res. Public Health* **2018**, *15*, 517. [CrossRef]

50. Michimi, A.; Wimberly, M.C. Associations of supermarket accessibility with obesity and fruit and vegetable consumption in the conterminous United States. *Int. J. Health Geogr.* **2010**, *9*, 49. [CrossRef]

51. Gorber, S.C.; Tremblay, M.; Moher, D.; Gorber, B. A comparison of direct vs. self-report measures for assessing height, weight and body mass index: A systematic review. *Obes. Rev.* **2007**, *8*, 307–326. [CrossRef]

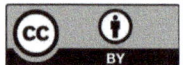

MDPI

St. Alban-Anlage 66

4052 Basel

Switzerland

Tel. +41 61 683 77 34

Fax +41 61 302 89 18

www.mdpi.com

*International Journal of Environmental Research and Public Health* Editorial Office

E-mail: ijerph@mdpi.com

www.mdpi.com/journal/ijerph

www.ingramcontent.com/pod-product-compliance
Lightning Source LLC
Chambersburg PA
CBHW041137120626
46547CB00020B/3018